Auditory Perception
An Analysis and Synthesis

This revised and updated Third Edition describes the nature of sound, how sound is analyzed by the auditory system, and the rules and principles governing our interpretation of auditory input. It covers many topics including sound and the auditory system, locating sound sources, the basis for loudness judgments, perception of acoustic sequences, perceptual restoration of obliterated sounds, speech production and perception, and the relation of hearing to perception in general. Whilst keeping the consistent style of the previous editions, many new features have been added, including suggestions for further reading at the end of each chapter, a section on functional imaging of the brain, expanded information on pitch and infrapitch, and additional coverage of speech processing. Advanced undergraduate and graduate students interested in auditory perception, behavioral sciences, psychology, audiology, architectural acoustics, and the hearing sciences will find this an excellent guide.

RICHARD M. WARREN is Research Professor and Distinguished Professor Emeritus in the Department of Psychology at the University of Wisconsin-Milwaukee. He is a Fellow of the Acoustical Society of America, American Psychological Association, and the Association for Psychological Science.

Auditory
Perception
An Analysis and
Synthesis

Third Edition

RICHARD M. WARREN

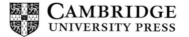

CAMBRIDGE
UNIVERSITY PRESS

CAMBRIDGE UNIVERSITY PRESS
Cambridge, New York, Melbourne, Madrid, Cape Town, Singapore, São Paulo, Delhi

Cambridge University Press
The Edinburgh Building, Cambridge CB2 8RU, UK

Published in the United States of America by Cambridge University Press, New York

www.cambridge.org
Information on this title: www.cambridge.org/9780521868709

First published 2008

Printed in the United Kingdom at the University Press, Cambridge

A catalogue record for this publication is available from the British Library

Library of Congress Cataloguing in Publication data
Warren, Richard M.
  Auditory perception : an analysis and synthesis / Richard M. Warren. – 3rd ed.
    p. ; cm.
  Includes bibliographical references and index.
  ISBN 978-0-521-86870-9 (hardback) – ISBN 978-0-521-68889-5 (pbk.) 1. Auditory
  perception. 2. Speech perception. I. Title.
  [DNLM : 1. Auditory Perception. 2. Speech Perception. WV 272 W2831a 2008]
  QP461.W27 2008
  152.1′5–dc22   2007050033

ISBN 978-0-521-86870-9 hardback
ISBN 978-0-521-68889-5 paperback

To Roslyn

Contents

Preface

As in the earlier editions, the present text emphasizes the interconnectedness of areas in auditory perception. These linkages are especially evident in the chapters dealing with acoustic sequences, pitch and infrapitch, loudness, and the restoration of portions of signals obliterated by extraneous sounds. In addition, the chapter on speech describes how processes employed for the perception of brief nonverbal sounds are used for the organization of syllables and words, along with an overlay of special linguistic mechanisms.

The basic format of the book remains unchanged, but all chapters have been updated. Among the additions are new sections in Chapter 1 describing the principles underlying functional imaging of the brain based on the hemodynamic techniques of fMRI and PET, and the electrodynamic techniques of EEG and MEG. New information concerning pitch and infrapitch appears in Chapter 3, and additional information concerning speech processing is incorporated into Chapter 7. Suggested additional reading now appears at the end of each chapter.

It is hoped that this text will be of value to research scientists and to professionals dealing with sound and hearing. No detailed specialized knowledge is assumed, since basic information necessary for understanding the material covered is provided. It may be used for advanced undergraduate and graduate courses in behavioral sciences, neurobiology, music, audio engineering, and the health sciences and professions.

My own research in perception was carried out at the following institutions: Brown University; New York University College of Medicine; Cambridge University; the Medical Research Council Applied Psychology Research Unit, Cambridge; Oxford University; the Laboratory of Psychology at the National Institute of Mental Health, Bethesda; and the University of Wisconsin-Milwaukee.

I acknowledge the debts to my graduate students over the years.

Dr. Peter W. Lenz has made essential contributions to all aspects of the research currently being carried out in our laboratory.

My debt to Jim Bashford is especially great: he has been my colleague and collaborator since the 1970s. Our back-and-forth discussions have played a basic role in designing and conducting the work in our laboratory.

I wish to thank Ms. Michelle L. Ullman for her valuable and thorough bibliographic work and in the preparation of the typescript.

I am grateful for the past research support by the National Research Council of the National Academy of Sciences, the National Science Foundation, the Air Force Office of Scientific Research, and the National Institutes of Health. My current support is from the National Institute on Deafness and Other Communication Disorders.

Finally, I acknowledge the essential role of Dr. Roslyn Pauker Warren, my colleague and wife. Without her, none of the editions of this book would have been started, and once started could not have been finished.

Please refer to www.cambridge.org/9780521868709 for audio demonstrations of some of the phenomena described in the text, that provide new insight into the mechanisms employed in auditory perception. The stimuli and descriptive narrative were produced by Dr. James A. Bashford, Jr.

1
_____

Sound and the auditory system

This chapter provides a brief introduction to the physical nature of sound, the manner in which it is transmitted and transformed within the ear, and the nature of auditory neural responses.

The nature of auditory stimuli

The sounds responsible for hearing consist of rapid changes in air pressure that can be produced in a variety of ways – for example, by vibrations of objects such as the tines of a tuning fork or the wings of an insect, by puffs of air released by a siren or our vocal cords, and by the noisy turbulence of air escaping from a small opening. Sound travels through the air at sea level at a velocity of about 335 meters per second, or 1,100 feet per second, for all but very great amplitudes (extent of pressure changes) and for all waveforms (patterns of pressure changes over time). Special interest is attached to periodic sounds, or sounds having a fixed waveform repeated at a fixed frequency. Frequency is measured in hertz (Hz), or numbers of repetitions of a waveform per second; thus, 1,000 Hz corresponds to 1,000 repetitions of a particular waveform per second. The time required for one complete statement of an iterated waveform is its period. Periodic sounds from about 20 through 16,000 Hz can produce a sensation of pitch and are called tones. For reasons to be discussed shortly, it is generally considered that the simplest type of periodic sound is a sine wave or pure tone (shown in Figure 1.1A), which has a sinusoidal change in pressure over time. A limitless number of other periodic waveforms exists, including square waves (Figure 1.1B) and pulse trains (Figure 1.1C). Periodic sounds need not have simple, symmetrical waveforms: Figure 1.1D shows a periodic sound

1

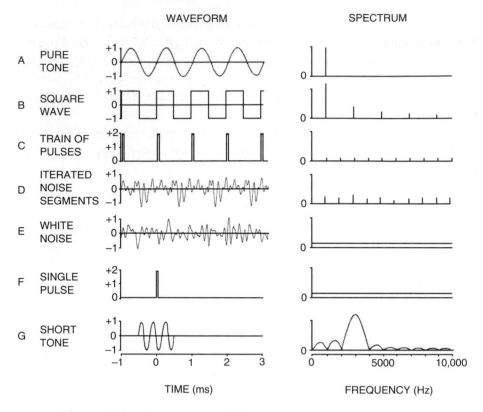

Figure 1.1 Waveforms and amplitude spectra. The waveforms A through E continue in time to produce the spectra as shown. Periodic waveforms A through D have line spectra, the others either continuous spectra (E and F), or a band spectrum (G). See the text for further discussion.

produced by iteration of a randomly generated waveform. The figure also depicts the waveforms of some nonperiodic sounds: white or Gaussian noise (Figure 1.1E), a single pulse (Figure 1.1F), and a short tone or tone burst (Figure 1.1G).

The waveforms shown in Figure 1.1 are time-domain representations in which both amplitude and time are depicted. Using a procedure developed by Joseph Fourier in the first half of the nineteenth century, one can represent any periodic sound in terms of a frequency-domain or spectral analysis in which a sound is described in terms of a harmonic sequence of sinusoidal components having appropriate frequency, amplitude, and phase relations. (Phase describes the portion of the period through which a waveform has advanced relative to an arbitrarily fixed reference time.) A sinusoidal or pure tone consists of a single spectral component, as shown in Figure 1.1A. The figure also shows the power spectra corresponding to the particular complex (nonsinusoidal) periodic sounds shown in Figures 1.1B, 1.1C, and 1.1D. Each of these sounds has a period of one millisecond, a fundamental frequency of 1,000 Hz (corresponding to the waveform repetition frequency), and harmonic components corresponding to integral multiples of the 1,000 Hz fundamental as indicated.

Frequency analysis is not restricted to periodic sounds: nonperiodic sounds also have a spectral composition as defined through use of a Fourier integral or Fourier transform (for details see Hartmann, 1998). Nonperiodic sounds have either continuous or band spectra rather than line spectra, as shown for the sounds depicted in Figures 1.1E, 1.1F, and 1.1G.

As we shall see, frequency analysis of both periodic and nonperiodic sounds is of particular importance in hearing, chiefly because a spectral analysis is performed within the ear leading to a selective stimulation of the auditory nerve fibers.

Although Figure 1.1 shows how particular waveforms can be analyzed in terms of spectral components, it is also possible to synthesize waveforms by adding together sinusoidal components of appropriate phase and amplitude. Figure 1.2 shows how a sawtooth waveform may be approximated closely by the mixing of only six harmonics having appropriate amplitude and phase.

The range of audible amplitude changes is very large. A sound producing discomfort may be as much as 10^6 times the amplitude level at threshold. Sound level can be measured as power as well as by amplitude or pressure at a particular point. Power usually can be considered as proportional to the square of the amplitude, so that discomfort occurs at a power level 10^{12} times the power threshold. The term "sound intensity" is, strictly speaking, the sound power arriving from a specified direction, and passing through a unit area perpendicular to that direction. However, the term "intensity" is often used interchangeably with "power," although the latter term has no directional specificity.

In order to span the large range of values needed to describe the levels of sound normally encountered, a logarithmic scale has been devised. The logarithm to the base 10 of the ratio of a particular sound power level to a reference power level defines the level of the sound in Bels (named in honor of Alexander Graham Bell). However, the Bel is a rather large unit, and it is conventional to use a unit 1/10 this size, the decibel (or dB) to express sound levels. The level in dB can be defined as:

$$dB = 10 \log_{10} (I_1/I_2)$$

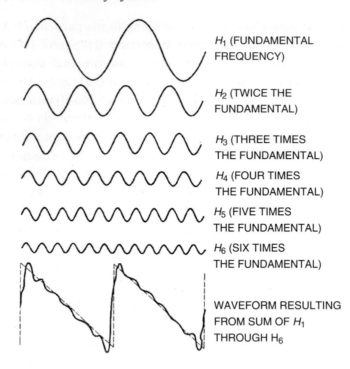

Figure 1.2 Synthesis of a complex waveform through addition of harmonically related sinusoidal components. The approximation of a sawtooth waveform could be made closer by the addition of higher harmonics of appropriate amplitude and phase. (From Brown and Deffenbacher, 1979.)

where I_1 is the intensity or power level of the particular sound of interest, and I_2 is the reference level expressed as sound intensity. One can also calculate decibels on the basis of pressure or amplitude units using the equation:

$$dB = 20 \log_{10} (P_1/P_2)$$

where P_1 is the relative pressure level being measured and P_2 is the reference pressure level. The standard reference pressure level is 0.0002 dyne/cm^2 (which is sometimes expressed in different units of 20 micropascals). The level in dB measured relative to this standard is called the Sound Pressure Level (or SPL). Sound-level meters are calibrated so that the numerical value of the SPL can be read out directly. There is another measure of sound level, also expressed in dB, called the Sensation Level (SL), which is used occasionally in psychoacoustics. When measuring SL, the level corresponding to the threshold of a sound for an individual listener is used as the reference level rather than the standard physical value employed for SPL, so that dB SL represents the level above an individual's threshold. Since SL is used relatively infrequently, dB will always refer to SPL unless otherwise specified.

To give some feeling for sound pressure levels in dB, the threshold of normal listeners for sinusoidal tones with frequencies between 1,000 and 4,000 Hz (the range exhibiting the lowest thresholds) is about 0 dB (the standard reference level); the ambient level (background noise) in radio and TV studios is about 30 dB, conversational speech about 65 dB, and the level inside a bus about 90 dB. Some rock bands achieve levels of 120 dB, which approaches the threshold for pain and can cause permanent damage to hearing following relatively brief exposures.

Experimenters can vary the relative intensities of spectral components by use of acoustic filters which, in analogy with light filters, pass only desired frequency components of a sound. A high-pass filter transmits only frequency components above a lower limit, and a low-pass filter transmits only frequencies below an upper limit. Bandpass filters (which transmit frequencies within a specified range) and band-reject filters (which block frequencies within a specified range) are available. The characteristics of high-pass and low-pass filters can be expressed in terms of both cut-off frequency (conventionally considered as the frequency at which the filter attenuation reduces power by half, or 3 dB), and the slope, or roll-off, which is usually expressed as dB/octave beyond the cut-off frequency (a decrease of one octave corresponds to halving the frequency). Bandpass filters are characterized by their bandwidth (the range in hertz between the upper and lower cut-off frequencies), and they can also be characterized by their "Q" (the bandwidth divided by the center frequency of the filter). In neurophysiological work, Q_{10} is sometimes used in which 10 dB downpoints are used to express the bandwidth rather than the conventional value of 3 dB. Filter types are shown in Figure 1.3.

Our auditory apparatus

The outer ear and the middle ear

It is convenient to consider the ear as consisting of three divisions. The outer ear, also called the pinna (plural "pinnae") or auricle, is shown in Figure 1.4. It appears to contribute to localization of sound sources by virtue of its direction-specific effect on the intensity of certain frequency components of sounds, as will be discussed in the next chapter. The human pinna is surrounded by a simple flange (the helix) which is extended considerably in some other mammals to form a conical structure functioning as a short version of the old-fashioned ear trumpet. These acoustic funnels can enhance sensitivity to high frequency sounds when pointed toward their source by controlling muscles, as well as being of help in locating the sound source.

After the acoustic transformation produced by reflections within our pinna, the sound passes through the ear canal (or external auditory meatus) which

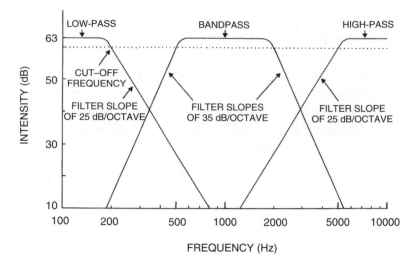

Figure 1.3 Characteristics of filters. Low-pass, high-pass, and bandpass filters are illustrated, along with filter slopes (dB/octave) and cut-off frequencies (frequencies at which there is a 3 dB reduction in intensity).

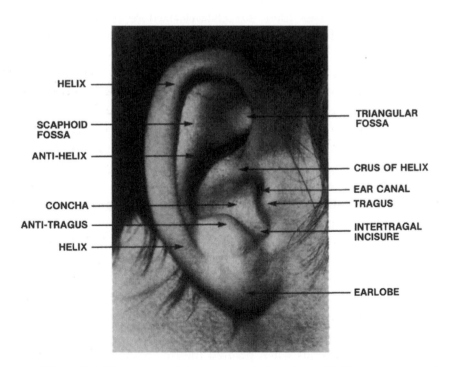

Figure 1.4 The outer ear (other names: pinna and auricle). The major anatomical features are shown.

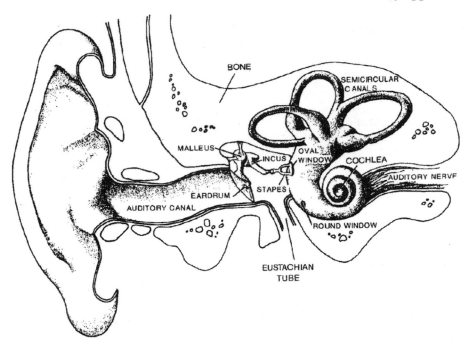

Figure 1.5 Diagram of the entire ear. The outer, middle, and inner ears are shown, along with adjacent structures. (Adapted from Lindsay and Norman, 1977.)

ends at the eardrum, or tympanum, as shown in Figure 1.5. This canal is more than a passive conduit. Its length is roughly 2.5 cm, and it behaves in some respects like a resonant tube, such as an organ pipe. The effect of this resonance is to amplify frequencies appreciably (5 dB or more) from about 2,000 through 5,500 Hz, with a maximum amplification of about 11 dB occurring at about 4,000 Hz (Wiener, 1947). The pressure changes at the end of the canal cause the eardrum (or tympanum) to vibrate. This vibration is picked up and transmitted by a chain of three small bones (or ossicles) located in the middle ear. The first of these bones, the malleus (or hammer) is attached to the tympanum, and its movement is transmitted to the incus (or anvil) and thence to the stapes (or stirrup). The stapes is connected to the oval window at the base of the fluid-filled cochlea. This window forms a boundary separating the middle and inner ear. The passage of sound through the cochlea is shown in Figure 1.6, and will be discussed subsequently.

The middle ear permits the airborne sound to be converted to liquid borne sound without the great loss which would otherwise occur. When sound in air impinges directly upon a liquid, a loss of about 30 dB (99.9 percent of the power) takes place, with most of the sound being reflected back into the air. Three physical principles act to increase the efficiency of the transmission of

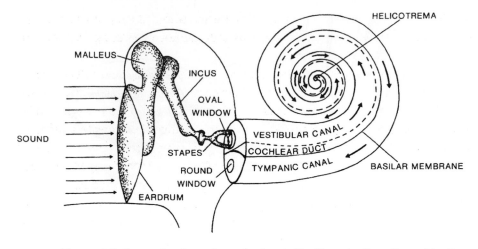

Figure 1.6 Conversion from air-conduction to liquid-conduction of sound by the ear. For details see the text. (Adapted from Lindsay and Norman, 1977.)

sound by the middle ear: (1) the curvature of the tympanum (which is somewhat conical in shape) causes it to act as a more efficient mechanical transformer (Tonndorf and Khanna, 1972); (2) the chain of three ossicles acts like a lever with a small mechanical advantage; and (3) the force applied to the larger area of the tympanic membrane, when transmitted to the much smaller area of the footplate of the stapes embedded in the oval window, produces a considerable mechanical advantage. This last factor is the most important of the three.

There are two muscles within the middle ear that can lessen the intensity of very strong stimuli and minimize the possibility of damage to the inner ear. One of these, the tensor tympani muscle, is attached to the malleus, and the other, the stapedius muscle, is attached to the stapes. These muscles are sometimes compared in their effect to the iris of the eye – a high level of stimulus intensity causes a reflex contraction of the muscles resulting in a decrease in stimulation. Once the threshold for initiating the reflex is reached, there is an attenuation up to about 0.6 or 0.7 dB for each 1 dB increase in the stimulus, with a maximum attenuation of perhaps 30 dB for low frequency sounds (the reduction in intensity is greatest for frequencies below 1,000 Hz). Middle ear muscle contraction can also reduce distortions which would otherwise occur from overloading the ossicular chain. A very few people can contract their middle ear muscles voluntarily, and thus attenuate even relatively faint sounds at will. For most of us the action is strictly reflexive, either in response to an external sound of 80 dB or more, or as an action that precedes the self-generation of sound in speaking or chewing food. The reflex activity of these muscles in response to external sound is very quick, perhaps 10 ms for very intense sounds, but this still cannot protect against sudden harmful sounds such as gunshots.

Are the intra-aural muscles more than an analog of the eye's iris? There have been some interesting speculations. Lawrence (1965) suggested that since animal studies have indicated that muscle activity is to some degree independent in the two ears, intermittent monaural changes in intensity and phase produced by muscle contraction can help in directing attention to sources at different azimuths under noisy conditions. Simmons (1964) considered that low frequency sounds produced by eating might mask high frequency environmental sounds of importance and that selective attenuation of these self-generated sounds by the intra-aural muscles could release these external sounds from masking and permit their detection.

Structure of the inner ear

The inner ear contains not only the receptors responsible for hearing, but also receptors involved in detecting acceleration and maintaining balance. The tortuous anatomical structure of the inner ear has led to its being called the labyrinth. The vestibule of the labyrinth contains the utricle and saccule which appear to be sensitive to linear acceleration of the head and to orientation in the gravitational field. There are also three bony semicircular canals, each canal lying in a plane that is at right angles to the other two, much as the floor and two adjacent walls of a room form three mutually perpendicular planes. This arrangement of the canals permits detection of the components of rotary acceleration in any of the planes (see Figure 1.5).

The bony spiral structure within the inner ear called the cochlea (from the Latin name for snail) contains the organ for hearing. This coiled tube consists of about 2.5 turns and has a length of about 3.5 cm. It is partitioned into three canals or ducts called scalae. Two of the scalae are joined: the scala vestibuli or vestibular canal (which has at its basal end the flexible oval window to which the stapes is attached) communicates (via a small opening called the helicotrema at the apex of the spiral) with the scala tympani or tympanic canal (which has the flexible round window at its basal end). These two scalae contain a fluid called perilymph, and when the oval window is flexed inward by the stapes, the almost incompressible perilymph causes the round window to flex outward. As shown in Figure 1.7, the scala vestibuli is bounded by Reissner's membrane and the scala tympani by the basilar membrane. Between these two membranes lies the scala media or cochlear duct, which has a closed end near the helicotrema and which contains a fluid called endolymph. A third fluid called cortilymph is found within the tunnel of Corti.

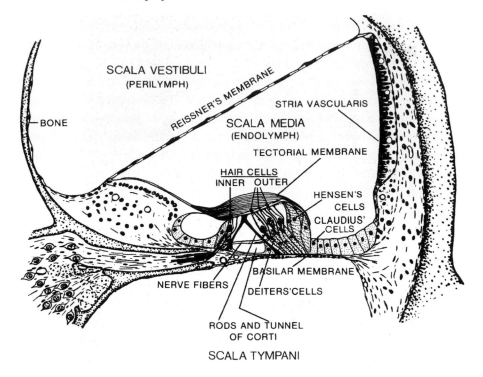

SCALA VESTIBULI
(PERILYMPH)

REISSNER'S MEMBRANE

STRIA VASCULARIS

BONE

SCALA MEDIA
(ENDOLYMPH)

TECTORIAL MEMBRANE

HAIR CELLS
INNER OUTER

HENSEN'S
CELLS

CLAUDIUS'
CELLS

BASILAR MEMBRANE

NERVE FIBERS

DEITERS'CELLS

RODS AND TUNNEL
OF CORTI

SCALA TYMPANI

Figure 1.7 Cross-section of the cochlea, showing the organ of Corti and associated structures. This diagram is based on the guinea pig, but is representative of the human inner ear as well. (Adapted from Davis, Benson, Covell, *et al.*, 1953.)

These fluids have different ionic compositions and different electric potentials which appear to play a role in the processes eventuating in the stimulation of the auditory nerve. A complex neuroepithelium called the organ of Corti lies on the basilar membrane and contains the hair cells that are responsible for stimulating the auditory nerve. As shown in Figure 1.8, the hair cells consist of two types: the outer hair cells, which are closer to the cochlear wall, and the inner hair cells, each topped by a cuticular plate containing stereocilia. The stereocilia are bathed in endolymph, whereas most of the receptor cell is surrounded by the cortilymph found in the extracellular spaces of the organ of Corti. There are about 12,000 outer hair cells, each containing about 100 to 200 stereocilia arranged in parallel rows. Within these rows, resembling a letter V or W, the longest stereocilia have their tips attached to the tectorial membrane (the consequences of this coupling of the basilar and tectorial membranes will be discussed shortly). There are about 3,500 inner hair cells forming a single row in the shape of a flattened letter U. Each inner hair cell contains about 50 stereocilia having tips that lie without attachment in a groove called Hensen's stripe on the underside of the tectorial membrane. The stereocilia of both the

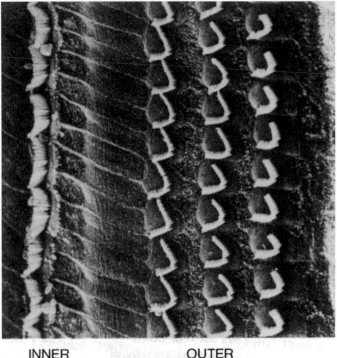

INNER   OUTER
HAIR CELLS   HAIR CELLS

Figure 1.8 Scanning electron micrograph of the top of the organ of Corti. The tectorial membrane has been removed to expose the stereocilia and upper surfaces of the outer hair cells (three rows) and the inner hair cells (one row). (Chinchilla photograph courtesy of Dr. Ivan Hunter-Duvar, Hospital for Sick Children, Toronto.)

inner and outer hair cells consist of a bundle of parallel actin fibers that are bonded together and are firmly rooted in the cuticular plate of the hair cell. The numerous stereocilia of an individual hair cell are cross-linked, so that they all tend to move together. The inner hair cells are the units primarily responsible for stimulating afferent fibers in the auditory nerve. Sound-induced movement of the stereocilia relative to the hair cell's cuticular plate produces a shearing deflection of these stereocilia. This results in electro-chemical changes in the receptor cells which, in turn, leads to stimulation of the associated auditory nerve fibers.

The adult basilar membrane is approximately 30 mm long. It is tapered, with a width of about 0.04 mm at the base increasing to 0.5 mm at the helicotrema (see Figure 1.9). In addition to becoming wider with increasing distance from the stapes and oval window, the basilar membrane decreases in its stiffness – the displacement to a constant force (its compliance) increases by a

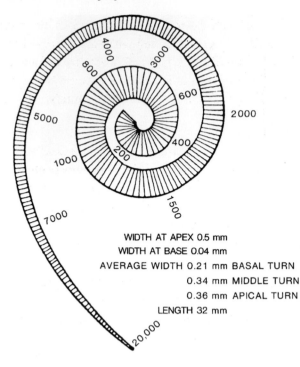

Figure 1.9 Diagram of the human basilar membrane, showing the approximate positions of maximal displacement to tones of different frequencies, and changes in width going from the base (near the stapes and oval window) to the apex (near the helicotrema). The ratio of width to length is exaggerated to show the variation in width more clearly. (From Stuhlman, 1943.)

factor of almost 100 in going from the basal end to the apex. These features appear to result in a "tuning" to different frequencies of sound along the basilar membrane. As shown in Figure 1.9, the region near the stapes shows maximum displacement amplitude and sensitivity to high frequencies, and the region near the helicotrema shows its greatest displacement and sensitivity to low frequencies. The frequency selectivity resembles a Fourier analysis of limited resolution. This is a topic of great importance to theories of hearing, and will be discussed in more detail in the section dealing with cochlear mechanics.

All of the blood reaching the cochlea comes through the internal auditory artery. Since there is no collateral source of blood, all structures within the cochlea degenerate if this blood supply is cut off. Capillaries are found below (not within) the basilar membrane and on the wall of the cochlear duct some distance from the auditory receptor cells, so that nutrients and metabolic products are transported by diffusion through the endolymph. This spatial separation of the capillaries reduces the sound associated with blood circulation at the location of the auditory receptors. Even with this increased distance from capillaries, there is still a relatively high level of low frequency noise at the receptors caused by blood flow (which is usually not heard because of the high threshold of the auditory system for low frequency sounds).

Neural structures and auditory pathways

Innervation of the auditory receptor cells is by the auditory nerve, which is also known as the cochlear branch of the vestibulocochlear (VIIIth) nerve. There are about 30,000 auditory nerve fibers associated with each inner ear. Their peripheral terminations consist of dendritic endings surrounding the inner and outer hair cells, and their central terminations are associated with neurons in the dorsal and ventral cochlear nuclei located within the lower brainstem.

The nerve fibers lose their myelin sheaths before entering the organ of Corti. They enter through openings near the inner hair cells called the habenula perforata, with about eight or nine fibers passing through each of the openings. Over 90 percent of these afferent fibers terminate on inner hair cells, with individual hair cells innervated by about eight separate fibers. The few remaining afferent fibers cross the tunnel of Corti, make a right-angle turn toward the basal end, and send out collateral branches which innervate the outer hair cells. About 10 outer cells are connected with each fiber, with each outer hair cell making contact with perhaps three or four separate fibers.

The first-order afferent or ascending auditory fibers all terminate at the cochlear nucleus. A number of different routes are available within the ascending pathway leading to the cortex. Some of the brainstem nuclei and their interconnections are shown in Figure 1.10. The ventral part of the cochlear nucleus sends second-order fibers to both the ipsilateral and the contralateral superior olive and the accessory superior olive. While not shown in the figure, there is ample neurophysiological and histological evidence that there are also some second-order fibers that cross over directly from one cochlear nucleus to the other (Shore, Godfrey, Helfert, et al., 1992), probably facilitating the cross-ear temporal comparisons that play an important role in localization of sources (see Chapter 2). The dorsal cochlear nucleus sends second-order axons to the contralateral lateral lemniscus and inferior colliculus. Some third-order neurons also reach the inferior colliculus after synapsing with second-order neurons in the dorsal nucleus of the lateral lemniscus. In addition, the inferior colliculus receives fibers from the contralateral accessory nucleus of the superior olive and both the ipsilateral superior and accessory olives. From the colliculus, fibers go both to the reticular formation and to the

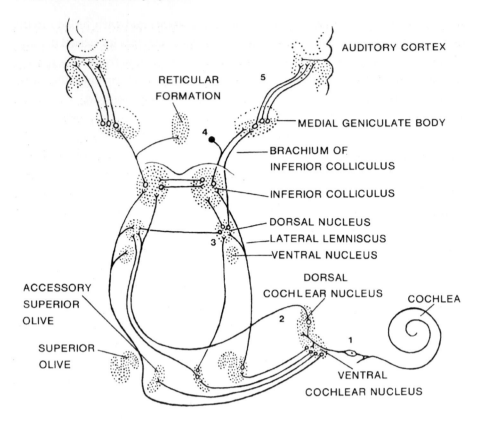

RETICULAR FORMATION

AUDITORY CORTEX

MEDIAL GENICULATE BODY

BRACHIUM OF INFERIOR COLLICULUS

INFERIOR COLLICULUS

DORSAL NUCLEUS
LATERAL LEMNISCUS
VENTRAL NUCLEUS

DORSAL COCHLEAR NUCLEUS

COCHLEA

ACCESSORY SUPERIOR OLIVE

SUPERIOR OLIVE

VENTRAL COCHLEAR NUCLEUS

Figure 1.10 Major structures in the ascending (afferent) chain from cochlea to cortex and some of the interconnections between structures. The numbers indicate the neuron levels (or orders). (From Gacek, 1972.)

medial geniculate. There are no connections between the two medial genicu-lates, so that all of the complex subcortical lateral interactions occur below this level. The auditory cortex is located within the temporal lobes. There is a lateral asymmetry in auditory cortical processing: the left hemisphere plays a domin-ant role in speech perception for most people, and other types of auditory processing also show evidence of dominance of one hemisphere or the other (Kimura, 1967; Møller, 2006). While information reaching one cochlea is trans-mitted to both hemispheres, under some conditions contralateral transmission seems favored over ipsilateral. (For a review of this literature, see Springer and Deutsch, 1993.) However, there is a richly innervated connection between hemispheres via the corpus callosum.

There are four or five synapses along the route from cochlea to cortex, with an increase in complexity of interconnections as we ascend the auditory pathway. In humans, the roughly 3,500 inner hair cells are responsible for stimulating the 30,000 afferent fibers within each of the two auditory nerves that feed into the roughly one million subcortical neurons on each side associated with the auditory pathway to the cortex. The cochlear nucleus has about 90,000 neurons, the superior olivary complex (together with the trapezoid body) 34,000, the lateral lemniscus 38,000, the inferior colliculus 400,000, the medial geniculate 500,000, and the auditory cortex 100 million (Worden, 1971).

Although the nature of interactions and processing of information along the afferent auditory pathway is still obscure, the large number of neurons within subcortical centers relative to the number of auditory nerve fibers indicates both the importance and complexity of subcortical processing. Hence, the conventional term of auditory "pathway" can be misleading, since it implies a passive conduit from receptor cells to cortex.

In addition to the afferent or ascending fibers carrying information from the organ of Corti, there are also efferent or descending fibers carrying impulses from higher centers down to their terminations on the inner and outer hair cells. The efferent fibers forming the olivocochlear bundle in the cochlear nerve have cell bodies located in the superior olivary regions (Rasmussen, 1946, 1953). Some of these cell bodies have fibers that are ipsilateral (uncrossed) and others have fibers that are contralateral (crossed) relative to the cochlea at which they terminate. These efferent fibers ramify extensively after entering the cochlea with the great majority of their terminations occurring at the outer hair cells. For the few efferents associated with the inner hair cells, it seems that contact generally is made through synapses with dendrites of afferent neurons, with only a small proportion of connections made directly with inner hair cells.

Brownell, Bader, Bertrand, and Ribaupierre (1985) showed that electrical stimulation of the outer hair cells could lead to their contraction, and Ashmore (1987) reported that this outer contraction occurred with an extremely short latency (120 μs). Therefore, it seems possible that the response of the inner hair cell receptors can be modulated by efferent stimulation of the outer hair cells for frequencies up to the kilohertz range. While it is of interest to study directly the effects produced by efferent stimulation of the outer hair cells, there are experimental difficulties, including the sensitivity of the efferent system to anesthesia. Despite these problems, Winslow and Sachs (1988) have provided neurophysiological evidence that the efferent olivocochlear bundle can improve the sensitivity of afferent auditory nerve fibers to tonal signals in the presence of interfering noise. This is consistent with the earlier behavioral report by Dewson (1968) that discrimination between two vowels in the presence of noise by monkeys was impaired by sectioning of the efferent olivocochlear bundle. It appears that efferent fibers release a neurotransmitter that modulates sensitivity of afferent nerve fibers (Puel, 1995), and also change the motility of the outer hair cells in a manner that alters the extent of vibration of the basilar membrane (Collet, Kemp, Veuillet, *et al.*, 1990).

Mechanics for stimulation within the inner ear

The mechanical responses within the inner ear leading to stimulation of the auditory receptor cells are quite complex. While our understanding of these processes has increased considerably in recent years, there are still aspects that remain puzzling and controversial.

In the nineteenth century, Helmholtz suggested that the inner ear performs a frequency (or Fourier) analysis of sounds, with different regions of the organ of Corti vibrating maximally to different frequency components. He considered that the spectrum was spread out along the basilar membrane, starting with the highest frequencies at the basal end, and the lowest frequencies at the apical end. The location of the stimulated nerve fibers, according to Helmholtz, signaled the frequency components of the sounds. His initial theory (presented in the first edition of his *Sensations of Tone* in 1863) suggested that the rods of Corti (also called pillars of Corti) located near the nerve fibers on the basilar membrane (see Figure 1.7) might furnish resonators for the spectral components by virtue of gradations in stiffness and tension. Subsequent studies indicated that the rods of Corti were absent in birds and amphibians; and this, together with new evidence showing that there was a graded increase in width of the basilar membrane in the direction of the apex (see Figure 1.9), caused Helmholtz to change his suggestion concerning the resonating elements. His second suggestion was that the basilar membrane itself was set into sympathetic vibration due to appropriately stretched and loaded radial fibers located within the membrane. These fibers, so the theory went, provided high frequency resonance at the basal end and low frequency resonance at the apical end (see Helmholtz, 1954, for a translation conformal with the 4th German edition, 1877). This second version of his place theory is the one generally remembered today, although we shall return later to his first theory involving the rods of Corti. In his revised place theory, Helmholtz did not propose that the resonance of a fiber within the basilar membrane was limited to a narrow range of frequencies, but that appreciable vibration of the fiber would still occur when the frequency was removed as much as a semitone (1/12-octave) from that producing maximal response.

Békésy, in a series of experiments having great impact on theories of cochlear mechanics for many years (for a summary see Békésy, 1960), claimed that although movement of the basilar membrane provided a basis for frequency analysis involving place of stimulation, the details were rather different than those envisioned by Helmholtz. Békésy examined preparations of the basilar membrane through a microscope and observed that when fine glass filaments with rounded tips were pressed against the membrane, a circular deformation was produced rather than the elliptical pattern that should result from the transverse tension postulated by Helmholtz. (However, Voldrich (1978) has questioned the validity of Békésy's observations.) Békésy also claimed that, when the basilar membrane was cut, the edges did not gape apart in a lens-shaped opening, as should occur if there were a lateral tension. Rather, the edges of the cut did not draw apart at all, indicating that there was little tension in any direction. Békésy likened the basilar membrane to a gelatinous sheet, and suggested that graded differences in the width and the stiffness of the basilar membrane are responsible for differences in the locus of maximal displacement by traveling waves. Perhaps the simplest type of traveling wave to visualize is one which sweeps down a rope attached to a fixed support at one end when it is given a shake at the other. However, a traveling wave on the basilar membrane has some features not found in this very simple model. The velocity of the traveling wave on the basilar membrane is not constant, changing from 105 m/s near the oval window, to about 10 m/s near the apex. The speed of sound in the cochlear liquids is very much faster, about 1,600 m/s (this difference is of significance in determining whether the traveling wave or the sound pressure wave is the stimulus for receptor cell transduction, as will be discussed subsequently). Thus, the traveling wave occurs later than the compression wave corresponding to sound transmission in the cochlear fluids. The traveling wave (see Figure 1.11) always moves in the direction from basal to apical end regardless of the direction of the compression wave. Even when the compression wave is made to travel in an antidromic direction from apex to base, the traveling wave still originates at the base and travels in the usual fashion toward the apex. Dallos (1978) has discussed in detail possible hydrodynamic principles governing production of the traveling wave by an exchange of energy between the basilar membrane and the surrounding fluids. The physical factors involved in the production of the traveling wave interact in an extremely complex fashion, making an exact analytic solution impossible. However, approximate solutions can be achieved by the introduction of several simplifying assumptions.

Since the maximal displacement of the basilar membrane occurs at different loci for different frequencies (as shown in Figure 1.9), the membrane itself functions as a filter producing a spectral analysis of sound. The basal end responds maximally to high frequencies, and these spectral elements are removed as components of the traveling wave as it continues its passage along

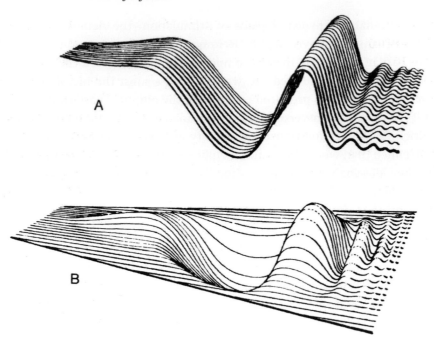

Figure 1.11 Two models of the traveling wave pattern along the basilar membrane produced by a single pulse: A represents the momentary displacement of a ribbon-like model; B represents a refinement of A in which displacement is shown for a ribbon attached at both edges. (From Tonndorf, 1960.)

the basilar membrane. The lower frequency components are present at loci responding maximally to higher frequencies, although these lower frequencies produce motions of relatively small magnitude at these positions. The first direct observations of traveling waves were made by Békésy, who used an optical microscope to view cochleas obtained from cadavers, as well as those obtained from a series of mammals ranging in size from a mouse to an elephant. Detection of motion using an optical microscope is limited to resolution of displacements of 1 μm or more, corresponding to very high sound intensities (120 dB and above). Also, Békésy's detailed observations were limited to the more accessible apical half of the basilar membrane. After his pioneering studies, more sensitive methods for measuring basilar membrane motion became available. One of these methods is the Mössbauer technique first employed in the study of cochlear mechanics by Johnstone and Boyle (1967) and Johnstone, Taylor, and Boyle (1970). In this procedure, a tiny bit of radioactive substance (a gamma-ray emitter) is placed on the basilar membrane, the added mass being considered small enough not to interfere appreciably with vibratory movement. The Doppler effect produced by motion of the gamma-ray source toward and away from the detector causes small frequency shifts. Usually cobalt-57 atoms locked into a crystalline lattice are used as the radioactive source. Decay of the cobalt-57 produces excited iron-57 atoms, which remain in the same lattice position, thus minimizing inertial recoil when the iron atom emits a gamma ray of characteristic fixed frequency and becomes stable iron-57. A screen of stable (nonexcited) iron-57 placed between emitter and detector serves as a very sharply tuned filter which absorbs the gamma rays when the emitter lying upon the basilar membrane is at rest. Vibratory motion of the basilar membrane results in Doppler shifts in frequency, which permit the radiation to pass through the filter to a detector. This ingenious technique was also used by Rhode (1971, 1973) to show that the mechanical properties of the basilar membrane are quite different in live and dead animals, with changes developing quite rapidly after death, bringing into question results reported by Békésy. Subsequently, Sellick, Patuzzi, and Johnstone (1982) used the Mössbauer technique to demonstrate that the mechanical response of the basilar membrane to sound deteriorates quite rapidly during the course of an experiment, so that caution must be used in extrapolating findings to intact animals. Another procedure employing the Doppler effect uses laser illumination of the basilar membrane (Kohllöffel, 1972a, 1972b, 1972c; Mammano and Ashmore, 1995; Cooper, 1999). Monochromatic light is split into two beams, a reference beam and a probe beam that has been reflected from a selected region of the basilar membrane set into vibration by an appropriate sound. The reflected light is subject to a Doppler shift in frequencies and, when combined with the stable reference beam, interference effects detected by an interferometer indicate the extent of displacement of the basilar membrane. In another procedure, Wilson and Johnstone (1975) used a very sensitive capacitance probe to measure the mechanical filter characteristics of the basilar membrane.

Although measurements of the filter characteristics of the basilar membrane have suggested to some investigators that its frequency resolution could account for the resolution observed for the electrophysiological responses of nerve fibers and psychophysical (behavioral) responses, a number of other factors could be involved in spectral resolution and response thresholds. These include lateral inhibition (or more accurately, lateral suppression) produced in regions surrounding those of maximal stimulation (Békésy, 1960; Houtgast, 1974a), leading to the "two-tone suppression" by which a louder tone suppresses the neural response to a fainter neighboring tone, thus enhancing the amplitude difference of the tones. It has also been suggested that spectral sharpening could be accomplished through interactions between waves produced along the basilar membrane through longitudinal coupling with the tectorial membrane (Zwislocki and Kletsky, 1979; Zwislocki, 1980). An especially interesting hypothesis that has received some recent support is that spectral resolution may involve stereocilia resonance – a mechanism reminiscent of Helmholtz's initial resonance theory (discussed earlier) involving resonance of rods (the rods of Corti) adjacent to the outer hair cells, rather than the hypothetical transverse fibers within the basilar membrane suggested in his later theory. Stereocilia resonance is suggested by the anatomical evidence that those cilia associated with the same hair cell are bonded to form stiff bundles (Flock, Flock, and Murray, 1977) – these bundles are tallest at the apex (the low frequency end) and shortest at the base (the high frequency end) of the cochlea (Lim, 1980), as would be expected for resonant bodies. Pujol, Lenoir, Ladrech, *et al.* (1992) have pointed out that although the inner hair cells do not vary much in length with position on the organ of Corti, the variation of size with position is considerable for outer hair cells. They have constructed what they have called a "xylophone-like" figure showing outer hair cell length as a function of estimated resonant frequency across mammalian species.

Evidence that hair cell resonance can occur without movement of the supporting structure was reported for the alligator lizard by Peake and Ling (1980). Although the basilar papilla (the reptilian homolog of the basilar membrane) of the reptile showed no traveling wave and no filtering characteristics when examined using the Mössbauer technique, there was a sharp frequency selectivity of hair cells and nerve fibers. Fettiplace and Crawford (1980) obtained intracellular recordings from single hair cells of another reptile (a turtle) and found sharp frequency selectivity. Cells were arranged tonotopically along the papilla, with sensitivity to the highest frequency found at the basal or stapedial end (as in mammals). As with the alligator lizard, there appeared to be no frequency selectivity of the structure supporting the hair cells – nevertheless the hair cells appeared to behave in their temporal characteristics as would be expected for simple tuned resonators.

Dancer (1992) has presented evidence involving phase lags and time delays indicating that the slow-moving traveling wave in mammals does not stimulate the hair cells, but rather that hair cells themselves act as tuned resonators (as demonstrated for reptiles), and that they respond directly to sound waves that are conducted at very high velocity through the fluid of the endolymph. What then is the role of the movement of the basilar membrane? One possibility was suggested by Braun (1994). After he examined anatomical, neurophysiological, and behavioral data for a number of mammalian species, he concluded that the functions of tuned resonance of the hair cells and of the basilar membrane are quite different. Braun considered that at low sound levels, the motility of the outer hair cell stereocilia provides an active response that amplifies the vibrations of the endolymph bathing both outer and inner hair cells. The induced movement of the adjacent inner hair cells could then stimulate the afferent fibers of the auditory nerve. The basilar membrane, according to Braun, plays no functional mechanical role at low levels of stimulation. However, at high stimulus levels, the movement of the basilar membrane function could act as a tuned absorber of excessive vibrational energy, preventing damage to the fragile stereocilia (that exhibit a passive resonance at these levels). Braun argued that the extremely low sound energy available at threshold is insufficient to move the relatively massive basilar membrane appreciably, while the slender and delicate stereocilia require very little energy to move at their particular resonant frequencies. Indeed, in terms of the energy required for stimulation at threshold, the ear is even more sensitive than the eye (which can require only 7 or 8 photons, each stimulating separate receptors, for flash detection in the dark adapted eye). Braun's hypothesis concerning vibrational damping by the basilar membrane at high stimulus levels could help explain how our hearing can cover the extremely great dynamic range of 120 dB (a power ratio of one trillion to one). This dynamic range is even greater than that of vision (roughly 80 or 90 dB) which, incidentally, also requires two separate peripheral processes (scotopic mediated by rod receptors, and photopic mediated by cone receptors) to cover its vast operational range extending from vision by reflected starlight on a moonless night to the viewing of a bright sunlit scene.

Detectable tone-like narrow band sounds can be emitted by the ear, indicating an active mechanical process, which is generally considered to involve motility of the outer hair cells. In one reported case, this "objective tinnitus" or ringing by the ear was loud enough to be heard by people nearby (Huizing and Spoor, 1973). Although reports of such emissions had been associated in the literature with hearing disorders (for discussion, see Dallos, 1981; Zurek, 1981), it is now accepted that tonal generation (albeit at a low level) occurs in people with normal hearing. Thus, Zurek (1981) found that of 32 persons with normal hearing, 16 had detectable acoustic emissions in one or both ears. It is tempting to hypothesize that tinnitus in general is caused by spontaneous acoustic emissions, but Bilger, Matthies, Hammel, and Demorest (1990) examined people suffering from tinnitus and found that only 5 percent demonstrated the objective presence of the sound that was heard. In addition to these spontaneously generated sounds, Kemp (1978) and others have observed and studied stimulated, or evoked, acoustic emissions consisting of a delayed replica or an acoustic echo generated by the ear following a brief stimulus. The delay between a brief click and the evoked sound can be much too long for an acoustic reflection, requiring an active process within the cochlea. In addition, following a short tone burst, a relatively long train of pressure fluctuations can be detected in the ear canal. For a comprehensive review of otoacoustic emissions, see Probst, Lonsbury-Martin, and Martin (1991).

The auditory-acoustic paradox: excellent discrimination from a poor instrument

In order for a microphone to be considered as a high-fidelity component of an audio system, it should produce a transduced signal that faithfully follows the waveform of sound, introducing no distortion of its own. Applying this criterion, the construction and functioning of the ear is extremely poor. The ear is not unique in this respect; characteristics which could be considered as serious flaws in a physical instrument are found in other sensory systems as well. Thus, Helmholtz listed and described in some detail the optical defects of the normal eye which include severe spherical aberration, chromatic aberration, light scattering by colloidal particles, inhomogeneities suspended in the ocular fluids, and inside-out retinal design (the blood vessels and nerves are in front of the light-sensitive receptor cells and cast shadows, rather than being located behind the receptors as in the octopus eye). He then stated that if an optician had tried to sell him an instrument with these defects, he would feel justified in blaming his carelessness in the strongest terms and returning the instrument (see Warren and Warren, 1968, pp. 73–80).

Comparable acoustical "defects" can be described for the performance of the ear. The pinna produces resonances and time delays that change the intensity and phase of spectral components in a manner which varies with azimuth and elevation of the source. The external ear canal operates as a resonant tube, selectively enhancing frequencies of about 3,000 or 4,000 Hz. The intra-aural muscles can produce frequency-selective amplitude reductions when they contract. The middle and inner ears are known to introduce distortions before neural transduction, so that sinusoidal stimuli at moderate intensities generate appreciable levels of extraneous sinusoidal frequencies at the receptor level (see Plomp, 1976; Kim, 1980; Dallos, 1981).

Helmholtz pointed out that the optical imperfections of the eye were the consequence of a design no better than it absolutely had to be (or, as he put it, one does not use a razor to cut firewood). Although optical defects correspond to the limits of tolerable distortion in vision, it appears that some acoustical distortions introduced by the ear serve actively to enhance auditory discrimination.

Although we can perceive relatively slight distortions and changes in spectral balance produced by loudspeakers and audio amplifiers, it is often not possible for us to detect the gross distortions and changes in spectral balance produced within our own ears. Acoustic distortions by the ear (which can be measured with appropriate techniques), if present consistently as part of the normal transduction process, are treated by the listener as nondistorted representations of the stimulus. Some acoustic transformations in spectral characteristics of a sound produced by pinna interaction, head shadows, and so on, are associated with the spatial location of the source (as discussed in some detail in Chapter 2). These position-dependent transformations do not interfere with identification of a sound, but they do contribute to spatial localization. Thus, some spectral changes cannot be perceived as such: they are interpreted as changes occurring in an external physical correlate (azimuth and elevation of the source) while the nature of the sound (its quality or timbre) appears to be unchanged.

Electrophysiological response of the cochlea and peripheral neural apparatus

Much of our knowledge concerning the nature of neurophysiological processing of acoustic information deals with events occurring within cochlear structures and first-order auditory neurons. We will deal first with the three types of electrical potentials generated by structures other than nerve fibers in the inner ear: the resting potential, the summating potential, and the cochlear microphonic.

The resting potential

In the absence of any stimulation by sound, DC (direct current) differences in resting potential are found between structures in the cochlea. Relative to the potential of both the perilymph and cortilymph, the endolymph of the scala media bathing the stereocilia of the hair cells has a potential of $+80$ mV. Since the resting potential within the hair cells is about -70 mV, there is a very high potential difference (that is, for structures within the body) of 150 mV across the cell membrane at the stereocilia. Mechanical deformation of the stereocilia during stimulation by sound opens ionic channels causing an abrupt decrease in the resting potential of the receptor cell, leading to the stimulation of the associated auditory nerve fibers. The stria vascularis lining the scala media seems to be implicated in maintaining the high endolymph potential necessary for stimulation of the receptor cells.

The summating potential

When stimulation by sound occurs, there is a DC change from the resting level, called the summating potential, which can be picked up by electrodes within and near the cochlea. The magnitude of the summating potential depends upon the locations of the measuring electrode and the

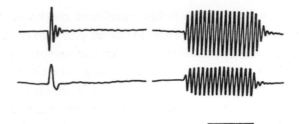

10 ms

Figure 1.12 Cochlear microphonic response to a click (left) and tone burst (right) in the guinea pig. The upper tracings represent the cochlear microphonic response measured with difference electrodes, the lower tracings depict the acoustic waveforms monitored at the eardrum. (From Dallos, 1973.)

reference electrode. At any particular location, the summating potential appears to be a complex function of both sound frequency and sound intensity. Despite the fact that the summating potential was discovered some time ago (Davis, Fernandez, and McAuliffe, 1950), there is still considerable uncertainty concerning the details of its nature. But there is general agreement that there are a number of different processes which summate to produce this potential (for details concerning possible factors and their interactions to produce the summating potential, see Møller, 2006).

The cochlear microphonic

The effect now called the cochlear microphonic was described by Wever and Bray in 1930. It was observed that if a sound was played in a cat's ear, an alternating current (AC) response could be picked up by an electrode placed at the round window of the cat. When this AC response was amplified and played back through a loudspeaker, a fairly faithful copy of the stimulus was produced. Thus, when someone spoke into the cat's ear in one room, the amplified potential changes within the cat's cochlea could be played back by a loudspeaker in another room to produce a quite intelligible message. Wever and Bray at first believed that they were measuring responses within the auditory nerve itself. However, the following year (1931) Lord Adrian reported some of his observations, which indicated that a large part of the response measured by Wever and Bray was due to what he called the "cochlear microphonic," with only a small contribution attributable to potential changes within the auditory nerve. The cochlear microphonic can be picked up at positions some distance from the cochlea, although the position generally employed is at or near the round window. Figure 1.12 shows how closely the cochlear microphonic follows the acoustic stimulus. In making the trace of the cochlear microphonic shown in the figure, "difference" electrodes were used, which were placed so as to make it possible to cancel out other types of potential changes. The cochlear microphonic appears without any latency (unlike neural responses), and the changes in the cochlear microphonic produced either by reduction of oxygen supply or by introduction of anesthesia are different from the changes produced in neural activity. The frequency-response limits of the cochlear microphonic to sinusoidal tones resemble the frequency limits of hearing of the animal under study, so that bats generate cochlear microphonics with frequencies well above the upper limits of response for humans. Studies with animals have shown that, when hair cells with maximum sensitivity to particular frequencies are destroyed by prolonged exposure to intense tones of these frequencies, cochlear microphonic responses to these frequencies are abolished. Detailed investigations using kanamysin, which selectively damages the outer hair cells, have shown that the integrity of the outer hair cells is required for normal cochlear microphonics, with inner hair cells playing a relatively minor role in the development of this response.

Whole-nerve action potential

When an electrode is placed near the cochlea and the indifferent or reference electrode at some remote site (such as the mouth or neck), the active electrode's response to sound reflects the effect of the whole-nerve response as well as the summating potential and the cochlear microphonic. If the reference electrode is placed appropriately, various procedures are available which are capable of canceling the potential changes attributable to summating potentials and cochlear microphonics (see Dallos, 1973). The isolated whole-nerve action potential reflects the integrated activity of individual fibers. An example of this action potential is shown in Figure 1.13. Usually, responses to clicks or to the onset of tone bursts are examined, since responses of individual nerve fibers consist of both negative and positive changes relative to their resting potential, and hence different nerve fibers can cancel each other when asynchronous responses are summed.

Single-unit receptor potentials

The gross potential changes within the cochlea in response to sound that have been described above (summating potential, cochlear microphonic, whole-nerve action potential) provide an environment in which further activity of single units in response to acoustic stimulation takes place. The first of these single-unit responses to sound is the receptor potential. The auditory receptor cells terminate in stereocilia which, as we have seen, are bent by the shearing forces produced by sound. This bending produces graded changes in receptor potential

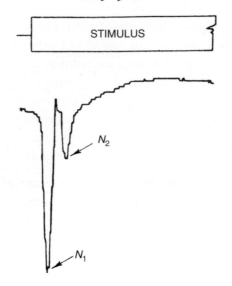

Figure 1.13 Whole-nerve action potential response at the onset of a tone burst of 8,000 Hz. The tracing represents the average of the potentials within the scala vestibuli and the scala tympani. The time separating N_1 from N_2 depends upon the stimulus level, and is usually between 1 and 2 ms. (From Dallos, 1973.)

(that is, changes in magnitude, which are monotonic functions of the angle of bending) that consist of both AC and DC components. The receptor potential acts upon the lower part of the receptor cell body containing presynaptic bars and possessing vesicles containing a chemical transmitter substance. Events associated with potential changes at the stereocilia cause release of this chemical transmitter, which diffuses to the nearby endings of auditory nerve fibers, where changes induced in membrane permeability lead to a "generator potential" change in the fiber. (For further discussion of the distinction between receptor potential and generator potential, see Davis, 1961, 1965; Dallos, 1978.)

Single-unit generator potentials

The initial segment of the auditory nerve axon exhibits a graded potential change reflecting the receptor potential. The generator potential is conducted with a decrement (that is, the potential change from the resting or baseline level decreases with distance from the synaptic endings near the hair cells). After passing out through the habenula perforata, the unmyelinated axon gains a myelin sheath, and it appears to be at this region that the all-or-none action potential is generated. Neural events beyond this point are quantized (all-or-none) and conducted without decrement, as the result of metabolic processes within the nerve fiber, to the synaptic ending of this first-order auditory neuron within the ipsilateral cochlear nucleus.

Action potentials of auditory nerve fibers

Using fine electrodes, it is possible to obtain responses from single fibers in the cochlear branch of the VIIIth nerve. Individual fibers have spontaneous discharge rates in the absence of sound varying from a few per second up to 100 per second or more. When the inner ear is stimulated by sound, the rate increases with intensity but cannot occur at rates greater than about 1,400 per second. The upper limit of response rate reflects the absolute refractory period (an interval following discharge during which intracellular processes ready the neuron for further response). The neural discharge measured by an electrode appears as a voltage spike of fixed amplitude and corresponds to a potential change sweeping along the fiber from cochlea to cochlear nucleus.

Individual nerve fibers exhibit frequency selectivity reflecting their particular place of origin on the organ of Corti, and the sinusoidal frequency corresponding to their greatest sensitivity (lowest threshold) is called the best or characteristic frequency. Neurons with highest characteristic frequencies are found near the surface of the auditory nerve bundle, with characteristic frequency decreasing regularly toward the center.

The frequency selectivity of an auditory nerve fiber is often shown as a "tuning curve" in which the ordinate represents the threshold in dB and the abscissa the frequency of the stimulating tone. Figure 1.14 shows a number of tuning curves for individual auditory nerve fibers with different characteristic frequencies measured in a single cat. While the typical form of a tuning curve has a gentle slope at the low frequency side of the characteristic frequency and a steep slope at the high frequency side, there are many other shapes. Some tuning curves are symmetrical, some have steeper slopes at the low frequency side, and a number of fibers show a break in the low frequency side of the tuning curve in which the slope becomes much less steep near the lower frequency limit of their response range. It seems that although tuning curves reflect the general filter characteristics of the basilar membrane at the position of the receptor cells associated with nerve fibers, this correspondence between basilar membrane response and tuning curves is far from exact. One difference is that tuning curves are often sharper (have steeper slopes) than the filter characteristics of the basilar membrane. When the stimulus is raised to supraliminal levels, we can examine the "response area," or range of frequencies and amplitudes to which a fiber responds. One useful measure within the response area is the response rate (spikes per second) of a single fiber measured for different frequencies at a fixed decibel level, with the process repeated at various intensity levels. These "isointensity contours" for a single fiber of a squirrel monkey are shown in Figure 1.15. It can be seen in this figure

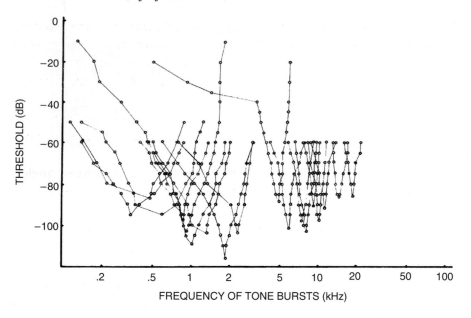

Figure 1.14 Tuning curves of individual auditory nerve fibers with different characteristic frequencies in a single cat. Each curve represents the intensity in decibels (relative to an arbitrary reference standard) needed to reach the response threshold of the fiber. (From Kiang, 1965.)

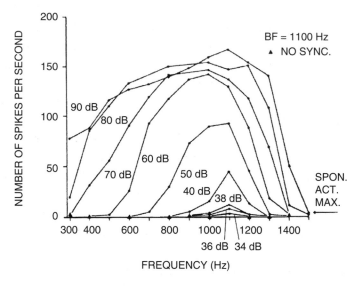

Figure 1.15 Isointensity contours for a single auditory nerve fiber of a squirrel monkey. The characteristic frequency or best frequency (BF) of this fiber is 1,100 Hz. The arrow at the lower right of the figure indicates the level of spontaneous activity, and the triangular data points near the bottom indicate the low level of activity at which there is no phase locking of spikes to the stimulus waveform. (From Rose, Hind, Anderson, and Brugge, 1971.)

that not only does the contour change with intensity, but the frequency producing the maximal response also changes. Considering only the response rate of the single fiber shown in this figure, it would not be possible to tell whether the stimulus were a relatively low intensity tone near the characteristic frequency or a relatively high intensity tone at a greater separation from the characteristic frequency. However, a single fiber may provide information identifying particular frequencies within its response area through phase locking.

Response spikes of the fiber tend to be locked to a particular phase angle of a sinusoidal stimulus. Thus, when a 200 Hz tone is used as the stimulus, and this frequency is within the response area of a single fiber, spikes picked up by the microelectrodes may be synchronous with a particular phase angle of the stimulus. The time between successive neural spikes is some integral multiple of the period of the 200 Hz sinusoid (5 ms), so that successive spikes can be separated by 5, 10, 15, or more ms. An individual nerve fiber generally does not discharge in a completely regular manner, so that there might be a 10 ms interval followed by a 20 ms interval followed by a 5 ms interval between successive spikes. However, if a recording of the pattern of firing is examined, it will be apparent that all periods between spikes are multiples of a 5 ms period. The phenomenon of phase locking seems to be a consequence of the mechanics of the cochlear events, discussed earlier, that produce the bending of the stereocilia that initiates the sequence of events leading to neural stimulation. As the frequency of the stimulating sinusoid is increased, phase locking can be observed up to about 4,000 or 5,000 Hz as long as the frequency is within the response area of the fiber. However, as has been pointed out earlier, fibers cannot discharge at intervals shorter than roughly 700 μs (microseconds), so that above about 1,400 Hz, a single fiber cannot respond to successive statements of a repeated waveform. But, if we consider the whole nerve, there will be some fibers responding to each repetition of the waveform. Hence, as suggested by Wever (1949), the rate at which "volleys" of neural firing occur can provide information concerning tonal frequency. The precision of locking to a particular phase angle decreases with frequency, and is effectively lost for sinusoids above approximately 4,000 Hz (periods below about 0.25 μs).

The extent of phase locking can be shown by interspike interval histograms. The histogram shown in Figure 1.16 is based on the responses of a squirrel monkey's single fiber to tones of the frequencies shown when presented for 1 s for a total of 10 times. The abscissa shows the time between successive spikes (discharges) of a single auditory fiber, and the ordinate shows the total number of occurrences of interspike intervals with this value. The same phase angle of

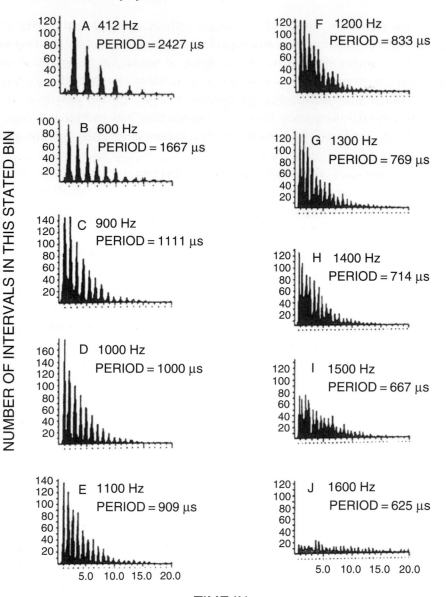

Figure 1.16 Interval histograms from a single auditory nerve fiber in a squirrel monkey. The abscissa gives the interval between successive spikes, with resolution into bins of 100 µs duration. Dots below the abscissa indicate integral multiples of the period for each frequency. For further details, see the text. (From Rose, Brugge, Anderson, and Hind, 1967.)

the sinusoid occurs at integral multiples of the sinusoid's period, and it can be seen that responses tended to occur at integral multiples of the particular period of the stimulus tone. For example, at 412 Hz, the periods between successive spikes generally were integral multiples of the tonal period of 2,427 µs (the time required for a single cycle of the 412 Hz tone), with more responses occurring at a value equal to the tonal period than for any multiple of this value. Evidence concerning the manner in which timing information encoded in the auditory nerve signal is maintained along the auditory pathway to the cortex has been summarized by Oertel (1999).

Investigation of human cortical function

When the signal processed by the brainstem nuclei reaches the auditory cortex, a flurry of local effects is initiated. There is an increase in blood flow to the region, accompanied by a greater uptake of glucose from the blood, and a greater conversion of oxyhemoglobin to deoxyhemoglobin. There is also increased intracellular and intercellular cortical activity producing electromagnetic effects detectable at the scalp.

These processes have led to two types of procedures used for studying the processing of auditory stimuli in the intact and healthy human cortex: hemodynamic, or blood flow measures that include functional magnetic resonance imaging (fMRI) and positron emission tomography (PET) scanning; and electromagnetic measures that include electroencephalography (EEG) and magnetoencephalography (MEG).

fMRI

Back in 1890, William James hypothesized that blood supply to the head would increase during mental activity, and described a fanciful experiment in which a subject would lie on a table that was delicately balanced so that it would tip to the head side during mental activity. A century later it became possible to measure blood flow in a rather more practical way.

Functional magnetic resonance imaging (fMRI) is based upon nuclear magnetic resonance (NMR), a property of some atomic nuclei that was discovered independently by E. M. Purcell and F. Bloch (for which they were jointly awarded a Nobel prize in 1952). Atomic nuclei with an odd number of nucleons (protons plus neutrons) each have an angular momentum, or spin, that results in a weak electromagnetic field with a characteristic resonant frequency.

When the fMRI procedure is used to study brain function, the subject's head is placed inside a coil producing a brief series of high-energy radio frequency (RF) bursts that are tuned to match the resonant frequency of hydrogen nuclei.

The nuclei absorb some of the energy of the bursts, and line up with the orientation of the field. When an individual pulse ceases, the nuclei lose their alignment and in doing so emit a weak decaying RF signal at their resonant frequency. This decaying signal can be detected either by the transmitter coil (which can also function as a receiver), or by a smaller surface coil placed on the region of the head closest to the auditory cortex. The nature of the emission-decay function is influenced by the composition of substances surrounding the emitting nuclei. The major factor determining the decay function is the Blood Oxygenation Level Dependent (BOLD) effect that reflects the increase in extent of oxygen uptake that accompanies an increase in local neural activity. Localization of the sites of activity along the mutually perpendicular x, y, and z axes in the brain is accomplished by producing three types of subtle gradient changes in the excitation pulses that influence the emission signal, and by processing the emission signal it is possible to determine the origin of the source to within 1–3 mm^3. Unfortunately, the use of fMRI to study the effects of auditory stimuli is made difficult by the intrinsically very loud noise produced by the scanning necessary to acquire the data for imaging. However, procedures have been developed to reduce this problem by "sparse" sampling during brief silent periods (Belin, Zatorre, Hoge, *et al.*, 1999; Hall, Haggard, Akeroyd, *et al.*, 1999).

PET

Positron emission tomography (PET) scanning involves introducing a short lived positron-emitting radioactive isotope into the bloodstream. The usual procedure involves the injection of a water solution containing the freshly prepared radioactive isotope of oxygen (^{15}O) incorporated in a metabolite mimic (deoxyglucose). The half-life of the isotope is only a few minutes, so it must be freshly prepared by appropriate equipment located near the PET scanner. During the first 30 s, the concentration of the isotope in the brain builds up and then rapidly decays, during which time the subject is performing some auditory task that results in the preferential uptake of the isotope by the neurons actively engaged in the task. When the ^{15}O decays, it emits a positron (an "antimatter" positively charged electron), which interacts with a nearby normal negatively charged electron; this results in their mutual annihilation and conversion of their mass to a pair of photons (gamma rays) traveling in opposite directions. Some of these pairs have both photons pass through the head without interacting with matter; they can then activate at the same time two of the coincidence detectors in a bank surrounding the head, each detector having a time-window of a few nanoseconds. The point of origin of the photons is located on the straight line between the pair of activated detectors.

By combining many of these lines, the locus of the ^{15}O uptake and associated increased metabolic activity can be computed in a manner similar to that employed for X-ray computer tomography (CT scans).

The spatial resolution of images produced by PET scans is poor. Since many of the gamma rays interact with matter within the head, health considerations prevent the use of the same subject for multiple runs. PET scans are normally used to supplement information produced by other scanning procedures.

EEG and MEG

By using a series of sensors placed over the scalp, the electroencephalogram (EEG) can record the electrical effects, and the magnetoencephalogram (MEG) can record the magnetic effects that accompany the neural activity produced by auditory stimuli. Both EEG and MEG are capable of recording events occurring during the initial neurophysiological responses to auditory stimuli, but they cannot localize the site of stimulation with the precision of the slower hemodynamic responses of fMRI and PET.

EEGs have a long history. The electrical activity of the exposed cerebral hemispheres of monkeys was described by Caton in 1875, and in 1913 Pravdich-Neminsky reported observations based on the evoked potentials in the dog. Berger began his studies of the human EEG in 1920, and was responsible for naming the effect. Since Berger's studies, there have been a great number of publications. It has been established that synchronous spiking of hundreds of thousand of neurons is required to produce effects large enough to be activated by detectors placed on the scalp. The cortical activities of columnar neural assemblies perpendicular to the scalp and of horizontally distributed units contribute to the EEG. The initial evoked responses have been observed in humans within 9–10 ms of the stimulus onset by EEG responses measured at the scalp (Starr and Don, 1988), and also by electrodes that had been implanted in the primary auditory cortex to determine the focus of severe epileptic seizures (Celesia, 1976). The EEG activity occurring between 10 and 40 ms (the so-called "middle latency" responses) reflects the acoustic nature of the stimulus, and the "late latency" responses from 50–300 ms after the onset of stimulation are attributed to higher-order processing. The extensive literature on the nature and interpretation of cortical EEG responses (and the less extensive MEG literature) has been reviewed and summarized by Näätänen and Winkler (1999).

Magnetoencephalography (MEG) does not have the long history of EEG. It is more difficult to employ, requiring a special magnetically shielded room to eliminate external magnetic fields, including that of the Earth. It also requires use of an extremely sensitive magnetometer, such as SQUID, that operates at low superconducting temperatures. Unlike EEG, MEG does not respond to responses of columnar-stacked neurons, but only to neurons having an orientation parallel to the surface of the head, with about 50,000 active neurons required to produce a measurable response. MEG has an advantage over EEG by not being subject to distortion by non-neuronal biosources, and of being capable of very high temporal resolution of less than 1 ms. MEG is not capable of accurate spatial localization, but this limitation can be overcome by its use in conjunction with data from fMRI.

Suggestions for further reading

For an excellent expanded coverage of most of the topics in this chapter along with disorders of the auditory system: Møller, A. R. 2006. *Hearing: Anatomy, Physiology, and Disorders of the Auditory System*, 2nd edition. San Diego, CA: Academic Press.

For a review of auditory physiology: Pickles, J. O. 1988. *An Introduction to the Physiology of Hearing*, 2nd edition. San Diego, CA: Academic Press.

For a detailed discussion of acoustics and its relation to hearing: Hartmann, W. M. 1998. *Signals, Sound, and Sensation*. New York: Springer-Verlag.

2

Spatial localization and binaural hearing

In Chapter 1 it was noted that the outer ear (pinna), ear canal, and middle ear modify and distort the acoustic signal before it reaches the inner ear. Although these changes would be considered serious defects if produced by microphones or other physical instruments, they can furnish valuable perceptual information. Thus, the complex acoustic changes produced by the pinnae when a source moves provide information concerning position, and result in perception of an unchanging sound at a changing location. This chapter discusses the effects produced by the pinnae, as well as other examples of how changes in acoustic input are not perceived as differences in the nature of the sound, but rather as differences in the location of the sound source relative to the listener's head.

Obviously, it often is important for us to know where the sound is originating, but there is another advantage associated with the ability to localize sound. As we shall see, mechanisms employed for localization allow us to hear signals which would otherwise be inaudible.

Any position in space can be specified relative to an observer by its azimuth (angle from straight ahead measured in the horizontal plane), elevation (angle from the horizontal measured in a vertical plane), and distance. Unfortunately, it is difficult to mimic the localization of sound sources in space using headphones because the sounds generated by them usually have apparent sources positioned within the listener's head (for reasons that will be discussed subsequently). These intracranial images can be made to move to the right or left by appropriate differences in the stimuli delivered to each ear, but such lateral images do not have either specific azimuth or elevation as do externalized sound images. It is conventional to use the term "lateralization" to describe intracranial sidedness of sound images produced through head-phones, and to use the term "localization" to describe positioning of exter-nalized images. The localization of a source in space involves both dichotic cues based upon differences in the input to each ear, and monoaural cues for which the stimulus to one ear alone can provide information concerning location of the source.

Binaural perception of azimuth

In 1876 and 1877, Lord Rayleigh demonstrated that the azimuth of the source of complex sounds such as voices could be identified accurately, as could high frequency sinusoidal tones. He attributed this localization ability to interaural intensity differences caused by the head's sound shadow. It was not until some 30 years later that Rayleigh (1907) appreciated that interaural phase differences could also be used for determining the azimuth of low frequency pure tones. He proposed at that time his influential "duplex" theory which considered that high frequencies are located laterally by interaural intensity differences while low frequencies are located laterally by interaural phase (or time) differences.

Figure 2.1 shows the analysis of Woodworth (1938) of how interaural path-length differences (leading to interaural time and phase differences) arise when a source is to the right or left of the medial plane. This figure shows the additional path length as due to two segments: a straight line portion, d_1, and the curved portion following the contour of the skull, d_2. The total increase in path distance to the further ear, ΔD, is described by the expression:

$$\Delta D = d_1 + d_2 = r(\theta + \sin \theta) \tag{2.1}$$

where r is the radius of a cross-section of the head considered as a circle and θ is the azimuth of a distant source measured in radians. This formula can be converted to give values for time delay, ΔT. If we consider that the radius of the head is 8.5 cm, and the speed of sound is 34,000 cm/s, then the difference in time of arrival of sound at the two ears is given by the expression:

$$\Delta T = 0.25 \, (\theta + \sin \theta) \, \text{ms} \tag{2.2}$$

Interaural phase differences can furnish cues to azimuth only at low fre-quencies. When a sinusoidal tone is about 650 Hz, its wavelength (about 50 cm) corresponds to about twice the path-length increment to the further ear with sources at azimuths of 90° or 270° from the medial plane. Hence, there will be a 180° interaural phase difference (that is, a pressure peak in one ear will occur

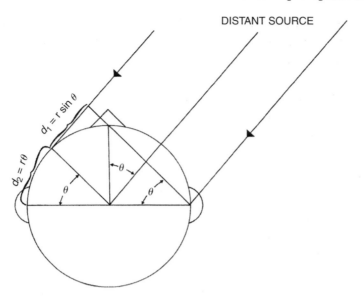

Figure 2.1 Path-length difference between the two ears corresponding to the azimuth of the source, θ. The additional distance to the further ear is shown as the sum of a straight line segment, d_1, and a curved segment following the contour of the head, d_2. The path-length difference can be used to calculate the difference in time of arrival of sound at the two ears, as described in the text. The effects of the pinnae are not considered in this model. (Adapted from Woodworth, 1938.)

at the same time as a pressure trough in the other) if the source is at 90° or 270°. When the sinusoidal frequencies are higher than about 1,300 Hz, multiple ambiguities occur with several azimuth angles corresponding to the same interaural phase difference, and phase no longer is a useful indicator of azimuth for sinusoidal tones.

Woodworth's model has been tested directly by measuring time differences for the arrival of clicks at the two ears (Feddersen, Sandel, Teas, and Jeffress, 1957), as shown in Figure 2.2. It can be seen that the values obtained agree very well with Woodworth's model. However, measurements using sinusoidal tones (see Abbagnaro, Bauer, and Torick, 1975; Kuhn, 1977) have indicated that Woodworth's assumption that interaural time delays (ITDs) are independent of frequency of tones is incorrect, especially for low frequencies, apparently due to interactions with sound diffracted by the head. Roth, Kochhar, and Hind (1980) have suggested that there might be two kinds of ITDs, one which they called "steady state" ITD and another which they called "group" ITD. They hypothesized that each of these time delays might be encoded by separate groups of neurons.

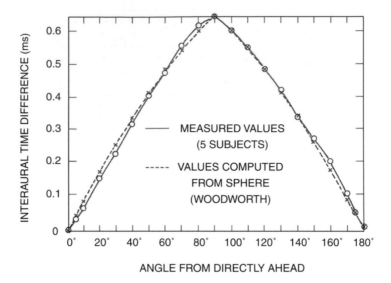

Figure 2.2 Interaural time differences for clicks as a function of azimuth. The solid line connects values as measured at the ears of actual heads, and the dashed line connects values calculated by Woodworth's procedure for a spherical head. (Adapted from Feddersen, Sandel, Teas, and Jeffress, 1957.)

There have been direct measures of the thresholds for detection of inter-aural time differences using sinusoidal tones of different frequencies delivered through headphones. Klumpp and Eady (1956) determined the minimal time delay permitting listeners to lateralize a sound correctly to the side of the leading ear 75 percent of the time. A minimum of about ten microseconds (10 μs) was found for a 1,000 Hz tone (this time difference corresponds to an azimuth of about 2° for an external source). The threshold rose to 24 μs at 1,300 Hz, and was not measurable (i.e., phase differences could not be detected at all) at 1,500 Hz and above. When frequencies were decreased from 1,000 Hz, there was a regular increase in interaural delay thresholds, reaching 75 μs at 90 Hz (the lowest frequency used).

As mentioned earlier, Rayleigh's duplex theory considered that sources of high frequency sounds can be located laterally through interaural intensity differences, so that when the frequency becomes too high for phase to operate, intensity comes into play. When a sphere has a diameter which is greater than roughly half the wavelength of a sinusoidal tone, it will cast an appreciable sound shadow. This shadow results in a detectable interaural intensity difference starting at about 1,000 Hz, with the interaural intensity difference increasing with frequency. Figure 2.3 shows measurements by Feddersen, Sandel, Teas, and Jeffress (1957) of interaural intensity differences as a

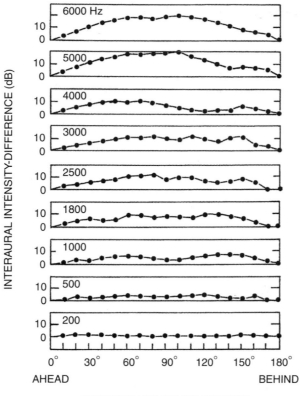

Figure 2.3 Interaural intensity differences measured as a function of azimuth for sinusoidal tones of different frequencies. It can be seen that there is no appreciable sound shadow cast by the head at 200 Hz, and a considerable shadow cast by the head at 6,000 Hz. The lack of symmetry in the front quadrant (0° to 90°) relative to the rear quadrant (90° to 180°) is attributable to the pinna. (Adapted from Feddersen, Sandel, Teas, and Jeffress, 1957.)

function of the azimuth of the source for frequencies ranging from 200 to 6,000 Hz. Were the head a sphere without pinnae, the curves would be symmetrical about 90°. However, the pinnae do produce sound shadows and resonances for high frequency tones (as will be discussed later) which enter into the asymmetries seen in this figure.

The accuracy of listeners' estimates of the azimuth of a loudspeaker producing pure tones was measured by Stevens and Newman (1936). Subjects were seated in a chair elevated above a roof to minimize sound reflections and approximate an anechoic (echo-free) environment, and measurements were made early in the morning to reduce extraneous sounds. When tone bursts (as well as noise and clicks) were delivered at various azimuths, a sizable number of front-back reversals were noted (that is, sources on the same side differing by plus or minus the same number of degrees from either 90° or from 270° were confused), but confusions of right and left were almost never made. The greatest errors occurred at about 3,000 Hz, with error scores dropping at higher and lower frequencies. Subsequently, Sandel, Teas, Feddersen, and Jeffress (1955) used listeners seated in an anechoic room with head movements restricted by a clamp. Broadband noise and sinusoidal tones were heard alternately, each fading in and out gradually to minimize transient clicks. Since broadband noise is localized with greater accuracy, it was used as an acoustic pointer, and was adjusted to correspond to the apparent azimuth of the tone. Sandel *et al.* (1955) reported that the tonal frequency producing poorest accuracy in localization was about 1,500 Hz, a value an octave lower than that reported by Stevens and Newman. As in the earlier study, front-back confusions were quite common. This is not surprising if we consider that the interaural time delays are equivalent for such positions. The question that needs answering seems to be how discrimination between positions in the front and back quadrants on the same side of the medial plane can be made at all.

There appears to be two main ways in which front-back errors can be minimized when dealing with real sources in everyday life: one involves asymmetrical effects of the pinnae which will be discussed subsequently, and the other involves head movements. Changes in time of arrival correlated with lateral head-turning can disambiguate the direction of continuing sounds. For example, if the sound is on the right side, rotation of the head to the right will decrease the interaural time difference for sources in the front quadrant and will increase the interaural time difference for sources in the back quadrant.

Minimal audible angle

Mills (1958, 1972) measured the minimum angle permitting lateral resolution of tones, calling it the minimal audible angle by analogy to the well-known minimum visual angle. Listeners sat in an anechoic chamber with the position of their head fixed by a restraining clamp. Pairs of sinusoidal tone pulses were presented, and listeners were requested to tell whether the second pulse came from the right or left of the first (the source was moved in the short interval separating the pulses). Figure 2.4 shows the results obtained. The minimal audible angle was the least when measured as variation from 0° (straight ahead). Since listeners tend to orient their head toward the source of a sound of interest, the source is usually brought into the region of most accurate localization. Also, it often is possible to fixate a sound source visually near the medial plane, so that the auditory cues to localization can be

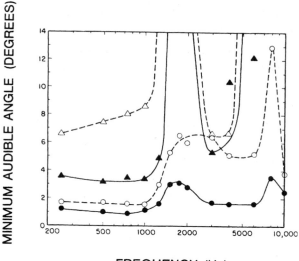

Figure 2.4 The minimum audible angle between successive pulses of a tone as a function of the frequency of the tone and the azimuth of the source (● 0°, ○ 30°, ▲ 60°, △ 75°). (From Mills, 1972.)

compared, and if appropriate, superseded by the more precise visual localization. In the medial plane, the minimum auditory angle is about one degree for high and low frequencies, being greater for frequencies from 1,500 to 2,000 Hz. (The minimum discriminable visual angle is about one minute of arc.) The high minimum auditory angle at midrange frequencies is in keeping with the duplex theory considering that judgments of azimuth are based on interaural phase differences at low frequencies and interaural intensity differences at high frequencies with neither cue acting effectively at midrange.

Binaural beats

When sinusoidal tones are mistuned slightly from unison and introduced separately into the two ears, binaural beats may be observed which are characterized by changing lateralization or fluctuation in loudness. For example, if a tone of 500 Hz is presented to one ear and 500.5 Hz to the other, a listener may hear a phantom source which moves from one side to the other and back again each 2 s, with any lateralization associated with the side of leading phase. Patterns of loudness maxima may also occur with beat periods longer than 1 s, but they are not very noticeable and show no consistent relation to phase angle. For fast rates of binaural beating (a few per second), lateralization shifts become difficult to hear, and listeners generally report a loudness fluctuation having a diffuse intracranial location (Lane, 1925). The upper frequency limit for the production of binaural beats by sinusoidal tones is uncertain. These beats are generally considered to be strongest for frequencies from about 300 to 600 Hz, becoming difficult to hear at 1,000 Hz. However, Wever (1949) claimed that by using "very slight frequency differences" he was able to obtain binaural beats (or lateralization shifts) up to 3,000 Hz. Wever also referred to an unpublished study by Loesch and Kapell indicating that subjects could hear binaural beats up to 2,500 Hz after about 10 hours of practice. Since there was evidence of increasing frequency limits with increasing practice time at the end of the experiment, Wever stated that "it seems certain" that further improvement would have occurred with further practice. It appears that the extent of practice and frequency separation (or beat rate) employed could be responsible for much of the variability in reports from different laboratories concerning the upper frequency limit for binaural beats.

Binaural beats were of importance in the development of the duplex theory of sound localization, since they helped convince Lord Rayleigh (1907) that interaural phase differences could indeed be detected. Rayleigh's earlier doubts appear to have been based upon the observation of Helmholtz and others that changing the phase relations between harmonic components of complex tones delivered to the same ear generally could not be detected.

Thus far, we have been considering the effect of time-of-arrival delays upon perception of laterality for sinusoidal tones. Rather different results are obtained when either brief clicks or extended complex sounds are heard.

Detection of interaural delays for clicks and for complex sounds

Klumpp and Eady (1956) obtained thresholds for detection of interaural time differences using a delay line to deliver a variety of different sounds through headphones.

We have already discussed their report that the lowest threshold value of 10 μs was obtained with a 1,000 Hz tone, with the detection of time delay becoming impossible at frequencies of 1,500 Hz and above. When they presented a single click with a nominal duration of 1 μs, an interaural delay threshold of 28 μs was found, but a 2 s burst consisting of 30 such clicks had a delay threshold of only 11 μs, indicating that integration of information from the individual clicks of a burst took place. When broadband noise was used, a threshold value of 10 μs was found, with approximately the same threshold observed for a 150–1,700 Hz noise band. Other noise bands with different bandwidths and frequency ranges had somewhat higher thresholds.

It might be thought that spectral components of noise below 1,500 Hz were required for detection of time differences, since Klumpp and Eady (1956) had found that phase differences for sinusoidal tones of 1,500 Hz and above were ineffective in producing lateralization. As discussed in Chapter 1, low frequency tones produce a phase locking of neural response, so that an interaural temporal comparison of fibers with the same low characteristic frequencies locked to the same phase angle could provide the temporal information for lateralization of broadband noise. However, Klumpp and Eady found that a narrow-band noise containing frequencies from about 3,000 to 3,300 Hz could be lateralized (although the threshold was at the relatively high value of 60 μs). It would appear that temporal information carried by the high frequency noise could be used for lateralization, despite the original formulation of the duplex theory that considered temporal information to be restricted to low frequency components. Henning (1974) provided an interesting demonstration of the nature of this temporal information. He introduced interaural time delays using a 3,900 Hz tone that was sinusoidally amplitude modulated at 300 Hz (that is, the amplitude envelope of the 3,900 Hz tone was varied in a sinusoidal fashion 300 times a second). Henning found that interaural time delays in the amplitude pattern could be detected with this stimulus at approximately the same threshold delay as found for a 300 Hz sinusoidal tone, despite the absence of any low frequency spectral components (spectrally, this amplitude modulated stimulus can be considered as consisting of three sinusoidal frequencies: the center frequency of 3,900 Hz, and two sidebands of 3,600 and 4,200 Hz respectively). McFadden and Pasanen (1975) used binaural beats to provide another demonstration that complex waveforms consisting of tones well above the classical limit of 1,000 Hz could give rise to dichotic temporal interactions. When a 3,000 Hz tone was presented to both ears and mixed with a 3,100 Hz tone at the left ear and a 3,101 Hz tone at the right ear, the difference in the interaural envelope frequencies (100 versus 101 Hz) produced binaural beating at a rate of 1/s. Binaural beats were noted even when the spectral components in the two ears were rather different as long as the envelopes were close in frequency. Thus 2,000 and 2,050 Hz in one ear would cause binaural beats of 1/s when heard with 3,000 and 3,051 Hz in the other ear.

Most experiments dealing with the limits for detection of interaural temporal delay have studied the lower limit for lateralization (the shortest detectable delay). But where does the upper limit lie? As we shall see, this limit is surprisingly high – at least one-half second for broadband noise delivered first to one ear and then to the other. At these long interaural delays, the sound is no longer lateralized to the leading ear.

As the interaural delay for broadband noise is increased from the threshold of about 10 μs reported by Klumpp and Eady (1956), an increase in the extent of lateralization is perceived for the fused single image up to delays of several hundred microseconds. The greatest possible delay attributable to interaural path-length differences is roughly 650 μs, and as would be expected, listeners hear a single lateral source at this delay. However, if the delay is increased to about 2,000 μs (2 ms), this sharp single lateral image starts to become diffuse (Bilsen and Goldstein, 1974). Blodgett, Wilbanks, and Jeffress (1956) reported that sidedness is lost for broadband noise with interaural delays of about 9.5 ms. The delay range producing diffuse lateralization is of interest because it appears possible to hear either lateralization to the leading ear or a pitch equivalent to that of a sinusoidal tone of $1/\tau$ Hz (where τ is the time delay in seconds), but not both. Fourcin (1965, 1970) used a variety of stimuli which permitted his listeners to hear this interaural delay pitch. The simplest condition involved broadband noise from two generators delivered to each ear. The noise from one generator was presented diotically (identical presentation in each ear), while the noise from the second generator had an interaural delay of a few milliseconds. Fourcin found that an interaural delay of τ s produced a pitch matching that of a sinusoidal tone of $1/\tau$ Hz. Later, Bilsen and Goldstein (1974) reported that it was possible to hear a faint pitch of $1/\tau$ Hz with noise from only a single source delivered to one ear several milliseconds after delivery to the other. (Pitches were produced for delays ranging from about 3 ms through 12 ms, corresponding to 333 and 83 Hz respectively.) Warren, Bashford, and Wrightson (1981) confirmed Bilsen and Goldstein's findings, but found that their subjects had an appreciably longer delay limit for the perception of pitch (50 ms delay corresponding to a pitch of 20 Hz). But, in addition, Warren *et al.* (1981) reported that an infrapitch periodicity could be detected at much longer interaural delays, up to a lower limit of at least 500 ms (corresponding to a repetition frequency of 2 Hz). These long delay periods could be matched in repetition time with periodic pulses delivered simultaneously to both ears (as could pitch-range interaural delays). In addition, for delays greater than 200 ms (corresponding to frequencies less than 5 Hz) the repetition period could be matched by the rate of finger tapping without the need for employing a second auditory stimulus. As we shall see in Chapter 3, mixing an ongoing diotic noise with its own restatement after a delay of 500 ms also can be perceived to repeat at 2 Hz, and the ability to detect such long-period repetition has implications for theories concerning neural periodicity analysis.

Curiously, although listeners can detect long interaural delays for broadband noise, they cannot tell which ear received the noise first. After perception of laterality was lost for delays greater than roughly 10 ms, the noise was heard as a spatial blur positioned symmetrically about the medial plane, and repetition was perceived as occurring within this space regardless of which ear received the noise first. A similar indefinite location has been reported for dichotic presentation of uncorrelated noises having equivalent long-term spectral characteristics (Kock, 1950; David, Guttman, and van Bergeijk, 1958; Warren and Bashford, 1976), with the percept described as resembling rain on a tin roof, or standing under a waterfall. Thus, although fusion into a single image does not take place either with long interaural delays of noise or with uncorrelated noises presented to each ear, neither is there an ability to hear two lateral inputs.

The following section deals with other examples of the loss of lateralization of monaural signals induced by contralateral sounds, and discusses evidence indicating that processing leading to delateralization corresponds to an early stage in auditory scene analysis that allows us to separate individual sources.

Contralateral induction

There have been several reports that monaural sounds seem to shift away from the stimulated side in the presence of qualitatively different sounds delivered to the other ear. Using headphones, Egan (1948) found monaural speech to be displaced toward the side of a contralateral noise, and Thurlow and Elfner (1959) found that a monaural tone would be "pulled in" toward the contralateral ear when it received a monaural tone of different frequency. Related pulling effects were found by Butler and Naunton (1962, 1964) when they stimulated listeners simultaneously with a monaural headphone and a moveable loudspeaker. Warren and Bashford (1976) considered that the shift in localization of a monaural sound induced by a qualitatively different contralateral sound provided a method for investigating the limiting conditions for binaural interactions. We developed a procedure for delateralizing a monaural signal completely using a contralateral noise of appropriate spectral composition and intensity, and found that this delateralization (which was called "contralateral induction") required that the noise have a spectrum and intensity such that the signal could be present as a masked component within the noise. Thus, operating in everyday life, contralateral induction can prevent mislocalization of a source that was above threshold at one ear, but masked by an extraneous sound at the other ear. In addition, it appears that contralateral induction represents a general early stage in binaural processing that can proceed further to yield a fused localized image under appropriate conditions.

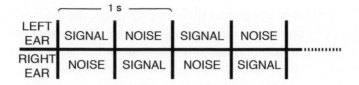

Figure 2.5 Alternating pattern of dichotic stimulation used to produce delateralization of the signal through contralateral induction. (From Warren and Bashford, 1976.)

The monaural signals used in the contralateral induction experiments were presented to one ear and a noise to the other, with the sides receiving signal and noise reversing each 500 ms, as shown in Figure 2.5. The noise was always at 80 dB SPL, and the listener could adjust the level of the signal.

For levels below the upper limit for contralateral induction, the monaural signal appeared to be stationary at a diffusely defined position symmetrical about the medial plane, whereas the noise was heard to switch from side to side each 500 ms. If the signal intensity was raised above the limit of contralateral induction, an abrupt change took place and the signal no longer appeared stationary, and was lateralized to the side of whichever ear was receiving the signal. The upper curves in Figure 2.6 show the upper limit of contralateral induction for tones from 200 through 8,000 Hz when alternated with: (1) broadband white noise; (2) one-third octave narrow-band noise centered at 1,000 Hz (slopes of 32 dB/octave); (3) band-reject white noise with a one-octave wide rejected band centered at 1,000 Hz (slopes of 80 dB/octave). It can be seen that curves for contralateral induction of the tones follow the spectral content of the contralateral noise, being relatively flat for the broadband noise, rising to a maximum at 1,000 Hz for the narrow-band noise, and showing a minimum at the frequencies of the missing band for the band-reject noise. The separations between the upper curves and the corresponding lower curves for detection thresholds for the tones represent the existence regions for contralateral induction. Figure 2.7, from the same study, shows contralateral induction limits for narrow-band filtered speech with center frequencies of 1,000 Hz and 3,000 Hz (bandwidth one-third octave, slopes 48 dB/octave) when presented with contralateral one-third octave noise bands having the center frequencies shown (slopes 32 dB/octave). It can be seen that, as with tonal signals, contralateral induction for narrow-band speech was maximum when the noise contained the same frequencies as the signals. As a consequence of this study, Warren and Bashford suggested the following rule: "If the peripheral neural units stimulated on the side receiving the louder noise include those corresponding to an ongoing contralateral signal, the

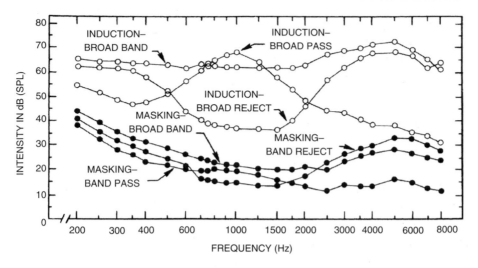

Figure 2.6 Upper intensity limit for delateralization (contralateral induction) of monaural tones presented with one of three contralateral 80 dB SPL noises: broadband noise; narrow-band (bandpass) noise centered at 1,000 Hz; and band-reject noise (rejected frequency band centered at 1,000 Hz). The detection thresholds in the presence of each type of noise are shown as well, and the differences between these masked detection thresholds and the upper limit of induction represent the range of intensities over which delateralization of the tones occurred. (From Warren and Bashford, 1976.)

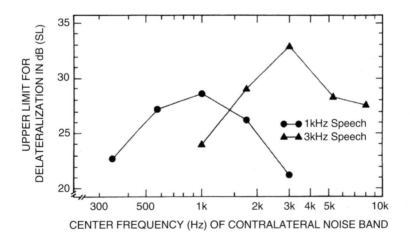

Figure 2.7 Upper intensity limit for delateralization (contralateral induction) of monaural filtered speech bands centered at 1,000 Hz and 3,000 Hz when presented with contralateral 80 dB SPL narrow-band noises of various center frequencies. Intensity of speech is given as sensation level (dB above threshold). (From Warren and Bashford, 1976.)

fainter signal is released from lateralization and moves to a diffuse position located symmetrically about the medial plane."

It was suggested that contralateral induction might correspond to an early stage common to all types of binaural interaction associated with sound localization. This stage involves a cross-ear comparison of power spectra which determines whether a sound present at one ear could be present at the other ear as well; if so, the sound is released from lateralization. The further processing of binaural input required to produce sharply localized images of external sources involves such factors as: (1) appropriate relative intensities at the two ears for each of the spectral components corresponding to a single source at a particular location; (2) appropriate phase or time-of-arrival relations at the two ears corresponding to the analysis described under (1); and (3) changes in (1) and (2) correlated with head movements.

It should be noted that these experiments dealing with contralateral induction have employed the simplest possible arrangement for dichotic interaction: only one sound at each ear. A number of other studies have employed more complex stimulus arrangements.

If separate sounds are introduced to each ear (as in contralateral induction experiments), but in addition one of these sounds is introduced to the other ear as well (i.e., one sound is monaural and the other diotic), or if each of the two sounds is delivered to both ears with interaural phase or time-of-arrival differences for at least one of these sounds, then processing beyond the stage of contralateral induction becomes possible, leading to "masking level differences." This topic has been the subject of considerable investigation.

Masking level differences

Irving Langmuir, a Nobel laureate in chemistry, was the leader of a World War II project on the detection of underwater sonar signals in the presence of noise. He and his associates noted that, when a tone and a masking noise appeared to be located at different azimuths because of interaural phase (or time-of-arrival) differences, the tone could be heard at levels as much as 15 dB below the limit of detectability found in the absence of interaural phase differences between signal and noise (Langmuir, Schaefer, Ferguson, and Hennelly, 1944). Hirsh (1948a, 1948b) independently made a similar discovery, and undertook the first systematic study of this effect, which came to be known as masking level differences (MLDs). In order to deal with Hirsh's studies and the many subsequent studies using a great variety of conditions, it is convenient to use the conventional system of notation: S denotes the signal, M is used for the masker, and subscripts are employed to indicate the relative

Table 2.1 *Masking level differences (MLDs) for various interaural differences (symbols are defined in the text)*

Interaural condition	MLD (compared to M_mS_m) (dB)
$M_\pi S_\pi$, M_0S_0, M_uS_m	0
M_uS_π	3
M_uS_0	4
$M_\pi S_m$	6
M_0S_m	9
$M_\pi S_0$	13
M_0S_π	15

From Green and Yost (1975).

interaural phases of S and M, with the subscript 0 used for no phase difference, and the subscript π for antiphasic or 180° phase difference. The subscript u is used with M to designate uncorrelated noise in each ear (that is, noise matched in long-term spectrum, but from independent sources). Some conditions used for S and M are summarized below.

S_0: signal presented binaurally with no interaural differences.
M_0: masker presented binaurally with no interaural differences.
S_m: signal presented to only one ear.
M_m: masker presented to only one ear.
S_π: signal presented to one ear 180° (π radians) out-of-phase relative to the signal presented to the other ear.
M_π: masker presented to one ear 180° (π radians) out-of-phase relative to the masker presented to the other ear.
M_u: maskers presented to the two ears consisting of uncorrelated noise having the same long-term spectrum.

Green and Yost (1975) summarized the typical experimental findings obtained over the years in Table 2.1, which is based on the use of a loud continuous broadband noise as M, and a brief (10–100 ms) 500 Hz sinusoid as S. The values listed for MLDs represent the differences in masked thresholds for the tone under the reference condition S_mM_m (signal and masker mixed and heard monaurally in the same ear) and the conditions specified in the table.

MLD studies generally use noise as M, and sinusoidal tones, speech, or pulse trains as S. Most studies have dealt with tonal signals, and it has been found that MLDs for tones decrease above 500 or 1,000 Hz, and for $M_\pi S_0$ and M_0S_π reach asymptotic values of about 3 dB above 1,500 Hz. Over the years, a considerable number of theories have been proposed for MLDs (for a review, see Green, 1976), some of which involve mechanisms employed for lateralization. There is good reason to believe that lateralization and MLDs are closely related, since differences in apparent positions of S and M are necessary for generation of MLDs.

While MLDs involve the use of headphones, a similar very sizable reduction in the masked threshold occurs under normal listening conditions (involving sources positioned in space) when a signal originating at one location is subject to interference from other sounds at other locations. The spatial separation of sound images resulting from binaural differences in acoustic input can allow us to hear signals which would otherwise be masked, as demonstrated by the increased intelligibility observed for stereo relative to one-channel recordings of speech under noisy conditions. The so-called "cocktail party effect," which permits us to attend to one of several competing conversations, depends in part on the ability to isolate the voice of interest on the basis of its spatial location.

Two types of temporal disparity

Tobias and Schubert (1959) compared the effects of different types of temporal disparity on lateralization. Short bursts of noise from 10 to 1,000 ms were used which could be gated to produce interaural onset disparities of 0 to 400 ms. The noise was passed through a delay line to produce a temporal disparity in fine structure (peaks and troughs in the waveform) which could be placed in opposition to the onset disparity (i.e., the ear hearing the noise starting first would have fine structure correspondence occurring later). Each cue operating alone (either onset disparity or fine structure disparity) could produce lateralization of short noise bursts to whichever side led in time. Subjects were required to adjust the fine structure disparity to cancel onset disparity so that the image was brought to the center of the head. As the noise burst durations were increased from 10 ms, briefer fine structure disparity was needed to offset the onset disparity. At the longer burst durations (300 ms or more), the onset disparity was of little importance for centering judgments, which were based essentially on interaural fine structure delays.

Hafter, Dye, and Gilkey (1979) studied the ability of listeners to lateralize a tone on the basis of phase differences in the absence of onset and offset disparities. The transients corresponding to the beginning and end of the tonal signals were masked by noise, so that only the interaural phase differences of the tones could be used for lateralization. It was found that when the duration of the tone was sufficient for it to escape being masked by the preceding and following noise, excellent lateralization performance was observed on the basis of interaural phase or temporal fine structure differences alone. Kunov and Abel (1981) eliminated transient cues in a different manner by using slow rise/decay times of their tonal signals. They found that rise/decay times of at least 200 ms were necessary to obtain lateralization judgments based solely upon phase.

Whereas these studies have dealt with different types of temporal cues to lateralization, another class of experiments has dealt with "time-intensity trading" in which time and intensity cues to sidedness were put in opposition.

Time-intensity trading

Using headphones, one can introduce interaural time differences indicating that a sound is on one side while interaural intensity differences indicate the sound is on the other side. (This happens when the side leading in time receives the fainter sound.) Among the early workers measuring the time (in milliseconds) per decibel required to produce a centered image with conflicting cues were Shaxby and Gage (1932), who worked with sinusoidal tones, and Harris (1960) who worked with filtered clicks. Considerable interest was given to this topic initially because of the hope that, since the latency of neural response was lower for sounds at higher intensity, there might be a single system based on interaural time differences responsible for lateralization. Thus, once acoustic intensity differences were translated to neural time differences, intensity might drop out as a separate factor, leaving lateralization based almost entirely upon interaural time differences.

However, subsequent studies by Whitworth and Jeffress (1961), Hafter and Jeffress (1968), and Hafter and Carrier (1972) have shown that separate images – one based on time and one based on intensity – may be perceived by listeners with sufficient training. It should be kept in mind that headphone-induced opposition of intensity and temporal cues is not found in nature, so that considerable experience was needed with these novel relations before separation of intensity from temporal contributions could be achieved by listeners. It would seem that experiments on time-intensity trading require an optimal amount of training – with too little, the necessary discriminations cannot be made; with too much, independent images are perceived for time and intensity. Even with optimal training, there is considerable variability among subjects concerning the relative importance given to time and intensity. Schröger (1996) has reviewed the literature using animals that had indicated that there are separate cortical cells sensitive to interaural time and interaural level, and has presented evidence involving auditory evoked potentials of human subjects that is in agreement with these animal studies.

Some cautions concerning interpretation of studies using headphones

Headphone experiments differ from normal listening conditions in important respects. With headphones, even when cues such as time and intensity are not deliberately placed in an anomalous relation (as in experiments with time-intensity trading), stimuli are abnormal and usually appear to have a source located within the listener's skull rather than out in the environment. When listening to external sources, extensive complex changes in the acoustic stimulus reaching the eardrums are produced by room acoustics, head shadows, pinnae reflections, the reflection and diffraction of the sound by the neck and torso, as well as by head movements. The nature of these changes varies with the listener's distance and orientation relative to the source. While it might be thought at first that perceptual interpretation would be simpler and more direct when these complex stimulus transformations are blocked, further consideration suggests that what appears to be of staggering complexity to an experimenter describing stimuli and their transformations corresponds to the norm that we have learned to deal with. Any change from this norm leads to unusual and conflicting information. Headphone sounds, especially when heard diotically without echoes, are in some ways more similar to self-generated sounds (e.g., our own voice, chewing sounds, coughing) localized within our head than they are to sounds with external origins. Hence, considerable caution must be used in applying results of experiments using headphones to localization of real sources in the environment, since *stabilizing and simplifying stimulus configurations may complicate and confuse perception*. Considering this rule in another way, since complex covariance of many stimulus attributes is normally associated with positional changes of an external source, changing only one attribute, while keeping others constant, can produce a conflict of cues and prevent perception of clear positional images. The extremely complex transformations produced by the pinnae, and required for optimal accuracy in localization, illustrate this principle.

Importance of the pinnae in sound localization

Charles Darwin considered that the pinnae were of little value for sound localization in humans, believing them to be vestigial remnants of more elaborate structures used for localizing sounds by other animals. However, Rayleigh (1907) considered that the pinnae permit us to distinguish between sounds originating in front and behind. Butler (1969) and Blauert (1969–1970), among others, have provided evidence that the pinnae furnish information

concerning the location of a source in the medial plane in terms of both front/
back position and elevation. These pinna cues appear to be primarily monaural, so that interaural comparison is not essential.

Batteau (1967, 1968) proposed a theory concerned with the effect of echoes
produced by the corrugations of the pinnae on the intensities of high frequency components (that is, above 6,000 Hz). He considered that these echo-
induced intensity transformations provided information concerning azimuth
as well as the elevation and front/back position in the medial plane. His conclusions were based upon measurements using a model constructed from a
cast of a human pinna, but enlarged to five times normal size. Microphones
placed at the entrance of the ear canal of the model measured echo delays
from various azimuth and elevation angles. After scaling down the results to
apply to the normal pinna, Batteau concluded that azimuth angles introduced
delays from 2 to 80 μs and elevation angles introduced delays from about 100
to 300 μs. Batteau then used casts of the listener's pinnae mounted on a stand,
with microphone inserts at the position of the ear canals (without a model of
the head between the pinnae). He found that, when sounds picked up by the
microphones were heard by the listener through headphones, it was possible
to create an externalized auditory image with accurate azimuth and elevation
relevant to the artificial pinnae. Removal of the pinnae leaving only the bare
microphones on the supporting stand destroyed localization ability. Batteau
claimed that pinna convolutions producing time delays are not a peculiarity of
human hearing – similar convolutions were found at the base of the ears of all
mammals he examined. It was also stated that all species of birds he examined
had hard acoustically reflecting feathers forming a "pinna-like structure"
surrounding the ear canal. There is evidence indicating that birds may utilize
additional physical principles for localization that are not available to mammals. Lewis and Coles (1980) stated that birds have an air-filled interaural
passage which could correspond to a pressure-difference sensing system
involving the acoustic coupling of the two tympanic membranes.

Freedman and Fisher (1968) continued Batteau's line of experimentation.
They found that it was not necessary to use the listener's own pinnae for
modifying the input to the pick-up microphones – casts of someone else's pinnae could enhance accuracy of localization to some extent. They also reported
that only a single pinna was necessary for localization and, when the distance
between the artificial pinnae was increased to double the normal interaural
distance (confounding binaural time differences and pinna cues), some localization was still associated with the acoustic effects produced by the pinnae.

Wright, Hebrank, and Wilson (1974) noted that questions had been raised
concerning the ability of listeners to detect the very short monaural time

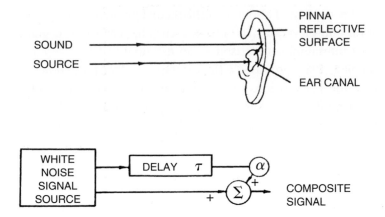

Figure 2.8 Diagram of the generation of a time delay for a composite signal produced by pinna reflection, and the electronic circuit used in experiments simulating delays produced by the pinna. (From Wright, Hebrank, and Wilson, 1974.)

delays required by Batteau's theory (see Davis, 1968), and they attempted to test for this ability directly. They found that monaural delay times of $20 \mu s$ were detected easily when the amplitude ratio of the delayed to the leading signal was greater than 0.67. A digital delay line was used to simulate the action of the pinna as shown in Figure 2.8, and Wright and his colleagues attributed the detection of delays to acoustic interaction resulting in high frequency attenuation for short delay times (see Figure 2.9 for representation of the high frequency reduction produced by a delay of $30 \mu s$). At longer delays, alternating peaks and troughs occur, with the peaks occurring in the rippled power spectrum at integral multiples of $1/\tau$ Hz, where τ represents the delay time in seconds.

While the study by Wright *et al.* (1974) dealt with a single delay for all frequencies, the pinna with its complex corregations (see Figure 1.4) generates many reflections and hence many frequency-specific time delays. These produce extremely complex spectral changes of a broadband sound at the entrance to the ear canal. These intricate changes, together with those produced by the head, are described as head-related transfer functions or HRTFs. They have values that vary with the azimuth and elevation of the sound source relative to the head and pinna. Differences in the shape of the pinna produce different HRTFs for individuals, and by synthesizing a HRTF matched to a particular listener's pinnae, Wightman and Kistler (1989a, 1989b) were able to produce external localization of a signal delivered through headphones rather than the intracranial image usually associated with headphones. Also,

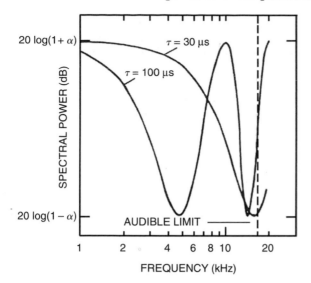

Figure 2.9 Spectral filtering produced by combining a broadband noise with a delay of itself. Delays less than 30 μs cause low-pass filtering and delays greater than 30 μs cause multiple spectral notches (α ratio of delayed to undelayed signal amplitude, τ time delay in μs). (From Wright, Hebrank, and Wilson, 1974.)

Wightman and Kistler reported that the simulated HRTF enabled listeners to locate the position of the corresponding external source with an accuracy corresponding to that obtained when listening to an external source under free-field (anechoic or echo-free) conditions.

In a study of the characteristics of signals responsible for external rather than intracranial sound images, Hartmann and Wittenberg (1996) started with a baseline stimulus delivered to the two ears through earphones that each simulated the effects of the HRTF upon a 1 s steady-state vowel ("ah") played through a loudspeaker at a 37° right azimuth in an anechoic room. Under baseline conditions, listeners could not distinguish earphone from loud-speaker stimulation. When selected acoustic characteristics of the stimulus delivered through the earphones were altered it was found that the external localization of the source depended upon the interaural phase relations of spectral components for frequencies below, but not above, 1,000 Hz, and that interaural level differences were of about equal importance for all frequencies. An interesting informal observation was reported involving stimuli that were delivered through a loudspeaker that was either directly in front of or directly behind the listener. The pinnae normally produce spectral differences for 0° and 180° azimuths, and listeners could detect the differences in timbre of the sound at each location – but only if the listener could not decide whether the source was in front or behind. If the appropriate direction was perceived, then timbre differences could not be heard, and the spectral differences were transformed into localization differences for a sound that seemed to have an unchanging timbre.

There have been a few studies concerning the effect of changing or eliminating pinna interaction with incident sound upon the detection of elevation. Roffler and Butler (1968) reported that, with normally positioned pinnae, listeners could identify with ease which source was radiating sound when two loudspeakers in the medial plane were separated in elevation by 11°. But performance in this task fell to chance level when they flattened and covered the pinnae using a plastic covering having an aperture over the opening of each ear canal. Gardner and Gardner (1973) studied the effect of occluding the cavities of the pinnae with plastic material on the ability to detect elevation in the medial plane. The accuracy of localization decreased with increased filling of the cavities, and no one portion of a pinna seemed more important than another.

Room acoustics

Plenge (1974) reasoned that listeners should not be able to localize sources within rooms unless they were familiar with both the nature of the sound and the acoustics of the room. He prepared two-channel recordings using microphones placed on a dummy head, and then played the recordings to listeners through stereo headphones. He claimed that his subjects could achieve external localization of sounds delivered through headphones when the stimulus resembled a familiar sound in a familiar room; otherwise, the source appeared to be located within the head, as is usually the case when listening through headphones. Plenge stated that only a few seconds of listening was sufficient for calibration of a room's acoustic properties, which were stored as long as the listener remained in the room and then cleared immediately upon leaving, so that the listener could recalibrate at once for a new acoustic environment.

Most experiments studying the cues employed for sound localization have attempted to eliminate or minimize the room-specific complex influence of echoes and reverberation by conducting experiments out of doors or in anechoic rooms. In order to study effects of enclosures on localization, Hartmann (1983) reported a systematic series of experiments in a special room having variable acoustics and determined the effects of changes in reverberation time upon the accuracy of localization for a number of different types of sound, including brief impulsive sounds, steady-state tones, and noise.

Auditory reorientation

In addition to the very rapid adjustment of listeners to the acoustics of a particular room described by Plenge (1974), there is evidence that listeners also can adapt to (or compensate for) long-term changes in auditory cues.

There have been reports going back to the last century that accurate directional localization may be found in complete or partial monaural deafness, indicating that a criterion shift or recalibration of the cues used to determine localization had taken place. Conductive deafness is of special interest, since it is possible to compensate for, or to remove, the blockage and restore normal hearing. If the blockage is due to a plug of cerumen (wax) in the ear canal, the procedure is especially simple and can be accomplished in a few minutes by syringing. Von Bezold (1890) reported that, when normal sensitivity was restored by removal of cerumen in one ear, there was a period of localization confusion lasting for a few weeks while adjustment to "normal" hearing took place. Bergman (1957) described the consequences of successful operations on people with conductive hearing losses involving the middle ear ossicles; along with an increase in acuity in one ear after the operation, there was a period of localization confusion which was not present before the operation.

Other experiments have reported that similar changes in localization could be produced experimentally by maintaining an artificial blockage in one ear for enough time to permit adjustment of localization to this condition, followed by confusion upon removal of this blockage (for summary of this literature, see Jongkees and van der Veer, 1957).

In addition to these dramatic changes in localization criteria, there is a slow recalibration that we have all experienced. During childhood, the dimensions of head and pinnae change, and our criteria for localization must change accordingly if accuracy is to be maintained.

There have been several experiments reported which have used "pseudophones" to alter localization cues. The first of these was by Thompson (1882), who was impressed both by Wheatstone's discovery of the stereoscope and Wheatstone's construction of a "pseudoscope" in which binocular cues to distance were inverted by interchanging inputs to the right and left eyes. Thompson designed an instrument he called the "pseudophone" which had reflecting flaps for directing sounds into the ears from front, back, above, or below. The experimenter could manipulate the flaps on pseudophones worn by blindfolded subjects, and so change the apparent position of sound sources. Young (1928) used a rather different type of a pseudophone consisting of two funnels mounted on the head which gathered sound that could be led to the ears through separate tubes. He studied the adaptation of localization to inversion produced by lateral cross-over of the sound-conducting tubes. Young's work was replicated and extended by Willey, Inglis, and Pearce (1937). These studies found that while listeners could learn to respond appropriately to the reversal of sides produced by the pseudophones, accurate localization of sound sources could not be accomplished even after periods as long as a week. The lack of complete adaptation, perhaps, was not too surprising since the pseudophones were quite different from pinnae, and the transformations produced by the apparatus were not a simple lateral inversion of normal input.

Held (1955) designed an electronic pseudophone employing hearing-aid microphones. These were mounted 20 cm apart on a bar that was attached to a headband worn by the subject. The bar formed an angle of 22° relative to the line joining the subject's ears, so that Held considered that he had shifted the interaural axis by 22°. The microphones were each used to power an ipsilateral earphone worn under a muff that served to attenuate the normal airborne stimulation. Listeners wearing this device for a day could adapt appropriately, and go through their normal daily activities without disorientation.

The ability to adapt to a changed correspondence of sensory input to environmental conditions is not restricted to hearing. As far back as 1879, Helmholtz wrote that "I have performed and described experiments in order to show that even with distorted retinal images (e.g., when looking through lenses, through converging, diverging, or laterally deflecting prisms) we quickly learn to overcome the illusion and to see again correctly ... " (see Warren and Warren, 1968, p. 237).

Changes in lateralization criteria can occur quite rapidly. Flügel (1920–1921) reported that after a short monaural exposure to a sinusoidal tone, a subsequent diotic tone that would normally appear to be in the medial plane would be shifted toward the previously unstimulated ear. He attributed this shift to a "local fatigue." However, this explanation was weakened by his observation that while a monaural poststimulus threshold elevation was restricted to the previous frequency, the poststimulus lateralization shift of binaural tones occurred with all frequencies. Bartlett and Mark (1922–1923) confirmed Flügel's observations, and then demonstrated that his explanation was inadequate. They found that similar after-effects were produced by listening to the same tone delivered to both ears at the same level, but with interaural phase differences causing the adapting tone to be lateralized. Following stimulation by this lateralized binaural tone, they found that a binaural test tone that was matched in level and phase at each ear was lateralized to the side opposite to that of the previous stimulus. Since the level of the adapting tone was the same at each ear, they concluded that the lateralization shift reflected an "error in judgment" rather than a change in sensitivity. This error in judgment was the result of the criterion for medial plane localization being shifted toward the side of the previously lateralized tone (assimilation). This caused a tone that would otherwise appear centered to be displaced toward the opposite side (contrast or negative after-effect). After-effects of a similar nature have been reported for a variety of perceptual judgments, not only in hearing, but with other perceptual modalities as well. Warren (1985) summarized this literature and suggested the following "criterion shift rule": *The criteria used for evaluating stimuli are displaced in the direction of simultaneous or recently experienced values.* This simple principle can help explain some of the experimental biases encountered in laboratory experiments, as well as a number of illusions occurring in speech perception. It has been suggested that the criterion shift rule reflects a continuing calibration of evaluative systems normally ensuring that behavioral responses remain appropriate to current conditions. Criterion shifts are discussed at greater length in Chapter 8.

Estimates of distance from the source

Experiments carried out many years ago demonstrated that under some conditions, listeners can estimate distances of sound sources with considerable accuracy (Matsumoto, 1897; Shutt 1898; Starch and Crawford, 1909). Other studies have shown that there is "loudness constancy" or "loudness invariance" by which listeners can compensate for changes produced by varying the distance of the listener from the source (Mohrmann, 1939; von Fieandt, 1951; Shigenaga, 1965). Let us consider the cues used by listeners in estimating the distance of a sound source.

Perhaps the most obvious cue associated with an increase in distance is a decrease in intensity. As a reasonably close approximation, the intensity of a sound reaching the listener directly from the source is inversely proportional to the square of its distance (the inverse square law), so that a twofold change in distance corresponds to a fourfold (6 dB) change in intensity. It has been recognized for a long time that intensity is a major cue to the distance of familiar sounds (see Thompson, 1882; Pierce, 1901). However, intensity is not the only cue to distance of a source; the ratio of direct to reverberant sound can be a quite important factor.

Since both reverberant and direct components can play a role in judgments of the distance of a source, a problem is encountered for experiments attempting to determine the ability of listeners to judge the manner in which sound varies with distance. If listeners are given the task of estimating the effect of, say, doubling distance, simply attenuating the signal creates a conflict of cues – the decreasing intensity of direct components (which arrive first) indicates an increase in distance, while the fixed ratio of direct to reverberant sound produced by attenuating the entire signal indicates an unchanging distance. However, there does appear to be a way of avoiding this dilemma, which permits a direct determination of the ability of listeners to estimate the manner in which intensity changes with distance without the influence of other cues, whether concordant or conflicting, to acoustic perspective. This can be accomplished by having the subjects generate the sounds themselves.

Warren (1968a) reported an experiment that required subjects to adjust their productions of various self-generated sounds (the vowel "ah," the consonant "sh," and a pitch-pipe note) so that the level at a target microphone ten feet away would remain unchanged when its distance was reduced to five feet. As will be discussed more fully in Chapter 4, the attenuations produced to compensate for halving the distance for all of the sounds were close to the theoretical value of 6 dB, ranging from 6 dB to 8 dB for sounds reaching a microphone directly from the source.

There have been a number of reports that when listeners are functioning as receivers rather than generators of sound, reverberation can function as an important cue to distance. When listening to external sources in rooms with normal acoustics, the ratio of direct to reverberant sound decreases with distance. In an experiment by Steinberg and Snow (1934), a person who was speaking at a fixed level moved back from a pick-up microphone while the gain was changed by the experimenter, so that the amplitude delivered to the listener through loudspeakers remained fixed. Even though the overall amplitude did not change, the talker seemed to recede from the listener, an effect attributed by Steinberg and Snow to a change in the relative proportions of direct and reverberant sound. Békésy (1938) reported similar results when he used equipment designed to change the ratio of direct to reverberant sound while keeping the overall amplitude fixed. Subsequently, Mershon and King (1975) and Butler, Levy, and Neff (1980) reported that noise generated under reverberant conditions seemed much further away than noise generated in an anechoic room.

Maxfield (1930, 1931) described the importance of matching what he called "acoustic perspective" to visual perspective in making sound movies. It was pointed out that since binaural suppression of echoes (which will be discussed shortly) was not possible with one-channel recordings, the overall level of reverberation must be decreased below the normal level to appear normal. He found it necessary to vary the proportion of direct to reverberant sound by appropriate positioning of the microphone when the camera position was changed in order to maintain realism: Maxfield gave an example of a long-shot sound track used with a close-camera shot which made it seem that the actors' voices were coming through an open window located behind them, rather than from their lips. He made the additional interesting observation that correct matching of acoustic and visual perspective influenced intelligibility – when a long-shot picture was seen, a long-shot sound track was more intelligible than a close-up sound track despite the fact that the increased reverberation would make it less intelligible if heard alone.

The delayed versions of a sound produced by echoes not only give rise to an acoustic perspective, but can also impart a pleasing "lively" character to voice and music (as opposed to an undesirable so-called "dead" character when echoes are much reduced). The ability of listeners to minimize interference of masking by echoes has been rediscovered many times, and it goes by a number of names including "precedence effect," "Haas effect," "law of the first wave front," and "first arrival effect" (see Gardner, 1968; Litovsky, Colburn, Yost, and Guzman, 1999 for reviews). Although reduction of masking caused by echoes works best with binaural listening, there is a considerable echo-suppression effect even without binaural differences. I have found that it is possible to demonstrate this single-channel suppression effect for speech by comparing a recording with a low normal reverberation with one that was identical, except that the reverberant sound preceded the direct sound (a condition that could never occur naturally). The reversed reverberation recording was derived from a master tape prepared in an acoustically dead studio with the microphone a few inches from the talker's mouth. This tape was played in a reversed direction into a room having normal reverberation characteristics. An omnidirectional pick-up microphone used for rerecording the speech was placed within two feet of the loudspeaker producing the reversed speech. When the backwards rerecording with the newly added reverberation was reversed once again on playback, the double reversal resulted in the speech being heard in the normal direction, but with reverberation preceding the voice. The slow build-up of reverberation preceding the sounds of speech and the abrupt drop in intensity at silent pauses seemed quite bizarre and was extremely noticeable. However, with a rerecording prepared from the same master tape in a fashion which was identical, except that the reverberation was added in the normal temporal direction, the reverberation was suppressed, resulting in speech having a barely perceptible reverberant quality.

Echo suppression is of little help in understanding a speaker when there are several simultaneous conservations going on along with other extraneous sounds: the so-called "cocktail party effect" (Cherry, 1953). Echoes of individual voices are masked by the babble, but it can be possible to direct one's attention to one of the speakers by ignoring the speech having different azimuths, timbres, and amplitudes. Interestingly, if one's own name or some other attention-capturing word is spoken by a nonattended speaker, it may be possible to become aware of the item and shift attention to the other speaker.

Gardner (1969) tested the ability of listeners to estimate their distance from the source of a voice in a large anechoic room at the Bell Telephone Laboratories. Echoes were effectively abolished by the use of sound absorbent wedges of appropriate composition and size that were placed along the walls, ceiling, and floor. Listeners and equipment were suspended between floor and ceiling on a wire-mesh support which did not reflect sound appreciably. When a voice was recorded and played back over loudspeakers at distances varying from 3 to 30 feet, estimates were independent of actual distance (probably due to the lack of reverberation that normally occurs in rooms and covaries with distance from the source). However, when a live voice was used, an accuracy better than chance in estimating actual distances was found, especially for distances of a few feet. Gardner speculated that the ability of the listener to estimate distance when close to the talker could have resulted from audibility of nonvocal breathing, acoustic cues to the degree of effort made in producing the level heard, detection of echoes from the talker's body during conversational interchanges, radiation of body heat, and olfactory cues. Incidentally, the acoustic cues of vocal effort are not necessary concomitants of changes in vocal level. Talley (1937) stated that professional actors in plays are capable of producing a special "audience speech" in which the fact that two people separated by a few feet on a stage are conversing at the level of a shout can be disguised by appropriate control of voice quality, so that the illusion is produced that they are communicating with each other rather than with the audience.

Another cue to distance comes into play outdoors with far-off sounds. Helmholtz (1954/1877) noted that consonants with their high frequencies did not carry very far, stating that, "it is interesting in calm weather to listen to the voices of the men who are descending from high hills to the plain. Words can no longer be recognized, or at most only such as are composed of M, N, and vowels as Mamma, Nein. But the vowels contained in the spoken word are easily distinguished. They form a strange series of alternations of quality and singular inflections of tone, wanting the thread which connects them into words and sentences." A more mundane example of the low-pass filtering of distant sounds is the transformation of explosive broadband thunderclaps to the deep rumble of a far-off storm. In keeping with these observations, Bloch (1893), after experiments with a variety of stimuli, concluded that sounds lacking high frequency components sounded farther away than sounds containing high frequencies. Also, Levy and Butler (1978) and Butler, Levy, and Neff (1980) reported that low-pass noise appeared farther away than high-pass noise. Coleman (1963) presented values for the absorption coefficient in dB/100 feet. for different frequencies, which showed that higher frequencies are attenuated much more than lower frequencies. He noted that this attenuation was highly dependent upon water-vapor content of the air, increasing with the humidity. The calculations he presented show that at "typical conditions" encountered in a temperate climate, components at 8,000 Hz may have an attenuation 3 dB greater than components at 1,000 Hz for each 100 feet of travel.

Sensory input and physical correlates

We have seen that changes in the nature of sensory input caused by shifts in the location of a source are perceived in terms of positional correlates, not in terms of the sensory changes themselves. As Helmholtz has stated "... we are exceedingly well trained in finding out by our sensations the objective nature of the objects around us, but ... we are completely unskilled in observing the sensations per se" (see Warren and Warren, 1968, p. 179). In keeping with Helmholtz's statement, evidence will be discussed in Chapter 4 indicating that, when attempts are made to have subjects estimate sensory magnitude directly by judging the relative loudness of sounds, responses are based upon experience with a familiar physical scale regularly associated with the extent of stimulation. Ordinarily, experience with localization serves as the physical correlate of loudness, and evidence will be presented indicating that judgments of relative loudness are based upon experience with the manner in which stimulation varies with distance from the source.

Suggestions for further reading

A standard text by an expert: Blauert, J. 1997. *Spatial Hearing: The Psychophysics of Human Sound Localization*. Cambridge, MA: MIT Press.

For a detailed discussion of selected topics: Gilkey, R., and Anderson, T. (eds.) 1997. *Binaural and Spatial Hearing in Real and Virtual Environments*. Hillsdale, NJ: Erlbaum.

3

Perception of acoustic repetition: pitch and infrapitch

This chapter reviews a classical problem, perception of tones, and suggests that our understanding of this topic may be enhanced by considering it as part of a larger topic: that of perception of acoustic repetition. As we shall see, periodic sounds repeated at tonal and infratonal frequencies appear to form a single perceptual continuum, with study in one range enhancing understanding in the other.

Terminology

Some terms used in psychoacoustics are ambiguous. The American National Standards Institute (ANSI, 1976/1999) booklet *Acoustical Terminology* defines some basic technical words as having two meanings, one applying to the stimulus and the other to the sensation produced by the stimulus. The confusion of terms describing stimuli and their sensory correlates is an old (and continuing) potential cause of serious conceptual confusions – a danger that in 1730 led Newton (1952, p. 124) to warn that it is incorrect to use such terms as red light or yellow light, since " ... the Rays to speak properly are not coloured." However, the ANSI definitions for the word "tone" reflect current usage, and state that the word can refer to: "(a) Sound wave capable of exciting an auditory sensation having pitch. (b) Sound sensation having pitch." A similar ambiguity involving use of the same term to denote both stimulus and sensation is stated formally in the ANSI definitions for the word "sound." The use of both of these terms will be restricted here to describe only the stimuli. The term *pitch* is defined as the attribute of auditory sensation which can be ordered on a scale extending from high to low.

The ANSI recommendation considers that the pitch of any particular sound can be described in terms of the frequency of a sinusoidal tone judged to have the same pitch, so that pitch is limited to the audible frequency range of sinusoidal tones extending from about 20 through 16,000 Hz. However, acoustic repetition of waveforms can be perceived as a global percept at rates well below the pitch limit for waveforms other than sinusoids, and we will name such periodic sounds as *infratones* or infratonal stimuli and their corresponding sensory attribute *infrapitch*. Thus, the topic of detectable acoustic periodicity repetition involves both tonal and infratonal sounds producing sensations of pitch and infrapitch, respectively. The term *iterance* will be used as a general term encompassing the perceptual attributes of both pitch and infrapitch.

Classical pitch studies

The ancient Greeks appreciated that sounds correspond to vibratory movement of the air, and analogies were made between sound vibrations and water waves (see Hunt, 1978). They had an interest in the nature of pitch and the basis for musical intervals, and Pythagoras in the sixth century BCE noted that simple integral ratios of the length of two vibrating strings corresponded to the common intervals (e.g., a ratio of 2:1 for an octave, a ratio of 3:2 for a fifth). In the seventeenth century, Galileo noted that if the Greeks had varied the pitches produced by a string by altering either the diameter or the tension rather than length, then the pitch would have been found proportional to the square root of the physical dimension, and the octave and fifth would correspond to ratios of 4:1 and 9:4 respectively. Galileo then described an elegant experiment demonstrating that the octave did indeed correspond to a frequency ratio of 2:1. He observed that when the rim of a goblet containing water was stroked, standing waves appeared on the surface of the liquid. By slight changes in the manner of stroking it was possible to have the pitch jump an octave and, when that occurred, the standing waves changed in length by a factor of precisely two. Galileo also noted that when a hard metal point was drawn over the surface of a soft brass plate, a particular pitch could be heard while, at the same time, a series of grooves with a periodic pattern (basically, a phonographic recording) appeared on the brass surface. With the appropriate velocity and pressure of the stylus, two sets of periodic patterns corresponding to the musical interval of a fifth were generated. When the spacings of the patterns were compared, Galileo found them to have the ratio of 3:2, indicating that this was the ratio of acoustic periodicities producing this interval.

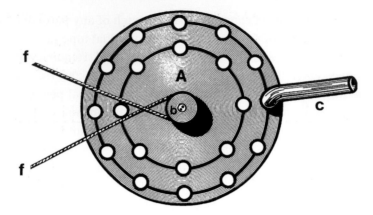

Figure 3.1 The acoustic siren as used in Seebeck's time. Compressed air passing through the tube (c) releases a puff of air each time it is aligned with a hole in the disk (A) which is rotated by a cord (f) passing over a grooved driveshaft (b). (From Helmholtz, 1954/1877.)

Modern experimental work on pitch perception may be considered to have started with Seebeck's experiments with a siren (see Figure 3.1). By forcing puffs of compressed air through holes in a disk rotating at a constant speed, periodic sounds consisting of a variety of puff-patterns were produced corresponding to the choice of distances separating the holes. For example, when the disk contained holes separated by the distances a, then b, then a, etc. (a, b, a, b, a, ...), the pitch heard was equivalent to that produced by a disk containing half the number of holes with a single distance c (equal to $a + b$) separating adjacent openings. When the distances a and b were made equal, the apparent period was halved, and the pitch increased by one octave. As a result of these experiments with repeated patterns consisting of two puffs, as well as more complex patterns, Seebeck (1841) concluded that the pitches heard corresponded to the period of the overall repeated pattern. Thus, it appeared to him that the number of complete statements of the periodic waveform per second determined the pitch. Ohm (1843) stated that Seebeck's contention that the pitches heard were based upon the repetition period of the overall pattern of puffs was incorrect, and that a Fourier analysis of the periodic signals into harmonic components took place with the pitch being determined by the frequency of the spectral fundamental. Seebeck (1843) countered by claiming that the spectral fundamental was not necessary for hearing a pitch equivalent to that frequency; he pointed out that, even when a spectral analysis showed that the fundamental was very weak or absent, the pitch of the fundamental (which corresponded to the waveform-repetition frequency) was still the

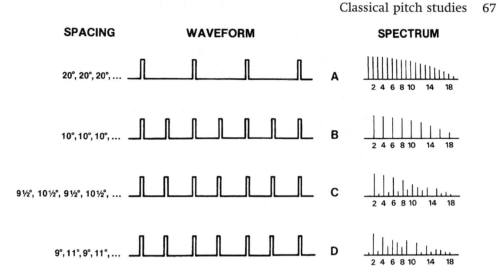

Figure 3.2 Seebeck's waveforms and their corresponding spectra. The spacing of the holes in the siren's disk producing these sounds is given in degrees. The numbers used to describe the harmonics of the line spectra shown on the right are based upon a waveform period corresponding to 20° (shown as A). (Adapted from Schouten, 1940a.)

dominant pitch heard. The spectra of some of the stimuli generated by Seebeck as summarized by Schouten (1940a) are illustrated in Figure 3.2. Seebeck suggested that the higher harmonic components might combine to cause the pitch corresponding to the fundamental to be heard, even when the fundamental was absent. As Schouten (1970) pointed out, this suggestion concerning the role of upper harmonics foreshadowed later nonspectral theories (including his own). In addition, there is more recent evidence that the stimuli employed by Seebeck (pulse trains with unequal alternate intervals) produce discharge patterns in auditory nerve fibers that are correlated with the pitches that are heard (see Evans, 1986).

Ohm (1844) had dismissed Seebeck's observations that a pitch could be heard corresponding to an absent or weak fundamental as merely an auditory illusion, to which Seebeck (1844) replied that the term "illusion" was inappropriate since only the ear could decide how tones should be heard. (For review of this controversy between Seebeck and Ohm, see Schouten (1970) and de Boer (1976).) In the second half of the nineteenth century, Helmholtz (1954/ 1877) backed Ohm's position in this controversy. Considering the ear to be an imperfect spectral analyzer, Helmholtz described distortion products which were capable of generating the fundamental frequency within the ear, even when missing as a Fourier component of a periodic stimulus. Helmholtz was well aware that a complex tone appears to have a single pitch rather than a cluster of pitches corresponding to the individual harmonics. He attributed the perception of a single pitch to the adoption by unskilled listeners of a "synthetic" mode of listening to the entire complex aggregate of components (resulting in a single pitch corresponding to the fundamental frequency and having a timbre, or quality, reflecting the harmonic composition), rather than an "analytical" mode available to skilled listeners in which the pitches of component harmonics could be abstracted. Helmholtz stated that unskilled listeners could be trained to hear individual lower harmonics in a complex tone "with comparative ease." One recommended procedure involved first playing the harmonic component by itself at a soft level, and then immediately substituting the complex tone at a louder level: the harmonic could then be heard to continue as a component within the complex tone.

Helmholtz's position that the analysis of complex tones into a harmonic series of sinusoidal components was responsible for the pitch of complex tones had great influence, largely because he also offered a plausible explanation of how this spectral analysis could be accomplished by the ear. As described in Chapter 1, he suggested that the cochlea acted as if it contained a set of graded resonators, each of which responded selectively to a particular component frequency. Low frequencies were considered to produce sympathetic vibrations at the apical end, and high frequencies at the basal end of the cochlea. His first version of the theory identified the rods of Corti as the resonant bodies, but this was later amended to consider resonating transverse fibers embedded in the basilar membrane as being responsible for spectral analysis. We have seen in Chapter 1 that Békésy modified the basis of Helmholtz's place theory from simple resonance to a traveling wave, with spectral analysis corresponding to the loci of maximal displacements produced by slow-velocity waves (much slower than sound waves) sweeping along the basilar membrane from base to apex. Chapter 1 also discussed recent evidence indicating that spectral analysis may involve not only the loci of maximal displacements along the basilar membrane, but also resonant tuning of the stereocilia of the receptor cells in a manner reminiscent of Helmholtz's first version of his resonance theory involving the sympathetic vibration of the rods of Corti.

There appears to be general agreement today that sound is subject to nonlinear distortions within the ear as Helmholtz had suggested. These distortions can introduce harmonic components when the stimulus consists of a sinusoidal tone, and can produce "combination tones" through the interaction of pairs of component frequencies. Among the more thoroughly studied combination tones are the simple difference tone $(f_2 - f_1)$, and the cubic difference tone $(2f_1 - f_2)$. Thus, sinusoidal tones of 900 Hz and 1,100 Hz can produce a simple difference tone of 200 Hz and a cubic difference tone of 700 Hz.

Whereas Helmholtz attributed the production of nonlinear distortion to the movements of the tympanic membrane and the ossicular chain within the middle ear, more recent evidence has emphasized nonlinearity within the inner ear (see Rhode and Robles, 1974; Plomp, 1976; Cooper and Rhode, 1993).

Nonlinear distortions and the spectral analyses leading to pitch perception occur within the ear prior to neural stimulation. In addition, a temporal analysis of recurrent patterns of neural response appears to be involved in the perception of pitch. Before dealing with the temporal analysis of acoustic repetition, let us consider the topics of masking and critical bands which can help in understanding the nature of both frequency (place) and temporal (periodicity) coding.

Masking

It is well known that a louder sound can, under some conditions, mask (or prevent us from hearing) an otherwise audible fainter sound. Masking is not only a topic of direct practical interest, but also has been used widely to further our understanding of auditory processing.

Wegel and Lane (1924) used pure tones ranging from 200 Hz through 3,500 Hz as maskers. The masker was presented at a fixed SPL, and the threshold for a second sinusoidal (masked) tone was determined for various frequencies. Figure 3.3 presents their masked threshold function (sometimes called a masked audiogram) for different frequencies with a 1,200 Hz masker at 80 dB SPL. It can be observed that higher thresholds (corresponding to greater masking) were obtained for frequencies which were above rather than below the masking tone (the so-called upward spread of masking). The masked audiogram for frequencies near and at intervals above the frequency of the masker is marked by discontinuities or notches. There is general agreement on the basis for the notch centered on the masker frequency of 1,200 Hz: when two tones close to each other in frequency are mixed, a single pitch of inter-mediate frequency is perceived, and the loudness fluctuations of first-order beats are heard. The beat rate is equal to the difference in frequencies of the tones, so that if the tones are 1,200 Hz and 1,206 Hz, beats are heard at the rate of six per second, with loudness minima occurring when the pressure crests of one sinusoidal waveform coincide with pressure troughs of the other. The threshold for detecting the addition of a sinusoidal tone having the same frequency and phase as the louder "masker" is the just noticeable difference (jnd), and has been used to measure jnds (see Reisz, 1928). The basis for the occurrence of notches at harmonics of the masker frequency is somewhat more controversial. Wegel and Lane attributed these dips to fluctuations in the

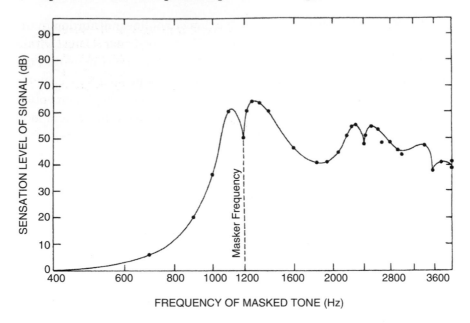

Figure 3.3 Masking of one tone by another. The 1,200 Hz masker has a fixed intensity (80 dB SPL), and the masked threshold is given as sensation level (or dB above unmasked threshold). (Adapted from Wegel and Lane, 1924.)

intensity of the masked tone caused by interactions with aural harmonics of the masker (that is, harmonic distortion products generated within the ear), and these notches in the masking function have been used to estimate the extent of harmonic distortion (Fletcher, 1930; Opheim and Flottorp, 1955; Lawrence and Yantis, 1956). However, this explanation has been criticized on a variety of grounds (see Chocholle and Legouix, 1957a, 1957b; Meyer, 1957). Plomp (1967b) studied the perceptual interaction of tones mistuned slightly from consonance, and provided evidence suggesting that higher-order beats (that is, beats involving mistuning from a consonance other than unison) are based upon detection of periodic fluctuations in the phase relations of the spectral components, even when these components are separated by several octaves. This comparison of temporal or phase information from widely separated cochlear loci could be responsible for the notches at harmonics of the lower frequency tone (2,400 Hz and 3,600 Hz) that appear in Figure 3.3.

The complicating effects of beats in masking experiments can be reduced by using narrow-band noise as the masker. Figure 3.4 shows masked audiograms measured by Egan and Hake (1950) using a narrow-band noise centered at 410 Hz presented at various intensity levels. The notches observed with tonal maskers, if present at all, are very much reduced in magnitude, and the tonal

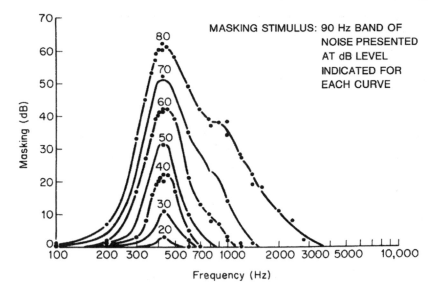

Figure 3.4 Masking of tones by different levels of a narrow-band noise centered at 410 Hz. (Adapted from Egan and Hake, 1950.)

threshold curves are almost symmetrical about the logarithm of the center frequency of the band of masking noise when it is present at its lowest intensity levels. An increase in the level of the masking noise band results in an asymmetrical spread of excitation along the basilar membrane, and produces an upward spread of masking that becomes quite pronounced at the highest intensity level, as can be seen in Figure 3.4.

In addition to simultaneous masking, there are two types of non-simultaneous masking. In "forward" masking, a louder preceding sound prevents detection of a brief faint sound. In "backward" masking, a brief faint sound is made inaudible by a louder subsequent sound. Both types of non-simultaneous masking usually have effective durations of less than 100 ms.

Forward masking may correspond in part to the time required for the receptors to regain their sensitivity and/or the persistence of activity after exposure to a louder sound. This time is quite short, usually only tens of milliseconds. Backward masking is more difficult to account for. One possible basis that has been suggested is that the subsequent louder sound produces neural activity which travels at a greater velocity and overtakes the fainter stimulus on the way to the central nervous system (R. L. Miller, 1947), thus effectively becoming a special case of simultaneous masking. It is also possible that central processing of the fainter sound takes an appreciable amount of time, and the louder sound disrupts the processing at some critical stage. (For a detailed discussion and comparison of the various types of masking, see Buus, 1997).

Critical bands

Fletcher (1940) interpreted earlier studies of masking as indicating that the basilar membrane operates as a bank of filters, each having a limited resolving power corresponding to what he called a "critical band." He considered that louder sounds could prevent detection of (or mask) fainter sounds when they stimulated the same critical bands. Fletcher attempted to measure widths of critical bands at various center frequencies by using noise to mask tonal signals. The long-term average power in a 1 Hz wide band within a broadband noise is called the "noise power density" and abbreviated as N_0. Fletcher started with broadband noise having a constant N_0 at all frequencies (that is, white or Gaussian noise), and measured the masked threshold for a tone presented along with the noise. He decreased the bandwidth of the noise keeping N_0 of the remaining noise fixed, and found that little or no effect was observed on the masked threshold when the frequencies removed from the noise were beyond a critical distance from the tone. Fletcher's conclusion that a narrow "critical band" is mainly responsible for masking is now generally accepted, and has proved extremely valuable in understanding the interaction of components having different frequencies. However, Fletcher made the further assumption that the total power of a noise within a critical band is the same as the power of a tone centered within that band at its masked threshold. This assumption has been questioned by Scharf (1970), who suggested that estimates of the width of the critical band based on the ratio of tonal power at masked threshold to N_0 are roughly 40 percent less than the width of the critical band measured by other methods involving direct frequency interactions on the basilar membrane. Values obtained using Fletcher's method are sometimes called "critical ratios," with the term "critical band" being reserved for values obtained with other procedures as shown in Figure 3.5. However, Spiegel (1981) has argued that Fletcher's method is valid when used with suitable precautions, either for pure tones masked with noise of various bandwidths, or for narrow-band noise masked with wider-band noise. The widths of critical bands have also been calculated in terms of equivalent rectangular bands (ERBs) (see Moore, 2003).

Greenwood (1961, 1990) has presented evidence that each critical band covers about the same distance on the basilar membrane in mammals, and has estimated the width corresponding to a critical band to be approximately 1 mm for humans.

Comodulation and masking reduction

As described in the previous section, when random or stochastic noise is presented along with a tone, only the spectral components of the noise that

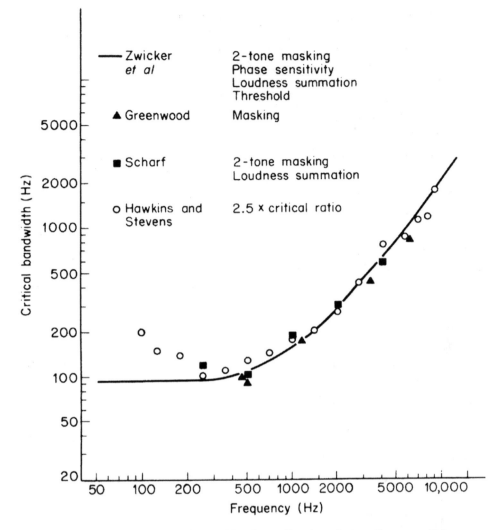

Figure 3.5 The width of critical bands as a function of center frequency. Values are presented from several sources. Data of Hawkins and Stevens were transformed by multiplying their values (considered as "critical ratios") by 2.5. (From Scharf, 1970.)

lie within a critical bandwidth of the tone have an appreciable effect in elevating the tone's threshold. Thus, if a tone is maintained at the center of a noise band having a uniform power density and the bandwidth of the noise is expanded from an initial value below a critical bandwidth, the threshold of the tone increases only until the boundaries of the critical band are reached – further increase of bandwidth has no appreciable effect. However, under certain conditions, the presence of noise beyond the limits of the critical band can *decrease* the threshold of the tone (Hall, Haggard, and Fernandes, 1984). This "comodulation masking release" (CMR) has been the subject of several studies. Usually, the tone is centered in one noise band (the target band) and the influence of a second noise band (the cue band) is investigated. CMR occurs when the target band and the cue band are comodulated – that is, when the amplitudes of the two bands fluctuate together. Comodulation of different frequency bands in everyday life usually indicates a common sound source, but there is an uncertainty concerning the mechanism by which the correlation of amplitude changes within the two noise bands reduces the threshold for the tone (for a summary and extended discussion of CMR, see Moore, 2003).

Place theory of pitch

Plomp (1968) and de Boer (1976) have pointed out that there are two classical place theories: one considers that there is a Fourier analysis of limited resolution along the basilar membrane, with lower frequencies stimulating the apical end and higher frequencies the basal end; the other considers that pitch is determined by the places stimulated. The first place theory is supported by overwhelming evidence; the second seems to be only partly true – that is, place is not the sole determinant of pitch. For a sinusoidal tone, the locus of maximum stimulation changes regularly with frequency only from about 50 through 16,000 Hz, so that place cannot account for low pitches from 20 through 50 Hz. In addition, the pitch of a sinusoidal tone does not change appreciably with amplitude despite the neurophysiological evidence that the place of maximal excitation does change appreciably, shifting toward the base of the cochlea as the level is increased. Measurements reported by Chatterjee and Zwislocki (1997) indicate that this shift can correspond to a distance equivalent to as much as one or two octaves over an 80 dB range. Further, the very small just noticeable differences (jnds) in frequency of sinusoidal tones are difficult to account for by spectral resolution along the basilar membrane. Figure 3.5 shows that at 500 Hz the critical bandwidth is about 100 Hz, yet jnds having values less than 1 Hz have been reported (Nordmark, 1968; Moore, 1974). Although there are mechanisms based on place which have been proposed for discriminating tones separated by considerably less than a critical band (Békésy, 1960; Tonndorf, 1970; Zwicker, 1970), they have difficulties handling jnds for pure tones as small as those reported by Nordmark and by Moore, as well as the relatively small changes in jnds with frequencies from about 500 Hz to 2,000 Hz.

Classical place theorists have encountered a number of problems in dealing with the pitch of complex tones. As we have seen, a single pitch corresponding to the spectral fundamental is generally heard despite the presence of harmonic components stimulating regions associated with other pitches. Also, the fundamental frequency still characterizes the pitch of a complex tone even when it is not present as a component of the stimulus. Helmholtz (1954/1877) described the generation of difference tones (that is, creation of frequencies corresponding to the difference between sinusoidal components) which could account for perception of the absent fundamental (although Helmholtz does not seem to have used difference tones explicitly as an explanation of this problem). However, Fletcher (1924) did claim that the distortion within the ear could produce a frequency corresponding to a missing fundamental – which thus would not be missing at the level of the receptor cells.

Experiments conducted after Fletcher made this claim have shown that a pitch corresponding to the missing fundamental is heard under conditions making it highly unlikely that the fundamental is generated within the ear. These experiments have led to the development of temporal or periodicity theories of pitch perception, which consider that iterated patterns of neural response can produce a sensation of pitch corresponding to the repetition frequency.

Periodicity theory of pitch

Schouten (1938) demonstrated in an elegant fashion that a pitch corresponding to the fundamental of a complex tone was heard even when this frequency was absent at the level of the receptor cells. He prepared a complex tone with a fundamental of 200 Hz, and first removed the fundamental by the addition of the appropriate intensity of a second 200 Hz sinusoidal tone that was 180° out of phase with the fundamental. Following this acoustic cancellation, a 206 Hz sinusoidal tone was added as a probe to determine whether the 200 Hz fundamental was present at the level of the receptor cells – if a 200 Hz tone were generated within the ear, it would interact with the probe to produce periodic fluctuations in amplitude (or beats) at the rate of 6 Hz. The probe verified the absence of the fundamental. Yet a pitch corresponding to the missing fundamental could be heard clearly, although the quality associated with this pitch was quite different from that of a sinusoidal tone corresponding to the fundamental. These observations led Schouten to his concept of "residue pitch" which will be discussed shortly.

Schouten's experiments, showing that the pitch of the missing fundamental is carried by higher harmonics, requires subjects skilled in matching the pitch of tones having different qualities. Licklider (1954) demonstrated the same basic phenomenon in a manner which did not require such skills. At a meeting of the Acoustical Society of America, he first let the audience hear a recognizable melody consisting of a sequence of complex tones lacking lower harmonics. In order to show that the melody was carried by the upper harmonics, he then added a band of low frequency noise of sufficient intensity to mask any distortion products corresponding to the fundamental and lower harmonics: the melody could still be heard quite clearly. Subsequent quantitative studies also have used low frequency masking noise to ensure that the spectral fundamental did not contribute to the pitch produced by higher harmonics of complex tones (Small and Campbell, 1961; Patterson, 1969).

Schouten's residue pitch

In a number of experiments, Schouten (1938, 1939, 1940a) verified and extended Seebeck's suggestion that higher harmonics of pulse trains could combine to produce the pitch of an absent fundamental.

Schouten first tried using an acoustic siren to generate pulses (as did Seebeck), and found that, while he could hear the auditory phenomena described by Seebeck, there was much variability in the stimulus and some undesired noise was produced. Schouten designed an "optical siren," in which rotating masks of different shapes determined the pattern of light reaching a photosensitive cell, which then controlled the waveform of a signal driving a loudspeaker. The optical siren could produce intact pulse trains, and the construction of appropriate masks permitted deletion of desired lower harmonics. (Fine adjustments in the masks were made with the help of a wave analyzer that measured the strength of individual spectral components.) As the result of his experiments, Schouten (1970) came to the following conclusions.

(1)   The ear follows Ohm's law (i.e., can hear out individual harmonics) for frequencies wider apart than, say, a full tone (12 percent). In a harmonic series, from 8 to 10 lower harmonics can be perceived by the unaided ear.

(2)   Higher harmonics are heard collectively as one subjective component (one percept) called the residue.

(3)   The residue has a sharp timbre.

(4)   The residue has a pitch equal to that of the fundamental tone. If both are present in one sound they can be distinguished by their timbre.

Schouten (1940a) realized that one possible objection to his explanation for residue pitch in terms of periodicity of the entire waveform could be that the difference between successive harmonics of a complex tone with a fundamental frequency of 200 Hz is also 200 Hz, and that this difference might be responsible for the pitch of the residue. He then produced a train of pulses of alternating polarity having a fundamental frequency of 200 Hz (see Figure 3.6).

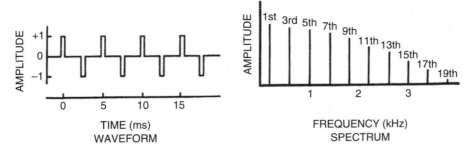

Figure 3.6 Waveform and odd-harmonic spectrum of a 200 Hz alternating polarity pulse train. The harmonic number of each spectral line is given. (Adapted from Schouten, 1940a.)

Any periodic sound consisting of alternate segments that are identical except for a polarity inversion has an acoustic fundamental corresponding to the repetition frequency of the entire waveform, but lacks even numbered harmonics (as illustrated in the spectrum shown in Figure 3.6). Hence, the spectral composition of the alternating polarity pulse train used by Schouten was 200, 600, 1,000, ... Hz. Schouten stated that a residue pitch could be heard when listening to this periodic stimulus without filtering, and that this pitch did not correspond to the difference frequency of 400 Hz, but to the waveform repetition frequency of 200 Hz. As we shall see, this choice of a 200 Hz fundamental was fortunate for his theory – had he lowered the fundamental frequency of the alternating polarity pulse train to 100 Hz, a pitch corresponding to the waveform repetition frequency would not have been heard (see Flanagan and Guttman, 1960a, 1960b; Flanagan, 1972; Warren and Wrightson, 1981; also see Figures 3.17, 3.18, and 3.19, and discussion in the accompanying text).

Pitch of inharmonic complexes

Schouten (1940b) provided another demonstration indicating that residue pitch was not due to the perception of difference tones corresponding to the frequency separation of neighboring spectral components. He started with a complex tone having a frequency of 200 Hz (components at 200, 400, 600, ... Hz) and increased the frequency of each component by 40 Hz (240, 440, 640, ... Hz). Although the frequency difference between components was 200 Hz for the latter stimulus, this was not the pitch heard: the pitch changed slightly but reliably to a little more than 200 Hz. This type of pitch shift was later studied in a detailed quantitative manner by de Boer (1956). De Boer first presented the five-component harmonic complex of 800, 1,000, 1,200, 1,400, 1,600 Hz, and observed that the fundamental of 200 Hz was heard, as would be

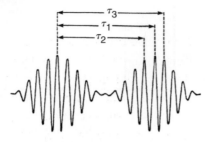

Figure 3.7 Behavior of a hypothetical pitch extractor that measures intervals between main peaks in a waveform. The waveform shown is that of a complex tone corresponding to the sinusoidal modulation of a carrier tone having a frequency ten times that of the modulation frequency. Some of the possible pitches are considered to be based on the intervals τ_1, τ_2, and τ_3. (Adapted from Schouten, Ritsma, and Cardozo, 1962.)

expected. When he increased each component by 50 Hz to produce the complex of 850, 1,050, 1,250, 1,450, 1,650 Hz, the pitch heard was increased to about 210 Hz. De Boer offered an explanation for the pitch shift in terms of a central pitch extractor which constructed a harmonic series most closely approximating the inharmonic complex. In the example given above, this would correspond to 833.3, 1,041.7, 1,250, 1,458.3, 1,666.7 Hz, with a missing fundamental of approximately 208.3 Hz (close to the experimentally found value). De Boer suggested that the pitch extractor employed place information for spectral components having low harmonic numbers that stimulated discrete loci, and temporal information for those components with high harmonic numbers that cannot be resolved by place of stimulation.

Schouten, Ritsma, and Cardozo (1962) proposed a somewhat different model. They took amplitude-modulated signals consisting of three harmonically related components, such as 1,800, 2,000, 2,200 Hz, and then shifted the frequency of each component by the same amount to produce an inharmonic sequence. Pitch shifts similar to those reported by de Boer for his five-component signals were observed. They also reported that while a harmonic three-component complex such as that described above (1,800, 2,000, 2,200 Hz) had a dominant pitch corresponding to the amplitude-modulation envelope (200 Hz), several fainter pitches could be heard as well (see Figure 3.7). Schouten and his associates suggested a model in which the ambiguity was attributed to a pitch processor that measured time intervals between peaks as shown in the figure. They noted that increasing component frequencies by a fixed amount did not change the envelope repetition frequency of 200 Hz but did change the fine structure within the envelope. Since the pitch does change, they reasoned that fine structure must enter into pitch judgments.

Spectral dominance

Since harmonic components of complex tones can generate a pitch matching that of the spectral fundamental, there have been attempts to determine which harmonics play the leading role in generating the pitch. Experiments by Ritsma (1962, 1963) suggested that components with low harmonic numbers play a dominant role. Subsequent experiments by Ritsma and by other investigators indicated that harmonic numbers from about three to five usually were the most important in establishing pitch (for reviews, see Ritsma, 1970; Plomp, 1976). However, the dominant harmonics change to some extent with fundamental frequency (Plomp, 1967a; Patterson and Wightman, 1976). In general, the dominant harmonics are resolvable along the basilar membrane and also overlap in critical bands, so that two types of temporal information as well as spatial information might be generated by these components, as will be discussed next.

Complex tones and local temporal patterns on the basilar membrane

In dealing with the possible bases for the residue pitch heard when all components were delivered to the same ear or ears, Schouten (1940c) considered the basilar membrane as a tuned resonator in which lower harmonics stimulated isolated regions without interaction with neighboring harmonics, while several of the higher harmonics stimulated the same region. Figure 3.8 shows the local pattern of excitation produced by a pulse train according to this model.

Plomp (1966) employed a more refined model of the basilar membrane response to a 200 Hz pulse train, using a set of 1/3-octave filters to approximate the width of critical bands. Figure 3.9 shows tracings obtained in our laboratory using Plomp's method with pulses of 100 μs duration and 1/3-octave filters having attenuations of 30 dB one octave from the center frequencies of the filters. The tracings resemble closely those obtained by Plomp for the same stimulus. The responses of the filters, of course, still are not intended to represent the actual patterns along the basilar membrane in a quantitative fashion. However, the tracings do illustrate clearly some effects of the bandpass filtering occurring within the cochlea.

Both Figures 3.8 and 3.9 provide an impressive indication that bursts of activity having a periodicity corresponding to the pulse rate occur at cochlear loci which respond to frequencies several times higher than the spectral fundamental. Even though it is tempting to consider that the periodic bursts of activity are responsible for the detection of a pulse-train periodicity,

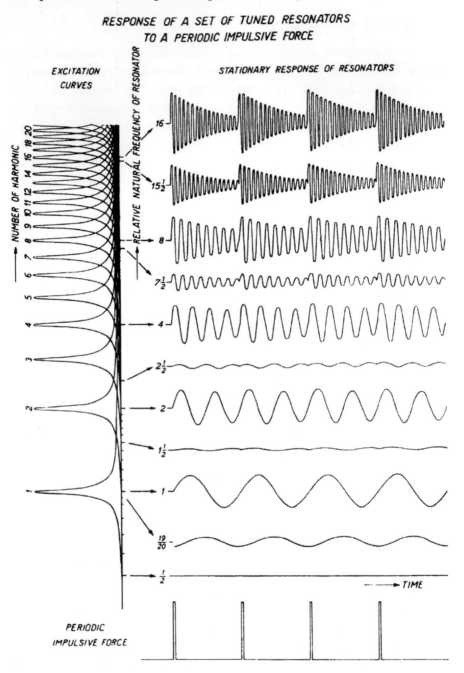

Figure 3.8 Response of tuned resonators to pulse trains. This diagram represents a model of how cochlear resonators could permit both the spectral resolution of lower harmonics and the interaction of higher harmonics to produce periodic waveforms having maxima corresponding to the period of the pulse train. (From Schouten, 1940c.)

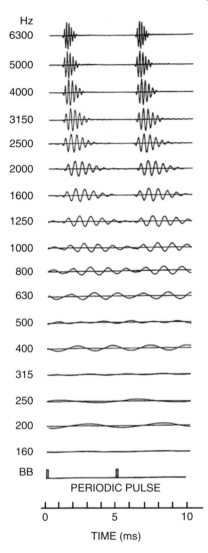

Figure 3.9 Demonstration of the nature of the basilar membrane's response to pulse trains based upon Plomp's procedure (see text). The pulse-train waveform is shown diagramatically in broadband form as BB at the bottom of the figure. Tracings are shown of the actual waveforms obtained as output from a set of 1/3-octave filters (center frequencies of 160, 200, 250, ..., 6,300 Hz) stimulated simultaneously by a 200 Hz pulse train. Spectral resolution of individual harmonics can be seen for the filters with lower center frequencies, as well as the emergence of pulsate patterns with repetition frequencies of 200 Hz for filters with the highest center frequencies. The same equipment and procedures were used in preparing the tracings for nonpulsate stimuli shown in Figures 3.1, 3.3, and 3.8.

nonpulsate complex tones (which also exhibit residue pitch) do not produce such bursts of activity, either broadband or when filtered. Indeed, the amplitude contours of individual critical bands of a complex tone need not be correlated in any way for them to be integrated into a unified percept of residue pitch.

Before attributing perceptual characteristics of specific sounds to their special acoustic properties, it is desirable to determine whether these characteristics are also exhibited by representative or generic stimuli lacking the special waveforms and spectral characteristics of specific types of sounds.

Let us turn for a moment to consideration of how the use of representative stimuli can help us understand the general principles governing the perception of periodic sounds.

Use of special versus model periodic stimuli

Periodic stimuli of a particular frequency can have an almost limitless number of waveforms and spectra. One of the most important special stimuli is the simple or pure tone, since it consists only of a single spectral component. These sinusoidal waveforms have proved invaluable in studying cochlear mechanics, neural physiology, and pitch perception. However, pure tones are encountered infrequently outside the laboratory, and all other periodic sounds have more than one spectral component. Also, the thresholds for pure tones become so high for frequencies less than 20 Hz that they are effectively inaudible; however, periodic waveforms having fundamental frequencies below 20 Hz can be heard if they have harmonics in the audible range.

In the nineteenth century, complex tones were generated by a siren or by a rotating Savart wheel (see Boring, 1942, p. 335), both of which could produce periodic pulses or clicks of any desired frequency. In the twentieth century, electronic pulse generators with adjustable frequency and pulse width or computer generated pulses were used frequently when complex tones with broad spectra were desired. If the width of the periodic pulse is narrow, the amplitude of higher harmonics decreases only slowly with harmonic number, as shown in Figure 3.10. However, the spectral alignment of the phases of spectral components of pulse trains produces unique patterns of auditory stimulation, as indicated in Figures 3.8 and 3.9. Also, at low tonal and infra-tonal frequencies, pulse trains are unique stimuli, sounding like a sequence of clicks separated by silence.

If we turn from pulses to familiar complex tones, such as the sounds employed in speech and music, we find that they each have special qualities and a limited range of repetition frequencies. Is there, then, any sound which can be considered as a model periodic stimulus?

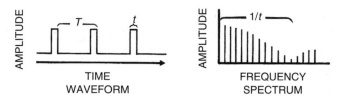

Figure 3.10 Amplitude spectra of pulse trains. The spacing between spectral lines shown in the figure on the right equals $1/T$ Hz, where T is the period in seconds of the waveform shown on the left. The spectral harmonic with minimal amplitude is the one closest to $1/t$ Hz, where t is the pulse duration (or pulse width) in seconds.

Iterated noise segments as representative or model periodic sounds

It has been suggested that iterated segments of Gaussian noise are useful as representative stimuli for studying the generic rules governing the perception of periodic sounds (Warren and Bashford, 1981). These stimuli have randomly determined waveforms and all harmonics of the fundamental repetition frequency lying in the audible range, with each harmonic having its own randomly determined amplitude and phase. Hence, they can be considered as exemplars of periodic stimuli with no *a priori* restrictions concerning the waveform or spectrum. As we shall see, it has been found that principles governing perception of these randomly derived periodic waveforms apply to special periodic sounds as well. However, specific classes of sounds (such as vowels, sinusoidal tones, pulse trains, square waves, etc.) can have additional properties superimposed upon the more general ones, so that it may be difficult to distinguish special from general perceptual characteristics.

Randomly derived periodic waveforms can be generated in a number of ways. In most of the studies described below, a segment of white or Gaussian noise ("frozen noise") was stored and iterated without pauses to produce "repeating frozen noise" or RFN. When, for example, the duration of the repeating noise segment is 5 ms, a complex tone is produced with a period of 5 ms and a frequency of 200 Hz. The pitch of a 200 Hz RFN is free from any hint of noise and matches that of a 200 Hz sinusoidal tone, but with a timbre that reflects the presence of higher harmonics. The dozens of harmonics of 200 Hz within the audible range are present and, as mentioned earlier, each of the harmonics has a randomly determined amplitude and phase so that each of the RFNs derived from independent 5 ms segments has an individual rich tonal quality.

It is of interest to compare the responses at different positions on the basilar membrane as simulated in Figure 3.9 for a 200 Hz pulse train with the equivalent simulation shown in Figure 3.11 for a 200 Hz RFN. For the

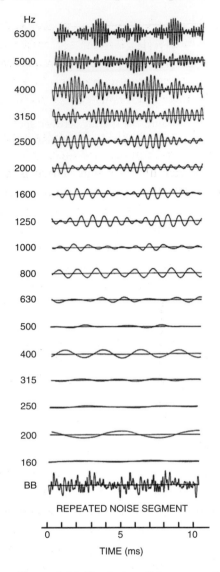

Figure 3.11 Simulation of the nature of the basilar membrane response to a model periodic sound. Two statements of a repeating white noise segment (period 5 ms, repetition frequency 200 Hz) are shown in unfiltered or broadband form in the bottom tracing labeled BB, with the tracings shown above obtained from the same set of 1/3-octave filters used with the pulse train in Figure 3.9. The center frequencies of the filters are shown to the left of each response curve. Spectral resolution of the sinusoidal waveforms of the individual lower harmonics can be seen, as well as a series of iterated complex patterns (each with a period of 5 ms) produced by individual filters with center frequencies above 800 Hz. For additional details, see the text.

1/3-octave bands with center frequencies below the fifth harmonic (1,000 Hz), spectral resolution of individual harmonics occurs for both the pulse train and the RFN, and their tracings appear quite similar. At center frequencies corresponding to the fifth harmonic and above, evidence of the interaction of neighboring harmonics within single 1/3-octave bands can be seen, and the response curves derived from pulse trains and RFNs differ. The waveform envelopes derived from pulse trains take on a characteristic pulsate structure, with synchronous bursts of activity corresponding to each pulse of the broadband stimulus at each of the higher filter settings. There is no such resemblance of the 1/3-octave bands of the RFN either to each other or to the broadband parent waveform. The waveforms of successive bands for the RFN above the fourth harmonic can be seen to have different randomly determined envelopes that trace the irregular peaks and troughs of the waveform. However, each of the 1/3-octave bands has the same period of 5 ms. Despite the lack of any interband correlation of waveform or fine structure, and by virtue of their common period, these RFN bands fuse seamlessly into a single pitch matching that of a 200 Hz sinusoidal tone.

The spectrally resolved lower harmonics are not required for hearing pitch. When the first ten harmonics of a 200 Hz RFN pulse train are removed by high-pass filtering, a residue pitch can be heard that matches that of the lower ten, but with a quite different timbre.

Pitch and infrapitch iterance

Frequency-dependent characteristics of repeating frozen noise segments can be heard with ease as a global percept or iterance encompassing the entire waveform over a range of approximately 15 octaves extending from about 0.5 Hz through 16,000 Hz. Five octaves of iterance (0.5 Hz through 20 Hz) lie below the pitch range. Figure 3.12 shows the perceptual characteristics for the RFNs having different fundamental frequencies along this continuum, as well as their possible neural bases. Although the boundaries for perceptual qualities and neural mechanisms for iterance are shown at discrete frequencies, it should be kept in mind that these boundaries actually represent gradual transitions occurring in the vicinity of the repetition frequencies indicated.

At fundamental frequencies above approximately 8,000 Hz, RFNs are equivalent to sinusoidal tones, since the harmonics of the fundamental lie beyond the nominal 16,000 Hz limit of audibility. At frequencies below 8,000 Hz, audible harmonics produce timbres that are different from that of a sinusoidal tone having the same frequency and pitch. Below about 1,000 Hz, these timbres become especially rich and distinctive (Warren and Bashford,

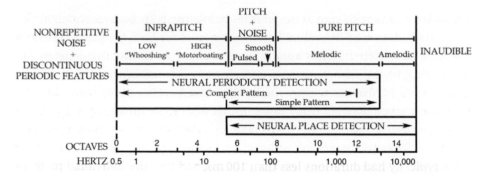

Figure 3.12 The iterance continuum. The figure represents the approximately 15 octaves over which global percepts can be heard for model periodic stimuli consisting of repeated segments derived from Gaussian (white) noise. Waveform repetition frequency is designated in hertz and also as the number of octaves above the lowest frequency for the perception of iterance encompassing the entire waveform. The upper portion of the figure describes the perceptual characteristics; transitions between the qualities given are gradual, with category boundaries at the approximate positions shown. Possible neurological mechanisms available for the detection of iterance at particular waveform repetition frequencies are also shown. For further description, see the text.

1981). Warren and Bashford also reported that from about 100 down to 20 Hz, RFNs have a hiss-like component that accompanies the pitch (the hiss can be eliminated by removing harmonics lying above 4,000 Hz). From about 100 through 70 Hz, the pitch seems continuous or smooth, and from about 70 through 20 Hz the pitch is heard as accented or pulsed. Pitch is absent for repetition frequencies below about 20 Hz. For the roughly five octaves of the infrapitch range extending from 20 Hz to 0.5 Hz (repetition periods from about 50 ms to 2 s), repeated noise segments are heard as global percepts that can be divided into two ranges (Guttman and Julesz, 1963). For the high infrapitch (HiIP) region from roughly 20 through 4 Hz, iterated noise segments have a clear staccato sound which they described as "motorboating." For the low infrapitch (LoIP) region from roughly 4 through 1 or 0.5 Hz, they described the perceptual quality as "whooshing." In keeping with the suggestion of Warren and Bashford (1981), RFNs in the HiIP and LoIP ranges are considered as "infratones" producing a detectable periodicity called "infrapitch." As with tonal RFNs having harmonics in the pitch range, different infratonal wave-forms having the same repetition frequency can be readily distinguished by their distinctive timbres. In the HiIP range it is not possible to detect con-stituent components or events, but in the LoIP range, after the initial global recognition of iterance, an assortment of components such as thumps, clanks, and rattles characteristic of individual RFNs can be heard to emerge (Warren and Bashford, 1981). (It may be of some interest to note that the durations of phonemes correspond to HiIP periods, and durations of syllables and words to LoIP periods.) It has been reported by Kaernbach (1992, 1993) that when listeners were instructed to tap to features heard in the whooshing range, there was considerable agreement in tap points by different listeners presented with the same RFNs. He also reported that the distinctive patterns within these RFNs typically had durations less than 100 ms, and that the individual patterns consisted of spectral components that could extend over a range from one to several critical bands.

When RFNs have repetition frequencies longer than 2 s (corresponding to repetition frequencies below the 0.5 Hz limit for the global percept of infrapitch), limited portions of the waveform can be heard to repeat with continued listening, and listeners can tap regularly in synchrony with these recurrent features. These repetitive events resemble the components that can be heard in the whooshing range, and are separated by featureless-seeming noise. Repetition of RFNs having periods of at least 20 s can be detected in this manner not only by laboratory personnel, but also by college students during a half-hour session in which they started with RFN in the HiIP range and then heard a series of successively increasing RFN periods (Warren, Bashford, Cooley, and Brubaker, 2001; see also Kaernbach, 2004). The ability to retain detailed auditory memory traces for long durations can make it possible to employ top-down syntactic and semantic context in speech, and also permits the recognition of repetition and variations from strict repetition of melodic themes in music. Cowan, Lichty, and Grove (1990) reported that the memory for unattended spoken syllables is at least 10 s, matching the neuromagnetic evidence described by Sams, Hari, Rif, and Knuutila (1993) that there is an auditory memory trace for a particular tone that persists for about 10 s. Using event-related brain potential measurements, Winkler, Korzyukov, Gumenyuk, et al. (2002) found that a memory trace of a particular tone could be detected for at least 30 s.

It is not necessary that the features of a long-period RFN that are heard to repeat represent some particularly unusual portion of the waveform – a crossmodal cue (a light flash) repeating synchronously at a randomly selected point along 10 s RFNs allowed listeners to tap to the same region that had been highlighted previously in the same experimental session, and also to tap to that region again after delays of 24 hours or more (Bashford, Brubaker, and Warren, 1993).

Let us examine the neural mechanisms shown in Figure 3.12 as subserving the perception of infrapitch. An RFN in the LoIP whooshing range having a repetition frequency of 2 Hz can be considered as a sequence of harmonic sinusoidal components with a fundamental frequency of 2 Hz and a 2 Hz separation between neighboring spectral components. The lowest harmonics cannot be heard, and the thousands of higher harmonics in the audible range are too closely spaced to be resolved along the basilar membrane (see Plomp, 1964, for limits of the ear's analyzing power). Many unresolved harmonics fall within a single critical band, and since these interacting harmonics have randomly determined relative phases and amplitudes, highly complex local patterns of stimulation are produced at every stimulated locus on the basilar membrane. Although the temporal patterns differ at separate loci, each of the complex patterns is repeated at the RFN repetition frequency of 2 Hz, as illustrated in Figure 3.13, and it is this cross-frequency equivalence that determines the ensemble of 2 Hz iterance that listeners hear.

Figure 3.13 shows the patterns corresponding to a 10 ms portion of the 500 ms period of a 2 Hz iterated pink noise segment. The noise segment was excised from pink noise bandpassed from 100 through 10,000 Hz. Since the long-term spectrum of the parent pink noise had equal power for each of the 1/3-octave bands (which approximate the critical bandwidths), the patterns at the lower frequencies shown in Figure 3.13 can be seen more clearly than they could be for white noise for which power is proportional to the center frequency of 1/3-octave bands. It should be kept in mind that the temporal patterns for the 2 Hz signal are quite long and complex, each being fifty times the 10 ms portion shown in the figure. Also, it should be noted that while not all audible 1/3-octave bands are depicted, independent patterns repeated each 500 ms would be created for each such band. It has been demonstrated that information concerning infrapitch periodicity is available along the entire length of the basilar membrane, for when a 1/3-octave filter was swept through a broadband infratonal RFN, the repetition frequency was heard at all center frequencies of the filter (Warren and Bashford, 1981). Identification of the 2 Hz repetition could be accomplished through the type of neural periodicity detection designated as "complex pattern" in Figure 3.12.

When a pitch-range RFN having a repetition frequency of about 20 Hz is heard at a moderate sound pressure level of 70 dB, the amplitudes of the fundamental and the first few harmonics are below the high thresholds for these low frequency sinusoidal components. However, the fourth to sixth harmonics would be at or above threshold and could be resolved along the basilar membrane. These spatially resolved sinusoidal components produce the local excitation maxima that provide the basis for the "neural place" cues to repetition frequency shown in Figure 3.12, and can provide information concerning frequencies of RFNs from the lower limit of pitch to the frequency

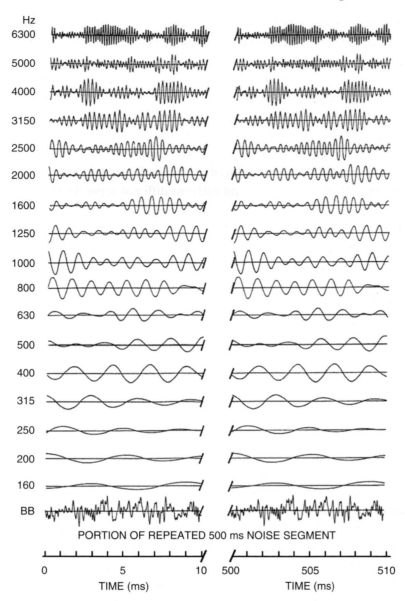

Figure 3.13 Simulation of the nature of the basilar membrane's response to an iterated 500 ms segment of pink noise (repetition frequency 2 Hz). The bottom of the figure shows 10 ms tracings of the unfiltered or broadband waveform (BB), with the tracings shown above obtained from the same set of 1/3-octave filters used with a pulse train in Figure 3.9. The remaining 490 ms of the period are not shown: the tracings in the figure recommence with the beginning of the next restatement of the iterated patterns. Each of the 1/3-octave filters generated a different complex 500 ms pattern.

limit for audibility at about 16,000 Hz. Nerve fibers originating at the places of excitation maxima may also provide neural periodicity information based on phase locking to resolved harmonics. This temporal cue, designated as "simple pattern" in Figure 3.12, can furnish information concerning RFN repetition from about 20 Hz to the roughly 4,000 or 4,500 Hz limit of phase locking (which is designated as the "melodic" pitch range in Figure 3.12 since it corresponds to the range of fundamental frequencies employed by orchestral instruments).

In addition to the phase-locked simple pattern, there is another class of temporal cues available for determining the iterance of both infrapitch and some pitch range RFNs. As discussed previously, when a nerve fiber's characteristic frequency is several times greater than the repetition frequency of an RFN, interaction of harmonics within the same critical band produces distinctive amplitude patterns that can modulate the responses of a nerve fiber. These local envelope patterns are designated as "complex pattern" in Figure 3.12, and are illustrated for a tonal RFN in Figure 3.11 and for an infratonal RFN in Figure 3.13. The complex patterns differ for individual critical bands, but they all are the same repetition period as the RFN. However, RFNs with a fundamental frequency above a few kilohertz cannot produce complex pattern cues to repetition frequency, since their few harmonics lying within the audible frequency range can be resolved and do not interact within the ear to produce these patterns.

Let us recapitulate the types of neural information available for the perception of iterance with our model of generic periodic stimuli consisting of RFNs that have unrestricted randomly determined relative amplitudes and phases for each of their harmonic components. There are three main types of neurophysiological cues shown in Figure 3.12 and listed below which, taken together, encompass the approximately 15 octaves of iterance encompassing waveform repetition frequencies from about 0.5 Hz to 16,000 Hz.

1.   Neural place information, requiring spectral resolution of the fundamental and/or lower harmonics and operating with RFN repetition frequencies from the lower limit of pitch at about 20 Hz up to the frequency limit of hearing at about 16,000 Hz. It is absent for infrapitch.

2.   Local complex pattern information produced by the interaction of unresolved harmonics. These patterns are carried by auditory nerve fibers having characteristic frequencies several times greater than the RFN frequency repetition. This mechanism operates over the entire infrapitch range, as well as the first seven octaves of RFN pitch from about 20 Hz to about 2,500 Hz (above this limit, harmonics are resolved).

3.   Phase-locked simple pattern information based upon the resolved spectral components of RFNs lying within the range from about 20 Hz to the upper limit of phase locking at about 4,000 or 4,500 Hz.

There is also a possibility (not depicted in Figure 3.12) that phase locking to local waveform envelope features rather than the fine structure components within an envelope may provide information concerning the RFN period up to the limit of audibility (see Burns and Viemeister, 1976).

If pitch and infrapitch represent regions of the same continuum, there may be infrapitch analogs of pitch-range phenomena. We have found that some phenomena that have been studied in the pitch range also occur with infrapitch. Echo pitch is one such phenomenon.

Echo pitch and infrapitch echo

When a noise is added to itself after a delay of τ seconds, this repetition is heard as a pitch equal to $1/\tau$ Hz for values of τ from 2×10^{-2} through 5×10^{-4} seconds (pitches from 50 through 2,000 Hz; see Bilsen and Ritsma, 1969–1970). Echo pitch is known by several other names including time difference tone, reflection tone, time-separation pitch, repetition pitch, and rippled-noise pitch. This last name refers to its rippled power spectrum with peaks occurring at integral multiples of $1/\tau$ Hz (see Figure 3.14A). The pitch heard with this rippled power spectrum is the same as that of a complex tone having harmonics positioned at the peaks of the rippling – however, echo pitch is considerably weaker than the pitch of a complex tone. While the rippled power spectrum shown in the figure corresponds to a mixture of undelayed and delayed noise having equal amplitudes, surprisingly a pitch can still be heard for differences in intensity up to about 20 dB between the delayed and undelayed sounds (Yost and Hill, 1978).

The detection of repetition for recycling frozen noise at frequencies below the pitch limit, as shown in Figure 3.12, led to the expectation that it might be possible to detect infrapitch echo at long repetition delays. The anticipated infrapitch echo was reported for delays as long as 0.5 s (Warren, Bashford, and Wrightson, 1979, 1980) and confirmed by Bilsen and Wieman (1980). At delays of 0.5 s, the spectral peaks of the rippled power spectrum are separated by 2 Hz, a spacing too close to permit resolution along the basilar membrane, so that infrapitch echo could only be detected by information provided through temporal analysis. Infrapitch echo resembled infrapitch RFNs as described by Guttman and Julesz (1963), but was considerably fainter (but, based on a suggestion by Bill Hartmann, detection of infrapitch echo was made easier by

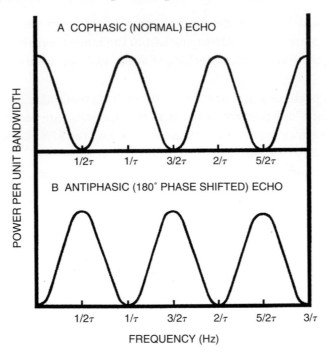

Figure 3.14 Rippled power spectra produced by adding a delayed restatement of broadband noise to itself. For further details, see the text.

1/3-octave filtering). Although infrapitch repetition could be heard over a wide range of center frequencies, it seemed clearest at center frequencies of about 1,000 to 2,000 Hz. As shown in Figure 3.15, subjects were able to match the periods of echo delays for broadband noise quite accurately to the repetition rates of periodic sounds for values of τ from 0.5 through 0.01 s, corresponding to repetition frequencies from 2 Hz through 100 Hz respectively. (Matches were made on the basis of pitch iterance at 50 Hz and above, and on the basis of infrapitch iterance from 2 Hz through 20 Hz.) At frequencies of 5 Hz and below, it was possible for subjects to dispense with a matching stimulus and indicate the repetition period of infrapitch echo by rhythmical tapping of a response key.

The nature of the infrapitch temporal analysis used for noise mixed with its echo may be clarified if we compare it with the infrapitch iterance of RFNs. We have seen that continued repetition of a segment of Gaussian noise A (that is, AAA ...) can be detected readily as a global "whooshing" pattern for periods of A as long as 1 or 2 s (Guttman and Julesz, 1963). In preliminary experiments, Warren, Bashford, and Wrightson (1980) found that multiple repetitions of the same waveform were not required. If a 500 ms segment of noise (A) was

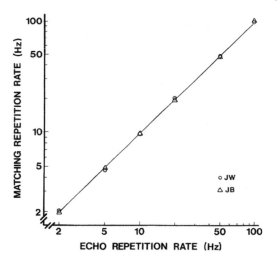

Figure 3.15 Apparent repetition rate of broadband noise mixed with its echo. Judgments of 50 and 100 Hz were made on the basis of pitch, and judgments of 2, 5, 10, and 20 Hz on the basis of infrapitch. For further description, see the text. (From Warren, Bashford, and Wrightson, 1980.)

repeated a single time, followed by a second 500 ms segment of noise (B) repeated once, then a third 500 ms segment of noise (C) repeated once, etc., to produce the stimulus AABBCC..., listeners could detect such a "pure" infrapitch echo based on these single repetitions with somewhat greater ease than they could detect mixed infrapitch echo. The classical mixed infrapitch echo can be considered to have the composition A + B, B + C, C + D, D + E, ... , where each letter corresponds to an independent noise segment. It can be seen that on the first appearance of C it is mixed with noise segment B, and on its single reappearance it is mixed with noise segment D. A mechanism is required for the extraction of temporal information corresponding to C from two uncorrelated maskers. A relatively simple mechanism involving recognition of the restatement of exceptional features associated with C might work for pure infrapitch echo, but would not work for mixed echo. Different exceptional features would be created by the mixture of C with B, and of C with D, and any unique characteristics of C by itself would be changed, and changed differently by its mixture with B and its mixture with D. A mechanism used for detection of infrapitch mixed echo needs to be capable of recognizing masked single repetitions of long-period random patterns. Mathematical models based upon autocorrectional analysis proposed by Licklider (1951) and Yost and Hill (1979) for pitch range stimuli could, in principle, work in the infrapitch range as well.

Reversing the polarity of the delayed noise (phase shifting by 180° to produce "antiphasic" echo) produced the rippled power spectrum shown in Figure 3.14B. Infrapitch repetition could be heard with equal ease for antiphasic and cophasic addition, and the apparent repetition frequency was $1/\tau$ Hz in both cases (Warren, Bashford, and Wrightson, 1980), so that the complex temporal pattern analysis was insensitive to polarity inversion in the infrapitch range. However, inverting the echo polarity in the pitch range has long been known to produce a marked effect: antiphasic echo pitch is weaker and has two simultaneous pitches, one about 10 percent higher and one about 10 percent lower than cophasic echo when the echo delay is approximately 4 ms (Fourcin, 1965; Bilsen, 1970; Yost, Hill, and Perez-Falcon, 1978). Warren, Bashford, and Wrightson (1980) found that the change from insensitivity to the phase of the echo in the infrapitch range to the phase sensitivity characteristic of the pitch range occurred at echo delays of about 30 ms, corresponding to roughly 35 Hz.

The spectral peaks of antiphasic echo pitch form an odd-harmonic sequence (i.e., frequencies 1, 3, 5, ... times the frequency of the lowest peak). Since the pitches that had been reported were, at least for a 4 ms delay, equal to the cophasic echo pitch of 250 Hz plus or minus roughly 10 percent, this presented a troublesome problem for classical pitch theories. Bilsen and Goldstein (1974) and Bilsen (1977) attempted to account for this puzzle by considering that a central pitch extractor uses the spectrally dominant region (the fourth and fifth peaks) of the antiphasic echo spectrum to calculate the fundamental of an all-harmonic sequence having successive harmonics closest to these two frequencies. This calculation results in two closest matches or "pseudofundamentals" corresponding to the dual antiphasic echo pitches perceived by listeners. However, there are serious problems with this spectral model. The peaks above the fifth lie above the dominant region used to calculate the pseudofundamentals and should have no influence upon pitch if this model is correct – yet when peaks above the seventh were removed by filtering, the deviation of the pitches heard from $1/\tau$ Hz decreased by about 35 percent (Warren and Bashford, 1988). This observation, together with the results obtained with other filtering conditions, led Warren and Bashford to conclude that broadband antiphasic echo pitch represented a weighted average of different local pitches occurring at different spectral regions. The deviations of these local pitches from the cophasic (normal) echo pitch of $1/\tau$ Hz was attributed to the changes in local delay times produced by the 180° phase change (which is equivalent to plus or minus half the period of the local frequency). Thus, the composite or total repetition delays occurring at different local positions along the basilar membrane is equal to the normal or cophasic delay of τ_1 plus or minus the contribution of half the period of τ_2 of the local frequency. This results in two local antiphasic echo pitches, EP_1 and EP_2, given by the equation:

$$EP_{1,2} = (1/\tau_1 \pm 2/\tau_2)\,\text{Hz} \tag{3.1}$$

As a result, as the echo delay time τ_1 becomes larger, the fixed contribution of the $\pm\tau_2$ component becomes proportionally less, providing a basis for why, as noted previously, cophasic and antiphasic infrapitch echoes produced by long delay periods were found to be indistinguishable.

Periodic signals with alternating polarity

Warren and Wrightson (1981) used noise segments as model periodic waveforms, and determined the apparent frequency when alternate statements of the waveform were reversed in polarity. These stimuli had the form $A_0, A_\pi, A_0, A_\pi, \ldots$ in which A_0 represents a waveform derived from noise, and A_π the same waveform that has been inverted in polarity (that is, phase-shifted by 180° or π radians). The overall repetition frequencies employed in the study ranged from 2 Hz through 1,935 Hz. An illustration of a stimulus waveform is given in Figure 3.16 for a 200 Hz signal.

If the waveform repetition period corresponding to $(A_0 + A_\pi)$ is τ seconds, then the fundamental frequency is $1/\tau$ Hz. As with all periodic sounds that consist of segments alternating in polarity but otherwise equivalent (square waves, symmetrical triangle waves, alternating polarity pulse trains, etc.), the spectrum contains only odd-numbered harmonics, so that the component frequencies are $1/\tau$, $3/\tau$, $5/\tau$, $\ldots$ Hz.

The results, obtained when the pitches of iterated noise segments in the tonal and infratonal frequency ranges were matched using adjustable unipolar pulse trains, are shown in Figure 3.17. Values obtained for the alternating polarity waveforms are indicated by squares, and values obtained for noise segments repeated without polarity inversions (used as an experimental control to determine the accuracy of frequency matching) are indicated by circles.

It can be seen that matches were accurate for the control stimuli at all frequencies. However, the alternating polarity noise segments were matched with unipolar pulse trains of the same waveform repetition frequency only at 200 Hz and above. At infratonal frequencies from 2 Hz through 20 Hz, they were matched with pulse trains having approximately twice the repetition frequency. Within the low pitch range between 20 and 200 Hz, the apparent frequency represented a compromise between these two modes of analysis.

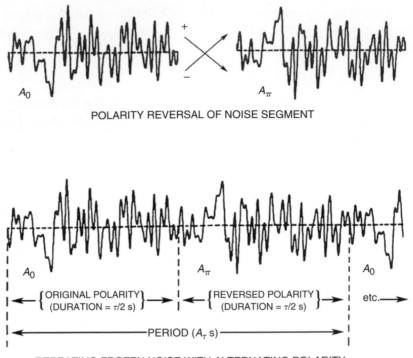

POLARITY REVERSAL OF NOISE SEGMENT

REPEATING FROZEN NOISE WITH ALTERNATING POLARITY

Figure 3.16 Representation of generic or model odd-harmonic periodic waveform having randomly determined amplitude and phase of spectral components. The overall period of τ s consists of two frozen noise segments of $\tau/2$ s duration. Each half-period represents a polarity-inverted version of the other, as with all odd-harmonic periodic sounds (e.g., square waves, symmetrical triangle waves, alternating polarity pulse trains). (From Warren and Wrightson, 1981.)

Figure 3.18 allows us to visualize why this shift in the apparent frequency function occurs. This figure illustrates the nature of patterns produced by a 200 Hz odd-harmonic stimulus when a series of 1/3-octave filters was used to approximate critical bands on the basilar membrane as in Figures 3.9 and 3.11. It can be seen that while the 200 Hz fundamental and the first few of the odd harmonics are resolved by this simulation of basilar membrane filtering, the higher harmonic components of this 200 Hz fundamental interact to generate iterated complex patterns. While these complex patterns appear to repeat twice within each 5 ms period, a close examination reveals that these two patterns are not exactly the same (the bases and consequences of these differences will be discussed later).

Whereas both complex patterns and spectral resolution of harmonics can be seen in Figure 3.18, both types of cues to acoustic repetition would not be

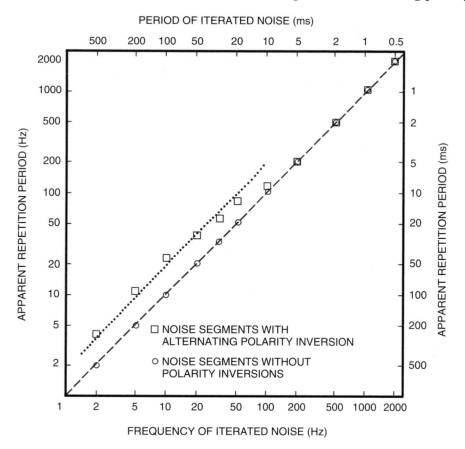

Figure 3.17 Apparent repetition rates of iterated noise segments with and without polarity inversion of alternate statements. The diagonal dashed line represents frequencies equal to the waveform repetition frequencies (and the spectral fundamentals). The dotted diagonal line represents polarity-insensitive apparent frequencies one octave higher than the waveform repetition frequencies. (From Warren and Wrightson, 1981.)

available for all of the repetition frequencies used by Warren and Wrightson as shown in Figure 3.17. When listeners in this study received the infrapitch stimuli consisting of odd harmonics of 2 Hz (a period, τ, of 0.5 s), the 4 Hz separation of neighboring harmonics did not permit spectral resolution, so that only complex temporal patterns were available as cues to repetition. As shown in Figure 3.17, listeners heard a repetition frequency close to 4 Hz, or twice that of this 2 Hz stimulus, indicating a perceptual similarity of adjacent half-period waveforms. In contrast, the 1,935 Hz alternating polarity stimulus has an almost 4,000 Hz separation of neighboring harmonics, permitting the spectral resolution of each of the few odd-harmonic frequencies within the

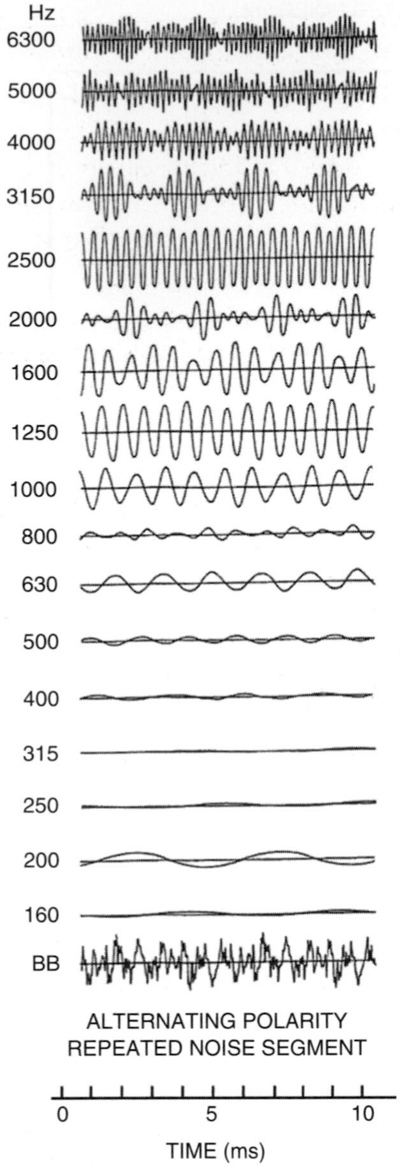

Figure 3.18 Simulation of the nature of basilar membrane responses to a model 200 Hz periodic waveform with alternating polarity (waveform repetition period of 5 ms), shown at the bottom of the figure in broadband form (as BB). The signal was derived from a 2.5 ms pink noise segment; the first half of the repeating pattern had the original polarity which was inverted for the second half. As with all alternating polarity waveforms (e.g., square waves, symmetrical triangle waves, alternating polarity pulse trains), the spectrum consisted of only odd numbered harmonics (i.e., 200, 600, 1,000, 1,400, ..., Hz). The response curves for the set of 1/3-octave filters (center frequencies shown on the left), demonstrate spectral resolution at the lower center frequencies, and complex periodic waveforms at the higher. Cursory examination shows that the tracings based on center frequencies of 2,000 Hz and above have successive 2.5 ms segments that are quite similar in structure. However, a detailed examination of expanded oscilloscope tracings reveals that the waveform period of 5 ms consists of two pseudoperiods, one less and one greater than 2.5 ms. For further details, see the text.

audible range, without any appreciable harmonic interaction within critical bands. As can be seen in Figure 3.17, the 1,935 Hz stimulus had a pitch corresponding to $1/\tau$ Hz (its fundamental frequency). At some region within the pitch range, a transition between the two analytical modes should occur. Figure 3.17 shows that this transition occurred at frequencies from approximately 30 to 100 Hz, with average matches between one and two times the spectral fundamental. There were also some reports of pitch ambiguity within this transitional range.

A close examination of Figure 3.18 indicates that while the odd-harmonic waveform is repeated every 5 ms for each 1/3-octave band, as noted earlier, the waveforms within adjacent 2.5 ms intervals, while similar, are not identical. These adjacent complex patterns form two alternating pseudoperiods, one slightly less, and the other slightly greater than 2.5 ms. These deviations from 2.5 ms change with the center frequency, and are produced by the 180° phase shift, which corresponds to $\pm 1/2$ the period of the center frequency of the particular 1/3-octave center frequency representing the approximate critical bandwidth. Thus, expressed as a general rule, the local pseudofundamental periods produced by an odd harmonic periodic signal when multiple harmonics are present in the same critical band are equal to twice the period of the signal (τ_1) plus or minus twice the period of the center frequency of the particular critical band (τ_2), so that the local pseudofundamental pitches, P_1 and P_2, are expressed by the equation:

$$P_{1,2} = (1/2\tau_1 \pm 1/2\tau_2) \text{ Hz} \tag{3.2}$$

In order to test the validity of this equation, Bashford and Warren (1990) presented four musicians with groups of three successive odd harmonics having equal amplitudes and randomly determined relative phases and had them match the pitches heard to the pitches of all-harmonic pulse trains. These triads had fundamental frequencies that varied in an unpredictable fashion within the range of 100 to 200 Hz. As shown in Figure 3.19, the center frequencies of the odd-harmonic triads ranged from the 5th to the 19th harmonic. The pair of thin vertical lines represents the frequencies of the pseudofundamentals as calculated using equation (3.2), disregarding whether or not the harmonic components could actually interact within the same critical band and so produce local pseudoperiods. It can be seen that the fundamental frequency of the spectrally resolved odd-harmonic triads dominated pitch matches up to the triad centered on the 9th harmonic. For the higher order odd-harmonic triads, harmonics could interact and produce local complex temporal patterns, and the pairs of dominant pitches heard corresponded to the pseudoperiods predicted by equation (3.2).

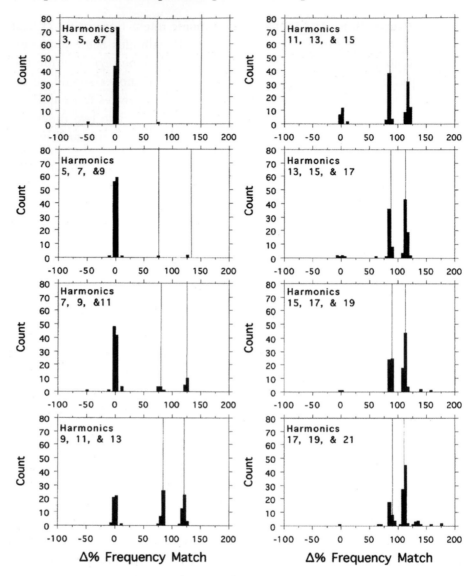

Figure 3.19 Frequency matches for groups of three successive odd harmonics. Each panel represents a total of 120 matches by four subjects for triads having fundamental frequencies that varied in an unpredictable fashion between 100 and 200 Hz. Frequency matches are scored as Δ% (the percentage increase or decrease relative to the fundamental frequency). The thin vertical lines in each panel represent the calculated local pseudoperiods, regardless of whether the odd-harmonic triads lie within the same critical band and could consequently interact to produce perceptual pseudoperiods. For further description, see the text.

Pitches produced by dichotic interactions

Houtsma and Goldstein (1972) presented two adjacent harmonics of a missing fundamental simultaneously for a duration of 500 ms, followed 250 ms later by a second 500 ms stimulus also consisting of two adjacent harmonics but with a different missing fundamental. These two missing fundamentals together corresponded to one of eight possible musical intervals, and their musically trained subjects were required to identify the interval, or, as it was considered, the two-note "melody." Houtsma and Goldstein found that this task could be accomplished not only when each component of the two-harmonic stimulus producing a missing fundamental note was delivered simultaneously to the same ear (monaural stimulation), but also when one harmonic of the two-harmonic complex was delivered to one ear at the same time that the remaining harmonic was delivered to the other ear (dichotic stimulation). However, this dichotic pitch is quite faint, and cannot be heard by everyone.

In addition to the creation of pitch through dichotic interactions of harmonics, there have also been reports of two types of rather faint dichotic pitches resulting from time delays between noise signals reaching the two ears. The first of these was described by Cramer and Huggins (1958). They presented broadband noise from a single generator to both ears, but introduced an interaural phase difference for a narrow frequency band lying below 1,000 Hz. This phase change over a small frequency range approximated a fixed time delay, and caused this frequency band to appear at the side of the leading ear while the rest of the noise was heard at the medial plane. The pitch perceived corresponded to that which would be heard if the laterally shifted band of noise was heard alone. However, there was no monaural spectral information: the input to each ear was broadband noise with no pitch, so that pitch emerged only following the binaural temporal processing that resulted in lateralization. Another type of dichotic pitch resulting from interaural time differences has been discussed in Chapter 2: when the interaural time delay of broadband noise exceeds the limit for lateralization for some of the spectral components, a faint pitch corresponding in Hertz to the reciprocal of the delay in seconds can be heard. The limits of the range of interaural time delays reported to produce such pitch extend from about 3 ms through 50 ms, corresponding to about 300 through about 20 Hz (Fourcin, 1970; Bilsen and Goldstein, 1974; Warren, Bashford, and Wrightson, 1981).

The existence of these three types of dichotic pitches demonstrates that it is possible to generate pitch through binaural interaction when information received at each ear alone is insufficient to establish the pitch heard.

Ear dominance for perception of pitch

While Houtsma and Goldstein (1972) demonstrated that dichotic information involving different pitches can be integrated to produce a third pitch, there have been experiments demonstrating that under some conditions there is a perceptual suppression of one of two tones presented dichotically. Deutsch has reported a number of illusions in which a lateral dominance is observed for the perception of different tones delivered to each ear simultaneously (Deutsch, 1974, 1975; Deutsch and Roll, 1976). She has observed that the dominant pitch is sometimes mislateralized, and has concluded that information concerning pitch and lateralization can be disassociated and processed independently at some stage (Deutsch, 1981). Efron and Yund (1976) have reported that lateral dominance for "dichotic chords" is not like that for monaural chords. For the monaural condition, relative intensities strongly influence the contribution of each component to perception; for the dichotic condition, there is a wide range of intensity mismatch over which lateral advantage can be maintained for a fainter tone.

Musical pitch and musical infrapitch (rhythm)

Musical pitch spans about seven octaves. The lowest note of a bass viol (also known as a double bass) at 41 Hz represents the lower limit, and the highest note of a piccolo (used rather infrequently) at about 4,500 Hz represents the upper limit of orchestral instruments. Of course, harmonics of the fundamental frequencies corresponding to musical notes may be present up to the approximately 16,000 Hz limit of hearing, and can enter into determining the quality of a tone. But why the rather low upper frequency limit for musical pitch? One possibility is that qualities of musical sounds depend to a large extent on their harmonic structure, and since there is little headroom left for audible harmonics above 4,000 or 5,000 Hz, these high pitches are not used in music and so seem amelodic. Another possibility is that place and simple phase-locked periodicity information occur together only from about 50 through roughly 4,500 Hz (see Figure 3.12), and melodic appreciation requires both types of information.

Musical intervals correspond to fixed ratios between the frequencies of notes. The basic unit is the octave (2:1), which is used in virtually all cultures having well-developed musical systems (see Helmholtz, 1954/1877). The division of the octave into smaller intervals is culture dependent. The music used in Western culture employs intervals for which the fundamental frequencies stand in the ratio of small integers: for example, fifths (frequency ratio of 2:3), fourths (frequency ratio of 3:4), major thirds (frequency ratio of 4:5). A pair of notes corresponding to one of these intervals seems consonant when sounded simultaneously by musical instruments, and one reason for this harmonious relation could involve the matching of frequencies for some of the harmonics from each note. Interestingly, the rules for consonance of pairs of complex tones do not seem to apply for pairs of pure tones. In a study by Plomp and Levelt (1965), two pure tones were generally rated as being dissonant when they fell within the same critical band, and being consonant when they were separated by more than a critical band. The sinusoidal tones falling within a single critical band produce beats and "roughness" which appear to be associated with dissonance, whereas a smooth-sounding consonance is heard when sinusoidal tones stimulate separate critical bands. In addition, there is some evidence that experience with conventional spacing of musical intervals may influence judgments of the extent of consonance of sinusoidal tone pairs (Ayres, Aeschbach, and Walker, 1980).

Rhythm in music involves the repetition of acoustic patterns at infratonal frequencies. These rhythmical patterns usually employ slowed down versions of the simple frequency ratios used for consonant musical intervals. It appears that music plays with variations from strict repetition not only in the pitch range, but in the infrapitch range as well. Musical rhythm can involve multiple infratonal periodicities having considerable complexity: percussive African polyrhythms use long-period sequences of sounds that can contain several harmonically related rhythmic frequencies, and listeners familiar with the conventions governing these complex patterns can attend either to the ensemble periodicity, or to one or another of the rhythmic components. However, unlike the case with mixed infratonal RFNs, the individual rhythmic percussive lines can be followed even when they deviate from harmonic relations with other lines. Some African music uses percussive "additive polyrhythms" in which the rhythm of each of the component inharmonic periodicities is perceived (see Sachs, 1953).

Deviations from strict periodicity in the pitch range

Although the ability to detect repetition (and deviation from exact repetition) of acoustic patterns is used for perception of rhythm and identification of melodic themes, this ability enters into other aspects of musical perception in a less obvious fashion. Attempts to produce a sustained note either vocally or by playing a musical instrument result in fluctuations in both frequency and amplitude. Although large fluctuations such as vibrato or tremelo are quite deliberate and noticeable, other involuntary smaller fluctuations are not detectable as such, but rather are heard as a "natural" quality. When a single period is excised from a recording of any musical instrument playing a particular note and iterated to produce a note unchanging in intensity and pitch, the instrument is no longer identifiable (unless it happens to be an organ). Robert Moog (the creator of the "Moog Synthesizer" designed to mimic individual musical instruments) had stated on several occasions that all instruments sound like an organ when a single period is excised and repeated without change. He believed that, "It is an inescapable fact that instruments sound the way they do because of the ways the waveform changes" (Dr. Robert Moog, personal communication).

The ability to detect slight fluctuations in amplitude and frequency can be demonstrated when a 1 s segment of a "steady" note produced by a musical instrument (other than an organ) or a 1 s segment of a "steady" vowel produced by a singer or speaker is stored digitally and reiterated without pauses. When played back, listeners then perceive a pattern of loudness and/or pitch fluctuation that repeats once a second. However, when the same 1 s segment is heard just once (that is, without repetition), the sound appears steady, and the perturbations from true periodicity contribute to the characteristic quality of the sound.

Some models for the pitch of complex tones

As we have seen, the loci of auditory stimulation (place information) and the rate at which patterns repeat (periodicity information) can establish the pitch(es) of a sound. There have been many theories and models concerning the manner in which place and periodicity cues are employed for pitch perception, some of which have been discussed earlier in this chapter, and a few others are described below.

A number of theories have considered that spatiotemporal patterns of stimulated regions along the basilar membrane determine the pitch heard. Thurlow (1963) has suggested that there can be vocal mediation of the spatial patterning in which the listener either covertly or overtly matches the pitch of the sound with his or her own production of a periodic vocal sound having matching harmonic components. (This vocal mediation mechanism would be limited by the pitch range of voice.)

Whitfield (1970) considered that peripheral spatial resolution leads to corresponding patterns of activity of discrete groups of neural units at more central locations, and that these patterns are responsible for pitch. Whitfield stated that experience with complex harmonic patterns could serve as the basis for pitch judgments; and that, even when components such as the fundamental are missing, the remaining information would be sufficient for recognition of the overall pattern and identification of the fundamental pitch.

Terhardt (1974) proposed a learning-matrix model for extracting "virtual pitch" through a comparison of a complex tone with traces acquired through experience with other complex tones. He considered that, over one's lifetime, individual harmonic components are each associated with subharmonics, and, when the matrix of subharmonics corresponding to a group of component frequencies interact, they produce a "virtual" low pitch characteristic of the complex.

Wightman's (1973) pattern-transformation model considers that the first stage in pitch processing is a rough spectral analysis accomplished through the peripheral auditory system, followed by a Fourier transform of the spectrum, with the final stage corresponding to a pitch extractor which calculates the lowest maximum in the derived function.

Goldstein's (1973) optimum-processor model considers that resolved harmonics produce an approximate or "noisy" central representation of their frequencies. A central processor then computes the harmonic numbers of these components and derives from this the fundamental frequency which corresponds to the perceived pitch. Goldstein (1978) stated that, while cochlear filtering is an essential stage in auditory frequency analysis, neural time-following determines the precision of pitch judgments.

A multilevel computer model for the pitch of complex tones has been formulated by Meddis and Hewitt (1991a, 1991b). The model considers that the pitch that is heard is based upon a number of successive processing stages. Some of these stages incorporate and modify earlier pitch models by other investigators.

Each of these models was designed to deal only with pitch perception, and cannot be extended readily to handle perception of infrapitch iterance. It would appear desirable to have a broader model or theory which can handle perception of acoustic iterance not only in the pitch range, but in the infra-pitch range as well. Such a theory need not consider a single mechanism operating over the entire range of detectable iterance – indeed, as discussed earlier in this chapter and summarized diagramatically in Figure 3.12, it appears likely that there are at least three neurophysiological mechanisms, some with overlapping frequency ranges, that are used for detection of iterance.

Suggestions for further reading

For a well-organized and clearly written discussion of pitch perception: Plomp, R. 1976. *Aspects of Tone Sensation: A Psychophysical Study.* New York: Academic Press.

For a more recent treatment of experiments and models for pitch perception:
Moore, B. C. J. 2003. *An Introduction to the Psychology of Hearing*, 5th edition.
London: Academic Press.

For detailed coverage of selected topics: Plack, C. J., Oxenham, A. J., Fay, R., and
Popper, A. N. (eds.) 2005. *Pitch: Neural Coding and Perception*. New York: Springer-
Verlag.

4

Judging auditory magnitudes:
the sone scale of loudness and
the mel scale of pitch

This chapter is concerned with the consequences of two broad principles applicable to hearing (as well as to perception in general): (1) there is an obligatory interpretation of sensory input in terms of events and conditions normally associated with stimulation; and (2) individuals are not aware of the nature of the neurophysiological responses to stimuli as such. The implications of these principles for the sone scale of loudness and the mel scale of pitch will be discussed, and evidence will be presented suggesting that the judgments used for the construction of these scales of sensory magnitude are based upon familiarity with physical scales correlated with the changes in stimulation.

Sensory input and perception

In the previous chapter on auditory localization, we saw how differences in acoustic input to the two ears are perceived in terms of associated external conditions and events without awareness of the aspects of sensory stimulation leading to this perception. Thus, when the sound radiated by a source reaches one ear before the other, listeners hear only a single sound located on the side of the leading ear: the difference in time of stimulation can be inferred by those having some knowledge of acoustics, but even then only one off-center sound is perceived. Also, we have seen that interaural spectral amplitude differences approximating those produced by the head and pinna for sources at different azimuths are perceived in an obligatory manner in terms of location rather than spectral mismatch.

Interpretation of sensory input in terms of environmental physical correlates is not, of course, unique to hearing. The disparity of retinal images resulting from the spatial separation of the eyes is not seen as a double image but, rather, in terms of an external correlate – the distance of the object represented by these images. Perception of depth is accomplished effortlessly without any awareness of differences in the retinal images. It is an intellectual exercise of some difficulty to use the laws of perspective to reason that objects are closer than the fixation distance determined by ocular vergence if they produce a crossed binocular disparity (i.e., a shift to the left for the right eye and a shift to the right for the left eye), and that they are further than the fixation distance if they produce an opposite uncrossed disparity.

A related perceptual principle is that aspects of sensory input which do not correspond to external events are difficult (and sometimes impossible) to detect. This principle appears to have received greater emphasis in studies dealing with vision than with hearing. Thus, the large visual gap or blind spot corresponding to the optic disc is quite difficult to perceive. Also, unlike the design of the octopus eye, having its retinal blood vessels behind the retina, our blood vessels are in front of the retina and their shadows can be seen by only some viewers, even with instructions and optimal viewing conditions. In hearing, we know that the reflex contraction of intra-aural muscles (the stapedius and the tensor tympani) produces a considerable change in the stimulus reaching the auditory receptors (see Chapter 1). Yet this alteration in amplitude and spectral profile is not perceived.

In keeping with these observations, we shall see that when subjects are required to estimate relative loudness they do not, and indeed they cannot, base their answers upon the quantitative nature of sensory processes. Instead, responses are based upon quantifiable physical dimensions familiar to subjects and associated with changes in stimulation.

The history of loudness measurement

The measurement of sensory intensity has had a long history of controversy. Fechner (1860) was the first to publish an equation relating sensory magnitude to physical intensity. His idea was simple: all just noticeable difference (jnd) steps are subjectively equal, and the magnitude of a particular sensation can be measured by adding up the number of jnd steps from threshold to the level of that sensation. Thus, a sensation 25 jnd steps above threshold would be half that corresponding to a sensation 50 jnd steps above threshold. Fechner claimed that if Weber's law were valid (this law states that the size of a jnd is proportional to the stimulus intensity), then it was possible to integrate the number of jnd steps above threshold and obtain the logarithmic relation:

$$S = k \log I + C \tag{4.1}$$

where S is the sensory magnitude, I is the stimulus intensity, and both k and C are constants.

Fechner claimed that sensory magnitude could not be measured directly, but only indirectly through the summing of jnd steps. Plateau (1872) did not accept Fechner's restriction, and described an unpublished experiment measuring visual magnitude that he carried out in approximately 1840, shortly before he went completely blind and ceased his work in vision. In that experiment, he asked eight artists to paint a gray midway between white and black, and found a close agreement in the reflectance of the mid-grays that were produced. He also observed that the same reflectance corresponded to mid-gray at different levels of illumination, so that at all absolute intensities of the stimuli, equal stimulus ratios produced equal sensation ratios. Plateau then expressed this simple relation in its mathematical form as the power function:

$$S = kI^n \tag{4.2}$$

where, as above, S equals sensory magnitude, I equals stimulus intensity, and both k and n are constants. In this 1872 paper, Plateau also suggested that since it is impossible to measure a single sensation level directly, his power function represented an indirect or relative measure based upon two contrasting levels. He went on to state that it was likely that pairs of contrasting levels of sound could be used to obtain an empirical loudness function.

There were only a few early attempts to measure loudness, probably because of the difficulty in achieving accurate control of relative stimulus intensities. One method used involved the impulsive sound produced by a weight striking a metal plate, with stimulus levels controlled by varying the distance the weight fell. Aside from the primitive nature and untested assumptions of such a procedure compared with the refined methods then available for controlling light sensitivity, there was another difficulty. This manner of controlling sound intensity introduced a physical magnitude associated with loudness magnitude, and it was found that subjects were influenced in their quantitative judgments of relative loudness by mental estimates of the relative distances traveled by the falling weight.

The first study of loudness using steady-state stimuli with precise amplitude control was carried out by Richardson and Ross (1930). Their stimuli were pure tones delivered through headphones. It was reported that loudness was a power function of the stimulus intensity over the entire 80 dB range that they employed, so that the relation between loudness judgments, L, and stimulus intensity, I, was expressed by the equation:

$$L = kI^n \tag{4.3}$$

where k and n are constants. Richardson and Ross stated that different power functions were obtained for each of their eleven subjects.

Following this pioneering work, a number of investigators in the early 1930s reported complex empirical functions for loudness judgments, and S. S. Stevens (1936), apparently unaware of Richardson and Ross's psychophysical power function, constructed his first "sone" scale of loudness intensity based upon these experimental values. This scale was presented in graphical form, and subsequently Stevens and Davis (1938) stated that this relation could be approximated by the equation:

$$L = I(10^{-5/2}I + 1)^{-2/3} \times 10^{-3} \text{ sones} \tag{4.4}$$

Throughout the 1940s and early 1950s many additional loudness measurements were reported, with little agreement of these studies with the original sone scale. The results of these studies were tabulated by S. S. Stevens in 1955. There was great variability in these reports, with the attenuation required for half-loudness ranging from 2.1 dB (62 percent of the standard's intensity) to 24 dB (0.4 percent of the standard's intensity). The distribution of values reported was skewed, probably reflecting the intrinsic asymmetry of the range available for responses: this potential response range for half-loudness was limited by the standard level at the upper end, and the threshold intensity (which could be as much as 80 or 90 dB below the standard) at the lower end. Stevens, faced with this mass of discrepant data, took a bold simplifying step. He was nonevaluative, and accepted all studies, gave each an equal weight, and calculated the median value reported for half-loudness. This value (-10 dB for half-loudness) was assumed to hold at all standard levels and was used for constructing a new sone scale of loudness. This revised sone scale was a power function having an exponent of 0.3. The last recommendation by Stevens (1972) was a minor change from -10 dB to -9 dB for half-loudness resulting in his third and final sone scale expressed by the function:

$$L = kI^{0.33} \tag{4.5}$$

Stevens (1961) considered the sensory organs as transducers converting energy in the environment to neural form, and stated that the input-output relations of these transducers determine the exponent of psychophysical functions.

He maintained this position over the years, and in a book published posthumously (Stevens, 1975), it was restated that the nature of built-in neural responses was responsible for sensory power functions. The numerous attempts that have been made to find neurophysiological responses that correspond to the psychophysical power function have been summarized by Smith (1988) and by Relkin and Ducet (1997). Despite these efforts, there has been no definitive demonstration that such a neurophysical relation exists.

It should be kept in mind that the sone scale is derived from experiments showing that the same fraction is chosen as half-loudness at all stimulus levels. The finding that equal stimulus ratios produce equal subjective ratios presents an unusual problem – an embarrassment of simplicity for the concept that sensory intensity judgments reflect built-in neurophysiological response functions. Even at the level of the auditory nerve, coding of amplitude is quite complex. Candidates proposed for neural signaling of an increase in amplitude are: increased firing rate of fibers, crossing the response threshold for less sensitive fibers, spread of excitation to fibers having characteristic frequencies that differ from the frequencies of the stimulus, and changes in the extent of phase-locking (for reviews of amplitude coding at the periphery, see Javel, 1986; Smith, 1988). How then can judgments emerge having a simple relation to a stimulus dimension? There is no convincing evidence that an isomorphism of neural response characteristics with the psychophysical power function is established either by further processing by the processing stations along the ascending pathways of the brainstem, or by the auditory cortex. Indeed, there is no need for such isomorphism: the central nervous system has the ability to process extremely complex neural input and produce evaluations and responses related simply to environmental events and conditions (indeed, that is a major function of the central nervous system). It is of cardinal importance to keep in mind that sensory input is a representation that need not resemble the environmental events and processes that it signifies any more than the letters forming the word "chair" need resemble the object it represents.

Loudness judgments and their relation to auditory localization: the physical correlate theory

As discussed in Chapter 2, intensity of sound is a major cue used by listeners to estimate the distance of a sound source; under conditions normally encountered, listeners can do this with considerable accuracy. Early in the last century, Gamble (1909) noted that changes in loudness and in distance seemed to be equivalent concepts for listeners hearing sounds at different intensities. She stated that, "judgments of 'nearer' and 'louder' and of 'farther' and 'softer' were practically interchangeable." Warren, Sersen, and Pores (1958) suggested that familiarity with the manner in which sound stimuli change with distance provides the basis for judgments of subjective magnitude, so that half-loudness judgments are equivalent to estimates of the effect of doubling distance from the source. This suggestion was part of a general theory (the "physical correlate theory") which considers judgments of sensory magnitudes to be equivalent to estimates of a physical attribute correlated with changes in stimulus magnitude (Warren, 1958).

Five consequences of the physical correlate theory as applied to loudness judgments are listed below. These quantitative consequences (or predictions) should be capable of being either verified or refuted experimentally.

1. Judgments of half-loudness and estimates of the effect of doubling the distance from the listener to the sound source should be equivalent when made under the same listening conditions by separate groups of subjects.

2. Under conditions designed to facilitate accurate estimates of the manner in which intensity changes with distance (see Chapter 2), twice-distance estimates (and hence half-loudness judgments) should be directly calculable from the inverse square law governing intensity changes with distance.

3. Since the degree of reverberation as well as intensity can change the apparent distance of the source of a sound having rapid dynamic changes such as speech (see Chapter 2), it should be possible to modify loudness judgments of speech in a predictable fashion by manipulation of the extent of reverberation.

4. People can operate not only as sound receivers, but also as sound generators, changing their speaking level in keeping with their distance from a targeted listener. Therefore, when a microphone serving as a target is kept in view, subjects should be able to adjust the amplitude of self-generated sounds so that the level measured at the microphone remains approximately constant when its distance is halved. The same change (approximately −6 dB) should be produced by a separate group seeing the target microphone at a fixed position and instructed to produce a sound first at one level and then at a level that is half as loud.

5. It should be possible to create new loudness functions by providing listeners with experience correlating new physical scales with changes in level of stimulation. Specifically, familiarity with measurement of intensity using sound-level meters should lead to a loudness scale based upon the decibel scale.

As we shall see, each of these anticipated consequences of the physical correlate theory has experimental support. Evidence will also be summarized indicating that familiar physical correlates are also used for judgments of sensory magnitudes for vision.

1.   *Equivalence of half-loudness and twice distance estimates*

In order to test directly the prediction of the physical correlate theory that judgments of half-loudness and twice distance from the source are equivalent, Warren, Sersen, and Pores (1958) asked one group of subjects to estimate half-loudness and a second group of subjects to estimate the effect of doubling their distance from the source. The groups were seated in a conference room, had instructions read to them (to familiarize them with the room acoustics), and were then blindfolded. Both groups heard the sounds delivered through a loudspeaker that was placed in a fixed position after they were blindfolded. The prediction was confirmed – the judgments of the effect of doubling the distance to the source and half-loudness were equivalent. Subsequently, Stevens and Guirao (1962) verified this equivalence. They used headphones rather than loudspeakers, and also reported that subjects chose equivalent attenuations for judgments of half-loudness and estimates of the effect of doubling distance. However, they concluded that their subjects became confused; when instructed to estimate the effect of doubling distance, they estimated half-loudness instead. They did not specify why they thought confusion occurred, but perhaps it was their use of headphones which would cause sounds to be localized within the head (see Chapter 2). But it was for this reason that Warren *et al.* used a loudspeaker to avoid intracranial localization, as well as blindfolds to prevent listeners from viewing the stationary sound source.

2.   *Loudness and the inverse square law*

The sound reaching a listener directly from the source can be isolated from the later-arriving reverberant components, and this "precedence effect" is used for determining the location of the source (see Chapter 2). The intensity of this direct sound follows the inverse square law. Hence, under conditions minimizing errors in estimating the effect of distance upon intensity, one-quarter intensity or −6 dB should correspond to estimates of the effect of doubling distance from the source, and consequently (according to the physical correlate theory) to judgments of half-loudness. However, Stevens' (1972) last recommendation for his sone scale (see equation (4.5)) had −9 dB rather than −6 dB corresponding to half-loudness. Warren (1970a) suggested that known systematic biases were present in most loudness experiments, and that by eliminating those biasing factors it might be possible to design bias-free conditions for testing predictions of the physical correlate theory.

We have seen that when Stevens (1955) proposed his sone power function for loudness, he pooled widely discrepant experimental values for half-loudness from different laboratories which ranged from -2.1 dB to -24 dB. This variability indicates a great sensitivity of loudness estimates to differences in experimental conditions. The range of available comparison levels is known to influence judgments, and a strong bias toward selecting values for half-loudness that lie in the middle of the available response range has been reported by Garner (1954). Also, an immediately prior judgment has a large "transfer" effect upon apparent loudness, and attempts to compensate for this by a balanced experimental design may not succeed because of asymmetrical transfer effects (Poulton and Freeman, 1966). In addition to these general biasing effects, there are a number of other factors associated with particular psychophysical methods capable of influencing loudness judgments (see Warren, 1977a, for a detailed discussion).

"Bias-free" (or, to borrow a term from physical science, "ideal") conditions were employed for testing quantitative predictions of the physical correlate theory. This procedure for obtaining bias-free judgments had been used previously for verifying predictions based upon the physical correlate theory for subjective visual magnitude judgments (see Warren, 1969, for review).

In order to obtain a bias-free value for half-loudness of a particular sound at some fixed level, several groups of subjects were required. Each individual in a group of 30 subjects made only a single judgment involving the fixed standard level and a particular comparison level (thus eliminating any influence of prior judgments and exposure to other levels of the stimulus). Subjects were allowed to switch freely between the standard and comparison stimuli to avoid classical time-order errors. After making their single judgment, they were no longer eligible for any other experiment dealing with subjective magnitudes. The same standard level was used with other groups receiving different comparison levels, permitting the construction of a loudness function for these amplitudes at that standard level. The process was then repeated using other standard levels of the same sound. There was still one major potential bias that could affect some (but not all) portions of the loudness function obtained with a particular standard level – that is, a response-range bias (see Woodworth, 1938; Garner, 1954). This bias can cause judgments above the middle of the range available for responses with a particular standard level to be under-estimated and judgments below the middle of the range to be overestimated relative to theory. Hence, when a standard level is assigned the value of 100, and a series of comparison levels produces a monotonic loudness function extending both above and below the middle of the available range, only the level corresponding to midrange (i.e., mean loudness judgments of 50) can be taken as free from known systematic biases, and hence a critical test of predictions based upon the physical correlate theory.

Although there are unique advantages for the single-judgment procedure in testing predictions of theory, there is a major practical drawback – it is quite inconvenient, requiring a considerable expenditure of time and large numbers of subjects (separate groups of subjects were used for each pairing of a standard level with a particular comparison level). Although the single judgments made by individuals within a group covered a wide range of responses, the use of large groups (at least 30 subjects) permitted replication of means and medians within a few percent. When this procedure was used earlier for a series of studies on visual magnitude judgments involving gray papers and colored papers, some 3,000 subjects were tested one at a time (for a review of these studies and others testing the physical correlate theory when applied to vision, see Warren, 1969). The subsequent series of studies involving single loudness judgments described below took several years and employed some 2,000 subjects, again tested one at a time.

Numerical loudness judgments were obtained for various attenuations of an 85 dB 1,000 Hz tone assigned a loudness of 100 (Warren, 1970a). Results are shown in Figure 4.1. Each data point corresponds to the mean of judgments by separate groups of 30 subjects, and the filled data points represent values that are not significantly different from the loudness of 50 (which is free from a potential asymmetrical response-range bias). It can be seen that the intersection of the monotonic loudness function with the midrange value of 50 occurred at a 6 dB attenuation (corresponding to 1/4 of the standard's intensity), in keeping with the physical correlate theory. Another series of experiments used Gaussian noise rather than tones (Warren, 1973a). Figure 4.1 shows that −6 dB corresponded to half-loudness of an 85 dB noise for presentation either through headphones or through loudspeakers. Loudspeakers were not used with tones because of standing waves associated with the reflection of steady-state tones from surfaces, even in sound-treated audiometric rooms. These standing waves result in differences in intensity at the two ears that change with head movements. Standing waves are not established for the constantly changing waveform of noise, and it can be seen in Figure 4.1 that the attenuation of −6 dB corresponding to theory was found for the midrange value of 50 not only with headphones (intracranial localization), but also with loudspeakers (external localization).

In another experiment measuring the loudness of noise shown in Figure 4.1, subjects listening through headphones were given a line labeled "louder sound" at one end and "silence" at the other. They indicated the loudness of a fainter comparison sound relative to an 85 dB standard by the position of a

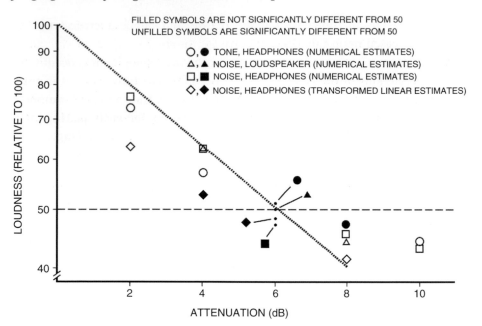

Figure 4.1 A test of loudness predictions of the physical correlate theory. Each data point represents the mean of first judgments of separate groups of 30 subjects. They were presented with an 85 dB standard stimulus consisting of either a 1,000 Hz tone or a broadband noise assigned a loudness value of 100 along with a comparison stimulus at one of the attenuations shown on the abscissa. They were allowed to switch freely between the two levels, made a single relative loudness judgment, and were dismissed. The horizontal dashed line corresponds to the value of 50 free from the classical response-range bias known to deflect judgments toward the mid-range, and the diagonal dotted line corresponds to loudness proportional to the square-root of the standard's intensity. The intersection of these two lines represents the "ideal" or bias-free condition testing the prediction of the theory. It can be seen that each of the four empirical loudness functions shown has a loudness of 50 (half-loudness) at an attenuation of 6 dB (one-quarter intensity) in keeping with theory. For further details and discussion, see the text. The figure first appeared in Warren (1981a) and is based upon data for tones from Warren (1970a) and for noise from Warren (1973a).

mark made upon this line, thus avoiding the use of numbers by the subjects (Warren, 1973a). Responses were scored as percentages of the distance along the line from the silence end to the louder sound end. The results are shown in Figure 4.1. It can be seen that the extent of asymmetrical range biases (as measured by deviations from the dashed diagonal line) differed for direct numerical judgments and those derived from marks on the line. But judgments at midrange values of 50 with both procedures corresponded to about −6 dB in keeping with theory.

Other series of experiments (not shown in the figure) using single loudness judgments found that −6 dB corresponded to half-loudness over the middle or moderate range of standard levels from approximately 45 through 90 dB for both 1,000 Hz pure tones (Warren, 1970a) and for broadband noise (Warren, 1973a). It also was reported that when various frequencies of pure tones were presented at moderate standard levels, −6 dB corresponded to half-loudness from 250 Hz to 8,000 Hz (Warren, 1970a).

3.   *Effects of reverberation on loudness functions*

Chapter 2 noted that reverberation can play a role in estimating the distance of a source from a listener: without changing the overall level, a speaker seems closer to the listener when the proportion of direct sound is increased, and further when the proportion of reverberant sound is increased (Steinberg and Snow, 1934; Békésy, 1938). As described in Chapter 2, when sound tracks were first coming into use in motion pictures, Maxfield (1930, 1931) reported that an illusion of realism required that normal or natural changes in the ratio of direct to reverberant components of a speaker's voice occur with changes in camera position – otherwise the speaker's voice became disconnected from the speaker's image.

Reverberation is an especially salient cue to distance for speech, with its brief silences and rapid transitions from one sound to the next (reverberation is much less obvious for the single continuous sounds of tones and noises usually employed in loudness studies). If loudness is based upon the physical correlate of distance, it follows that simply attenuating the overall level of speech without a concomitant increase in the proportion of reverberant components would cause the sound to seem closer (and hence louder), requiring a greater attenuation for half-loudness judgments. In keeping with this analysis, Pollack (1952) found that speech required a greater attenuation for half-loudness judgments than did steady-state sounds. Warren, Sersen, and Pores (1958) confirmed Pollack's finding that half-loudness judgments with speech required a greater attenuation than did tone. Warren *et al.* tested a second group of subjects under the identical conditions they used for the loudness group, except that subjects were instructed to estimate the effect of doubling distance from the hidden loudspeaker. It was found that estimates of the effect of doubling distance required greater attenuation for speech than for tone, and that the extent of this increase was equivalent to that observed for half-loudness.

In order to confirm that the loudness function for speech is based upon direct sound, but modified by reverberant components, the extent of reverberation was varied in a series of experiments (Warren, 1973b). Rather than

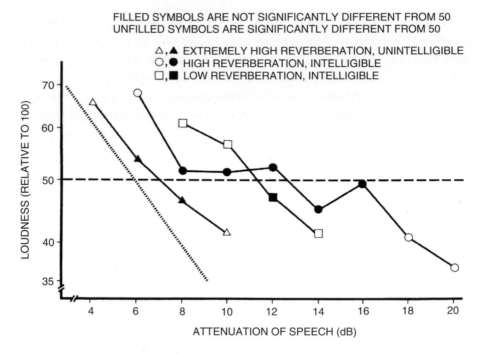

Figure 4.2 Confirmation of the effects of reverberation on loudness functions for speech. Numerical judgments of loudness are shown for the same recorded speech passage heard under three different degrees of reverberation. Each standard was presented at 85 dB and assigned a loudness value of 100. The horizontal dashed line corresponds to the midrange value of 50, and the diagonal dotted line corresponds to loudness proportional to the square root of the stimulus intensity. Each data point represents the mean of first numerical judgments from a separate group of 30 subjects listening through headphones (total of 480 subjects). For further discussion, see the text. The figure first appeared in Warren (1981a), and is based upon data from Warren (1973b).

employing the psychophysical procedures employed in the early studies by Pollack and by Warren *et al.* that involved potential procedural biases, these experiments employed the bias-free single judgment procedure for half-loudness determination described earlier. The stimulus was a recording of a speech passage read for this study by a professional announcer in an acoustically "dead" radio studio (i.e., one with low reverberation time). To ensure that there was little distraction produced by content, the passage had little intrinsic interest. The intensity change required for half-loudness judgments was about −12 dB as shown by the square symbols in Figure 4.2. These results are quite different from those obtained with tone and with noise (see Figure 4.1), in keeping with the earlier reports that greater attenuation was required for half-loudness judgments with speech.

Although the ratio of direct to reverberant sound can influence loudness judgments, the level of reverberant sound produced by multiple reflections does not change in any systematic fashion with the distance from the source in enclosures such as rooms and lecture halls. Hence, reverberant sound heard by itself does not provide distance cues that can be used as the physical correlate of loudness, and judgments of the relative loudness of different intensity levels of a voice lacking appreciable direct components should be indeterminate and cluster about the middle of the available response range. This prediction was tested in the second experiment of the series.

Loudness judgments were obtained for a highly reverberant (but still intelligible) rerecording of the same speech recording used in the previous experiment. The results obtained are summarized by the circular symbols in Figure 4.2. As predicted, the lack of appreciable direct components had a profound effect – loudness judgments did not change with intensity over a wide range of comparison levels. As indicated by the figure, there were no significant differences from the half-loudness value of 50 for attenuations ranging from 8 dB through 16 dB.

In the third and final part of this study, extremely reverberant speech was employed for loudness judgments. This stimulus was prepared through successive re-recordings, each made under highly reverberant conditions. After six such re-recordings, the original single voice could no longer be distinguished – the speech was a completely unintelligible noise, sounding like the babble of voices in a large terminal. As shown by the triangular symbols in Figure 4.2, the loudness function obtained with this stimulus resembled the function for Gaussian noise (see Figure 4.1) more closely than either of the other two loudness functions based upon the same speech passage.

To summarize this work with recorded voices, it appears that loudness is not determined by amplitude alone. Reverberation can play an important role in judging half-loudness of speech, and the manipulation of reverberation produces effects consistent with its role in modifying the apparent distance from the source.

4.   *Loudness of self-generated sound*

While loudness experiments usually employ subjects operating as sound receivers, subjects can also estimate loudness while operating as sound generators. Loudness experiments based on self-generated sound have unique characteristics of especial interest. The experimenter is not faced with troublesome choices concerning the psychophysical methods to be employed for presenting stimuli to the subject, along with problems concerning possible biases associated with each of these procedures. When the subjects serve as sound sources rather than as passive receivers, then all level adjustments are done by the subjects using their self-contained equipment. It is necessary only to instruct them to produce a sound at a steady level and then at a second steady level, say, one-half that of the first. Any sound that can be generated at different levels by the subject and held steady for a few seconds can be used as a stimulus. Most importantly for testing the physical correlate theory, the ratio of direct to reverberant sound does not influence judgments of loudness for self-generated sounds, since this ratio does not change with intensity when the subject estimating loudness is also the source.

The first study of the loudness of self-generated sounds was that of Lane, Catania, and Stevens (1961). They had subjects produce the vowel "ah," and found that "autophonic" judgments of half-subjective magnitude corresponded to a reduction of approximately 6 dB, as would be predicted by the physical correlate theory. However, since this attenuation differed from the value of 9 or 10 dB for half-loudness according to the sone scale, Lane *et al.* reasoned that autophonic judgments could not be based upon loudness, but upon some factor associated with production. They concluded that this factor used to estimate the magnitude of self-generated sound was the magnitude of muscular effort.

In order to test whether the 6 dB reduction for half-autophonic level was based upon muscular effort or upon loudness, Warren (1962) obtained autophonic magnitude judgments using three different types of self-generated sounds: the voiced speech sound "ah" used by Lane *et al.*, the unvoiced fricative consonant "sh," and a note produced by blowing air through a reed pitchpipe. Subjects were required to produce a sound at a steady "moderate level" of their choosing, and then another at a level they considered to be one-half. Production of each of these three sounds was governed by different physical principles and involved different muscular efforts. Hence, it may be concluded that an agreement in the attenuation corresponding to half-level for each of the sounds would indicate that autophonic judgments were based upon sound that was produced (and hence loudness) rather than muscular effort. It was found that equivalent attenuations (approximately 7 dB) were required for half-level judgments for the three types of sounds – a value close to the 6 dB attenuation reported by Lane *et al.* for half-autophonic level with "ah."

Speakers normally adjust the level of sounds they produce to compensate for the distance separating them from a target listener. In order to determine whether judgments of half-loudness of self-generated sound are equivalent to estimates of the attenuation needed to compensate for the effect of halving the distance to a target, the same three sounds ("ah," "sh," and a pitch-pipe note) used for the judgments of autophonic level were employed with a separate group of subjects (Warren, 1968a). Each of the participants was seated in front of a long table with a microphone in view at a distance of ten feet. They were told to adjust the level they produced for each of these sounds so that the intensity reaching the microphone did not change when its distance was moved by the experimenter from ten to five feet (these distances were marked off by a tape measure lying in view on the table). The relative levels of the sounds as generated were determined using a second microphone in a fixed position that was out of the subject's view. It was found that the attenuations in sound productions chosen to compensate for this two-fold change in target distance for the three sounds ranged from 6 to 8 dB, in agreement both with the actual manner in which the sound reaching the target microphone directly varied with its distance, and with the half-autophonic judgments reported earlier (Warren, 1962) for subjects generating the same three sounds.

5.   *A new physical correlate can result in a new loudness scale*

When subjects participate in loudness experiments, they probably are making judgments of a sort they have never made before. The previous sections have described evidence indicating that quantitative loudness judgments are based upon the physical correlate of distance. Reports from several laboratories have indicated that when subjects are familiar with another physical scale associated with the level of stimulation, they can use this scale as the basis for their quantitative loudness estimates. Thus, subjects familiar with the decibel scale used it as their physical correlate for subjective magnitude judgments. Ham and Parkinson (1932) observed that familiarity with decibel measurements resulted in loudness functions based on this logarithmic scale of sound level. The experimenters were forced to abandon the use of subjects having experience with sound measurement and switch instead to college students without such experience for their formal experiments. Laird, Taylor, and Wille (1932) encountered the same problem. They reported that subjects who were familiar with calibration of audiometers would choose approximately one-half the decibel level when asked to judge half-loudness, so that 30 dB was selected as half-loudness of a 60 dB standard (a thousand-fold reduction in intensity). They stated that it was not possible for their subjects to ignore their experience with decibel levels.

Finally, Rowley and Studebaker (1969) used graduate students in audiology as their subjects, and despite repeated attempts by the experimenters to explain that they were interested in the subjective magnitude of loudness and not estimates of the physical level in decibels, their subjects could not abandon their use of the decibel scale as the physical correlate for their loudness judgments.

A similar observation was reported for half-brightness judgments made while viewing large contiguous standard and comparison fields with eyes adapted to the ambient illumination (Warren and Warren, 1958). Half-brightness judgments by college students approximated 25 percent of the standard's intensity (a reduction of 6 dB), in keeping with distance as the physical correlate, for intensities ranging from 8.6×10^{-4} to 87 millilamberts (spanning the range from dim scotopic vision mediated by retinal rods to bright photopic vision mediated by retinal cones). However, an individual who had considerable experience using photometers (that use a linear rather than the logarithmic decibel scale) chose 50 percent intensity for half-brightness judgments at all standard levels, even though he was told repeatedly that he should judge relative subjective brightness, not relative luminance.

Thus, it appears that distance is used as the physical correlate for both loudness and brightness in the absence of familiarity with a physical scale that measures stimulus magnitudes directly – once such a scale becomes familiar, it supplants distance as the basis for subjective magnitude judgments.

The mel scale of pitch magnitude

Tones have been characterized not only by the psychological magnitude of loudness, but also by the psychological magnitude of pitch. Stevens, Volkmann, and Newman (1937) constructed the mel scale for quantifying the pitch of sinusoidal tones based upon estimates of half-pitch for frequencies of standards ranging from 125 through 12,000 Hz. Their results are shown by the triangular symbols in Figure 4.3. For the middle of the range, values of roughly half-frequency were generally selected as half-pitch. Wever (1949) noted this tendency to choose half-frequency as half-pitch; and stated that, for frequencies ranging from 1.25 Hz to 5,000 Hz, half-pitch judgments could be explained as the direct appreciation of frequency differences, so that two intervals of pitch that seemed equal contained the same number of hertz. However, Wever did not suggest why this simple relation was found by Stevens, Volkmann, and Newman (1937).

In an article, entitled "A replication of the mel scale of pitch" Siegel (1965) published additional data on half-pitch judgments. He employed sinusoidal tones as did Stevens et al. (1937), and a somewhat broader range of standard frequencies extending from 92 Hz to 9,200 Hz. It can be seen in Figure 4.3 that his results for half-pitch (shown by circular symbols) are even closer to half-frequency than those of Stevens et al. Excluding judgments at the ends of the frequency range (standard frequencies of 92 Hz and 9,200 Hz), the half-pitch judgments averaged 48.9 percent; when judgments at the extremes of the

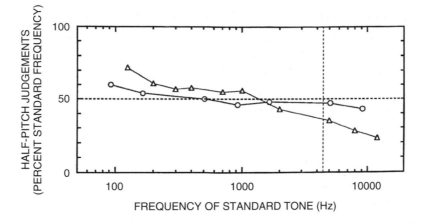

Figure 4.3 Percent of the standard's frequency selected as half-pitch. The horizontal broken line at 50 percent corresponds to the physical correlate of subjective magnitude judgments one octave below the standard. The broken vertical line at 4,500 Hz corresponds to the highest note produced by an orchestral instrument. The triangles represent data reported by Stevens, Volkmann, and Newman (1937), and the circles represent data reported by Siegel (1965).

range are included, the average for all seven standard frequencies is 49.7 percent. Curiously, Siegel made no mention of the fact that these half-pitch judgments corresponded to half-frequency, but restricted his discussion to the relation of his values to those of the mel scale.

A basis for half-frequency, or the octave, serving as the physical correlate for half-pitch judgments and the derived mel scale is furnished by Helmholtz's statement that the " ... musical scale is as it were the divided rod, by which we measure progressions in pitch, as rhythm measures progression in time." Helmholtz pointed out that the basic unit of musical scales is the octave, and that this interval is used in the music of virtually all cultures. For tones, the octave is the only interval that is completely consonant – the harmonics of a higher octave are also harmonics of a lower one, so that they blend perfectly with no discordant beats. Figure 4.3 shows that deviation from the approximately one octave decrease in frequency for half-pitch occurs at the limits of the mel scale. This deviation appears to be linked to experience with musical intervals.

The vertical dotted line in Figure 4.3 shows the upper limit of the musical scale at roughly 4,500 Hz. The ability to recognize the octave and other musical intervals is generally limited to notes lying within the range of notes used by orchestral instruments. Bachem (1948) used subjects with absolute pitch (the ability to identify a note heard alone without the help of a reference note) and found that they could not identify notes above the orchestral limit. He stated that these subjects reported that the concept of musical pitch seemed to be without meaning at these high frequencies. In another experiment, Ward (1954) used musicians, each of whom played at least two instruments, and had them estimate the octaves of pure tones. While this task was done with accuracy within the musical range by all, when the frequency was raised above the highest note of a piccolo, only two of the nine subjects could estimate octaves. Ward found out that these two had experience with oscillators generating pure tones, and he determined that they could estimate octaves accurately up to the limit of audible frequencies. Without such special training, the octave could not be used as the basis for half-pitch judgments above the musical range. As for the deviation from the octave relation for half-pitch judgments of the lowest standard frequencies used for construction of the mel scale, one octave below this value is close to the limit of 41 Hz for orchestral instruments (see Chapter 3).

In their article proposing the mel scale, Stevens, Volkmann, and Newman (1937) reported an interesting observation concerning the responses of a trained musician who served as one of their subjects and who gave half-pitch judgments differing from those of the rest of the group. The musician stated that it was very difficult for him to avoid using the octave or some other familiar musical interval in judging half-pitch, and he consciously tried to avoid such settings. However, the other subjects did not try to avoid the octave, and appeared to base their judgments on this interval for frequencies within the musical pitch range.

Greenwood (1997) criticized the mel scale on methodological as well as other grounds, and reported a previously unpublished experiment that he and M. Israel carried out in 1956 in S. S. Stevens' laboratory. Greenwood stated that when their subjects were asked to equisect the difference in pitch between two sinusoidal tones, the resulting pair of subjectively equal pitch intervals corresponded to physically equal pitch ratios.

Some conclusions and inferences

If it is accepted that quantitative estimates of sensory magnitudes are based upon learned associations with some quantifiable physical scale, can it still be maintained that the sone scale of loudness and the mel scale of pitch measure sensory magnitudes? The answer must be yes, if we also accept the operational definitions employed by S. S. Stevens – that is, the scales are defined by listeners' responses concerning loudness and pitch obtained under particular specified conditions. However, defining the scales operationally leaves unanswered questions concerning the bases employed for listeners' responses. The hope expressed by Stevens, and by others engaged in the measurement of sensation, has been that a neurophysiological correlate would be found that could explain the simple rule that equal stimulus ratios produce equal subjective ratios (and the psychophysical power function derived from this rule), as well as the attenuation required for judgments of half sensory-magnitude used for determining the exponent of the power function. This hoped for correspondence has not been found. The alternative physical cor-relate theory considers that judgments of sensory magnitudes are based upon estimates of associated physical magnitudes, and offers an explanation for the empirical psychophysical power function, as well as predicting the exponent of the power function under familiar conditions that permit accurate estimates of the magnitude of the physical correlate. This chapter has discussed evidence concerning this theory as applied to loudness and pitch.

This physical correlate theory is a corollary of the broader principle that there is an obligatory interpretation of sensory input in terms of the conditions and events associated with stimulation. Examples of this principle occur throughout this book.

Suggestions for further reading

Stevens, S.S. 1955. The measurement of loudness. *Journal of the Acoustical Society of America*, **27**, 815–829.

A posthumous publication summarizing his experiments and theories:
    Stevens, S.S. 1975. *Psychophysics: Introduction to its Perceptual, Neural, and Social Prospects*. G. Stevens (ed.). New York: Wiley.

A detailed summary of my experiments on loudness of tones, noise,
    and speech: Warren, R.M. 1977a. Subjective loudness and its physical
    correlate. *Acustica*, **37**, 334–346.

A review of experiments dealing with quantitative judgments involving the
    other distance sense: Warren, R.M. 1969. Visual intensity judgments: An
    empirical rule and a theory. *Psychological Review*, **76**, 16–30.

An evaluative review of the history of measurement of subjective magnitudes
    including brightness, loudness, pitch, taste, and heaviness: Warren, R.M.
    1981a. Measurement of sensory intensity. *Behavioral and Brain Sciences*, **4**,
    175–189; open peer commentary, 189–213; author's response and
    references, 213–223.

5

Perception of acoustic sequences

The comprehension of speech and the appreciation of music require listeners to distinguish between different arrangements of component sounds. It is often assumed that the temporal resolution of successive items is required for these tasks, and that a blurring and perceptual inability to distinguish between permuted orders takes place if sounds follow each other too rapidly. However, there is evidence indicating that this common-sense assumption is false. When components follow each other at rates that are too rapid to permit the identification of order or even the sounds themselves, changes in their arrangement can be recognized readily. This chapter examines the rules governing the perception of sequences and other stimulus patterns, and how they apply to the special continua of speech and music.

Rate at which component sounds occur in speech and music

Speech is often considered to consist of a sequence of acoustic units called phones, which correspond to linguistic units called phonemes (the nature of phonemes will be discussed in some detail in Chapter 7). Phonemes occur at rates averaging more than 10 per second, with the order of these components defining syllables and words. Conversational English contains on average about 135 words per minute, and since the average word has about 5 phonemes, this corresponds to an average duration of about 90 ms per phoneme (Efron, 1963). It should be kept in mind that individual phonemes vary greatly in duration, and that the boundaries separating temporally contiguous phonemes are often not sharply defined. Oral reading is more rapid than spontaneous speech, and this higher rate of about 170 words per minute corresponds to about 70 ms per phoneme. Joos (1948) stated that at average phoneme durations of about 50 ms, intelligibility of speech starts to decline. However, devices have been used that accelerate recorded speech without introducing the pitch change that would result from simply increasing the playback speed. Foulke and Sticht (1969) have summarized evidence that some comprehension of this "compressed speech" is still possible at rates exceeding 400 words per minute, or an average of about 30 ms per phoneme.

Notes forming melodies usually occur at rates approximating those of syllables in speech rather than those of phonemes. Fraisse (1963) has stated that although the rate at which notes of a melodic theme are played varies considerably depending upon the composer and the piece (and presumably the performer as well), the fastest rate within the normal range corresponds to about 150 ms per note. While notes can and do occur at faster rates, they then appear to function as ornaments or embellishments which, while recognizable, do not contribute to either the melody or the harmony. Some composers employ rates of less than 50 ms per note, and this rapid rate produces an effect that has been described as a "flickering or rustling" (Winckel, 1967).

Since temporal ordering of individual sounds is considered to play a basic role in speech and music, a considerable interest has been shown in determining the thresholds for identification of order in acoustic sequences.

Identification of components and their order

Hirsh (1959) stated that it is necessary to identify phonemes and their orders before words can be recognized. In order to investigate the minimum separation necessary for identification of order, he used pairs of sounds selected from a variety of hisses, tones, and clicks. It was found that differences in onsets of about 20 ms allowed 75 percent correct responses of order with practiced subjects (termination of the two sounds occurred simultaneously). Hirsh cited the word pair "mitts" and "mist" as an example of word discrimination based upon temporal order identification. Since a hiss resembles the fricative sound /s/, and a click the brief sound bursts of the plosive /t/, he suggested that the ability to distinguish whether a click comes before or after a hiss in his temporal resolution experiments was an "experimental analog" of the "mitts"/"mist" distinction.

Following Hirsh's experiment, Broadbent and Ladefoged (1959) used pairs of sounds selected from hiss, buzz, and pip (tone). They found that initially, individuals could not name the order of successive sounds each lasting 150 ms, but after some experience with the task, the order could be named accurately at 30 ms durations (approximating the value reported earlier by Hirsh for practiced observers). Broadbent and Ladefoged commented that temporal ordering seemed to be made on the basis of "quality" rather than " ... a difference of a type normally described as a difference in perceived order." (We shall return to their prescient comment concerning sound quality when we describe the distinction between pattern recognition and the naming of order.)

Hirsh and Sherrick (1961) continued the investigation of thresholds for order identification using bings (pulses sent through a circuit resonant at 666 Hz) and bongs (like bings, but the circuit was resonant at 278 Hz). These sounds were described as resembling xylophone notes of high and low pitch, respectively. In one experiment, they found that when the bings and bongs were delivered sequentially to the same ear (conditions similar to the earlier studies of Hirsh and of Ladefoged and Broadbent), discrimination of order by trained subjects was possible down to a temporal separation of about 20 ms. Hirsh and Sherrick also reported that the thresholds for perception of order for pairs consisting of successive stimuli were approximately the same whether the two events were light flashes in different parts of the visual field, two vibrations (one to each hand), or two different types of stimuli delivered to separate sensory modalities. They concluded that the value of 20 ms is a fundamental limit for perception of order, which is independent of the modality employed.

Values close to those reported by Hirsh for temporal resolution of pairs of nonspeech sounds have been reported by other laboratories. Both Kinney (1961) and Fay (1966) found that resolution was possible at about 30 ms separation. Fay commented that, since both Kinney's and his experiments employed "untrained" subjects, practice could well result in improvement to the 20 ms value of Hirsh (1959). Fay also used pairs of recorded sustained speech sounds, and found that his unpracticed subjects could identify the order for some phoneme pairs with excellent resolution (e.g., 10 ms for /v/ and /l/), while other phoneme pairs were even more difficult to resolve than pairs of tones (e.g., /m/ and /n/ could not be ordered at onset disparities of 70 ms).

However, considerable caution should be used in extending observations made with two-item sequences to the identification of order in extended sequences – the initial and terminal sounds of sequences, whether consisting of two items or many items, are identified with especial ease (Warren, 1972, 1974a; Warren and Sherman, 1974). In order to study the ability to identify the order of items in sequences consisting of several items without the special salience of the first and last items, the procedure of recycling or looping of sequences of several different sounds was introduced by Warren (1968b) and

Warren, Obusek, Farmer, and Warren (1969). Continuing repetition of the sounds in the same order permits a limited number of sounds (usually three or four) to be used to produce relatively simple patterns of indefinite duration. As with nonrepeating sequences, the first and last sounds heard can be identified with especial ease, but this does not help in determining their location relative to the other items when the sequence is repeated without pauses. Recycling sequences of two sounds represent a simple alternation with only one possible arrangement, sequences of three sounds have two possible arrangements, and four sounds have six possible arrangements (a repeating sequence of n sounds has factorial $[n - 1]$ arrangements).

Identification of the order of components for extended sequences of unrelated sounds and for steady-state phonemes

The first studies to use recycling sequences reported a quite surprising inability of listeners to identify the order of components (Warren, 1968b; Warren, Obusek, Farmer, and Warren, 1969; Warren and Warren, 1970). For example, in one experiment listeners heard a sequence of four sounds consisting of successive steady statements of a hiss, a tone, a buzz, and the speech sound "ee." Each item lasted 200 ms, and the sounds were played over and over in the same order. It was found that the listeners could not name the temporal arrangement even though the duration was well above the classical limit for detection of order. In another experiment, a recycling sequence was employed consisting of four isochronous digits (one, three, eight, two, one, three, ...), with each complete statement of the four numbers taking 800 ms. In order to avoid any transitional cues to order, each digit was recorded separately. Despite the fact that each of the words was itself complex, so that presumably phonemic orders had to be established within each digit, correct identification was accomplished with ease by all listeners. When the four items consisted of single speech sounds (four 200 ms steady-state vowels) rather than the multiphonemic digits, the task was more difficult, but performance was still significantly above chance. The task became considerably easier when each of these steady-state vowels was reduced to 150 ms with 50 ms of silence separating items; and it was easiest of all when the vowels also possessed the onset and decay characteristics of natural productions. (Again, each vowel lasted about 150 ms with 50 ms silences without transitional cues linking successive phonemes.) Subsequent work by Thomas, Hill, Carroll, and Garcia (1970) and by Thomas, Cetti, and Chase (1971) indicated that the threshold for naming order within a recycling sequence of four concatenated steady-state vowels was 125 ms, with the threshold dropping to 100 ms when brief silent intervals were inserted between the steady-state vowels. Cole and

Scott (1973) and Dorman, Cutting, and Raphael (1975) found that introduction of normal articulatory transitions linking successive items facilitated identification of order with recycling phonemic sequences. And finally, Cullinan, Erdos, Schaefer, and Tekieli (1977) used recycling sequences containing items consisting of either four vowels or of four two-item consonant-vowel syllables. They reported lower thresholds for the syllables, despite the fact that each item consisted of two phonemes rather than one. They attributed the lower threshold for the syllables to their closer resemblance to the phonetic sequences occurring in normal speech. However, none of their stimuli yielded thresholds below the limit of 100 ms per item that had been reported earlier for sequences of vowels.

Identification of order within tonal sequences

Successive tones of different frequencies form sequences having special interest for two reasons: (1) it is possible to control the extent of frequency differences between sounds so that the items can be made nearly identical or very different; (2) tonal sequences are related to melodic perception and music.

It has been known for some time that perceptual splitting of a pair of interleaved melodies can occur when each is played in a different frequency range. Two separate melodies can be heard under these conditions as a result of the domination of pitch contiguity over temporal contiguity (Ortmann, 1926). Interleaving of melodic lines has been used by Baroque composers, such as Bach and Telemann, so that a single instrument can seem to produce two simultaneous melodies. This melodic segregation has been called "implied polyphony" by Bukofzer (1947) and "compound melodic line" by Piston (1947), each of whom gave examples of its use in Baroque compositions. Dowling (1973) has named this separation "melodic fission." A demonstration of the separation of simultaneous melodies was given at a meeting in Teddington, England, by Warren (1968b) who played a piano recording by Professor Gregoria Suchy playing "God Save the Queen" and "America the Beautiful" with the notes from each melody alternated. Neither of the interleaved melodies could be recognized when both were played in the same frequency range, even with instructions to try to link together alternate notes. But when the notes of each melody were played in separate octaves, it was easy to recognize each. It was suggested by Warren (1968b) that the interleaved melodies, as well as voices occurring at the same time, form "parallel auditory continua" that remain perceptually separated without the possibility of temporal cross-linking. This concept was applied to nonmelodic tonal sequences by Bregman and Campbell (1971). They used recycling sequences consisting of six brief tones, interleaving the three in a cluster of high frequencies with the three in a cluster of low frequencies. As with the alternating notes of melodies, they found that it was easier to identify the order of tones within the same frequency range than across frequency ranges, and called the process "primary auditory stream segregation," which was subsequently shortened to "streaming" (see Bregman, 1990).

Limits of stream segregation as an explanatory principle

Before dealing further with the important problem of perception of sequences of sounds which are all within the same continuum or stream (as in tones or speech), let us return to the difficulty reported by our laboratory for identifying the order within recycling sequences of unrelated sounds that are not in the same stream, such as 200 ms items consisting of hisses, tones, and buzzes. Bregman and Campbell (1971) and Bregman (1990) considered that each of the items in these recycling sequences of four sounds formed a separate auditory stream with its own repetition, resulting in an inability to distinguish between permuted orders. However, experiments have shown that this is not the case: as we shall see, listeners can distinguish between these different arrangements not only at 200 ms per item, but down to 5 or 10 ms per item. Although it may not be possible to identify the orders of items in such sequences, different arrangements of the same items are not perceptually equivalent, but form readily distinguishable patterns. It is only the naming of the order of components that requires long item durations, and there is evidence indicating that the rate-determining stage in identification of order is the time required for providing verbal labels for each of the sounds.

Identification of order and verbal labeling

Of course, it is easy to name the order of sounds within a recycled sequence if the durations of items are sufficiently long. For example, if a repeating sequence consisting of hisses, tones, and buzzes is heard with each sound lasting 1 s, virtually everyone can call out the correct order. This achievement hardly seems surprising since listeners have ample time to name each sound before it terminates. However, when separate groups of 30 listeners were presented with isochronous sequences of four unrelated sounds repeated without pauses and allowed to listen for as long as they wished before calling out the order, the threshold for order identification was surprisingly high: item durations had to be between 450 and 670 ms before the proportion of correct responses was significantly above chance level. This threshold for identifying order fell to between 200 and 300 ms when different groups of subjects responded by arranging the order of cards, each bearing the name of one of the four items (Warren and Obusek, 1972). Card-ordering permitted listeners to break the task into parts by arranging the cards to record a series of pairwise decisions involving contiguous items. The task of identifying order was somewhat easier when the number of items was reduced to three (for which there are only two possible arrangements). With three-item sequences, subjects can choose one of the sounds as an anchor, and make a single decision concerning which of the remaining two components follows this sound. The problem is then completely solved; the remaining sound must precede the anchor. Using this procedure with an unlimited time for responding and name-cards to facilitate the task, the threshold was found to be about 200 ms per item with untrained subjects (Warren and Ackroff, 1976a).

Why does the lower limit for identification of order for unrelated sounds occur at approximately 200 ms per item or about five items per second? A possible answer is indicated by an observation by Helmholtz (1954/1887). Helmholtz was listening to pairs of sinusoidal tones mistuned from unison, and trying to determine the time required to count a fixed number of beats (the number of beats per second is a measure of the frequency difference). Counting beats, even subvocally, involves attaching a verbal label (a number) to each sound as it occurs, and Helmholtz reported that at rates above five per second, "they are too rapid for accuracy." Garner (1951), apparently unaware of Helmholtz's finding, reported the same limit for counting identical events (in this case, tone bursts) presented in long sequences.

It was suggested by Warren (1974a) that it is the time required for verbal labeling of an ongoing stimulus that sets the limiting rate of item presentation, not only for counting successive items, but for the naming of order within sequences of sounds. Successful performances for both of these tasks was considered to require that the verbal encoding of one item be completed before the onset of the next.

Single statements of short sequences may not require labeling of each item as it occurs. It was reported by Garner (1951) that low numbers of identical tone-bursts (up to about four to six) could be counted at twice the presentation rate required for higher numbers of tone-bursts; and Warren (1972) reported that when 3 s of silence separated repetitions of sequences containing three or four unrelated 200 ms sounds, the order of items could be named during the silent interval. Apparently, a read-out from short-term storage occurred between repetitions – a task that was facilitated by the special ease of identifying initial and terminal sounds in sequences (Warren, 1972).

Naming the order of items in recycling sequences consisting of vowels and of monosyllabic words (such as one-syllable digits) is especially interesting. Rapid verbal encoding would be anticipated since not only are the listeners very familiar with these sounds but, perhaps more importantly, the sound is the name: that is, the names of the sounds, and the sounds of the names, are the same. As noted earlier, recycling sequences consisting of four vowels can be ordered, under optimal conditions, at a presentation rate of about 100 ms per item, and when each of four items in an iterated sequence consisted of a word (a digit), naming of order was at least as easy as with four recycled vowels, even though the average duration of phonemes in the digits was well below 100 ms.

Teranishi (1977) measured the minimum item durations permitting the identification of order within various four-item recycling sequences consisting either of nonrelated sounds or of Japanese vowels. He independently arrived at the same explanation proposed by Warren (1974a): that is, the time required for naming component sounds is the rate-determining step in the identification of order, and that the order of sequences of vowels can be identified at high presentation rates because the sounds themselves are their verbal labels.

If verbal encoding time sets the limit for naming of order within auditory sequences, we would expect similar limits set by verbal encoding time for visual sequences. Terence O'Brien and Anne Treisman in 1970 determined the threshold for discrimination of order for three visual items, such as successive geometrical figures or successive colors, when recycled in a three-channel tachistoscope (personal communication). They found the same threshold that has been reported for recycled three-item auditory sequences of nonrelated sounds – that is, 200 ms per item (see also Holcombe, Kanwisher, and Treisman, 2001). Sperling and Reeves (1980) presented a rapid string of digits on a screen and reported that although their subjects could perceive the digits, they could not tell their order. They stated that this difficulty was "analogous" to that reported by Warren for sequences of sounds.

Need for verbal labeling for serial order retention in memory experiments

There have been several studies in the field of memory dealing with verbal encoding and the accuracy of recalling the serial order of sequential items. Paivio and Csapo (1969) presented sequences consisting of printed words or pictures of familiar objects. When the presentation rate was too rapid to permit naming of pictured items (but not the printed words), the pictures could be recalled as accurately as the words, but only the word sequences permitted retention of order information. When the presentation rate was slowed so that the objects in the pictures could be named, tasks requiring temporal ordering of the pictures could be handled readily. Del Castillo and Gumenik (1972) used drawings of objects and found that the "nameability" of depicted objects and the presentation rate both influenced recall of order in a manner consistent with the hypothesis that accurate ordering by subjects requires that the items be named at the time of presentation. Similar observations were made by Philipchalk and Rowe (1971) who compared recall of order for sequences consisting of familiar sounds with recall of order for sequences consisting of words, and found that performance was poorer for the sequences of nonverbal sounds. Finally, Rowe and Cake (1977) used a variety of presentation rates and compared ordered recall for sequences of sounds, and sequences of the verbal labels for these same sounds. They found that, for their seven-item sequences, performance was poorer for the sounds than for the words at interstimulus intervals of 500 ms, with this difference disappearing at interstimulus intervals of 1 s. They extended their study to serial probe, probe recognition, and running memory span, and found the words superior to the sounds in the recency component of the serial position curve in all cases. They concluded that their results supported the theory that verbal encoding facili-tates ordering and conflicted with explanations based on higher-order pro-cessing strategies or retrieval problems. These results are consistent with Paivio's (1971) two-process theory of memory (which emphasizes differences between verbal and nonverbal encoding of information), as well as with the hypothesis that the rate-limiting process for identification of order with extended sequences of sounds involves the verbal encoding time for individual components.

Identification of patterns without discrimination of order: global pattern recognition

In the 1970s, evidence became available indicating that it was possible to discriminate between permuted orders of two brief sounds well below the limit of 20 ms cited by Hirsh (1959) for the naming of order. Patterson and Green (1970) used pairs of brief click-like sounds called Huffman sequences which have identical power spectra but different phase spectra, so that the only difference between members of a pair is in the temporal domain. They reported that Huffman sequences permitted discrimination between temporal arrangements down to 2.5 ms. Yund and Efron (1974) found that listeners could discriminate between permuted orders of a two-item sequence (such as two tones of different frequencies) down to temporal separations of only 1 or 2 ms. Efron (1973) emphasized that such "micropatterns" were not perceived as a succession of discrete items, but rather as unitary perceptual events, with different qualities associated with the different orders.

The ability to discriminate between permuted arrangements of sounds at durations well below the limit permitting unaided identification of order has also been reported for recycling sequences. Wilcox, Neisser, and Roberts (1972) first reported that trained listeners could tell whether pairs of recycling sequences consisting of the same four sounds had identical or permuted arrangements at durations below the threshold for order identification. Subsequently, Warren (1974b) reported similar results for untrained listeners.

Using simple stimuli (recycling and nonrecycling sequences consisting of three different types of sound), Warren (1974a) found that following training, not only could subjects discriminate readily between permuted orders down to 5 ms per item, but also that it was easy to teach them the names and order of components within these sequences. Further, as we shall see, incidental learning of the arrangements of brief items can occur when subjects have had practice with the same sequences at longer item durations.

In one experiment within this study, subjects heard pairs of recycling three-item sequences (2,500 Hz sine-wave, 1,000 Hz square-wave, white noise) with members of each pair consisting of the same items that were arranged either in identical or permuted order. After little training, subjects were able to achieve nearly perfect discrimination performance at all item durations (5 through 400 ms). Whereas subjects were able to name order without training at the longest item duration, at the shorter durations (30 ms per item and below), without training listeners could not even identify the component sounds, much less distinguish their order. When asked how they discriminated between the permuted orders of the briefest sounds, none of the listeners mentioned a resolution into component items, and all answers referred to some overall quality, such as "One sounds more like a cricket." Another experiment in this study used nonrecycling (one-shot) two-item and four-item sequences, and attempted to teach listeners to name the order of permuted arrangements at brief item durations with both types of sequences. Following training, the items and their orders could be named accurately at durations down to 10 ms per item. Of course, the naming of order was not a direct identification of components and their orders, but a rote response of a taught verbal label – an incorrect identification of order could have been learned just as easily. However, it is possible for listeners to learn the order of very brief items without receiving instruction.

Inadvertent learning of the arrangement of items can occur in experiments designed to measure thresholds for order identification. This rote description of items in their proper order can occur when listeners, who have heard sequences having long durations for which unaided naming of order is possible, are then presented with sequences of the same items with shorter durations. When isochronous sequences differ slightly in the duration of their components (up to item duration ratios of 2:1) they may be recognized as having the same or different arrangements, so that the verbal description of the components and their order within the longer sequence may be transferred to the shorter. Through a series of successive transfers to even briefer items, a level can be reached which is well below the threshold possible without prior experience. Using this procedure for threshold training, it was found possible to obtain correct identification of order in recycling three-item sequences down to 10 ms per item without communicating information concerning order to the subjects in any direct fashion (Warren, 1974a).

Extent of temporal mismatch permitting global pattern recognition

An experiment was undertaken to determine the extent of mismatch of item durations required to prevent recognition of identical orders within recycled four-item sequences of the same sounds (Warren, 1974b). In order to avoid inadvertent learning of order-equivalence at different item durations, groups of college students were used having no prior experience with experiments dealing with sequences. Subjects were presented with one recycling sequence consisting of tone, noise, extended vowel "ee," and buzz, and a second sequence consisting of either the identical order of the same items or the same items with the order of noise and buzz interchanged. The first sequence (A) always had item durations of 200 ms, and the second sequence (B) had item durations ranging from 127 through 600 ms, as shown in Figure 5.1. Separate groups of 30 subjects were used for each of the eight durations of the second sequence, and each subject made only two judgments: one same-or-different order judgment involving identical arrangement of components, and one same-or-different order judgment involving permuted arrangement of components (total of 60 judgments obtained for each duration of the second stimulus). Figure 5.1 shows that the accuracy of judgments was highest at 200 and 215 ms item durations of the second sequence, and that accuracy decreased monotonically below 200 ms and above 215 ms item durations. The decrease in accuracy at longer item durations is of interest, since direct naming of order became possible at the longest item durations. However, since one of the sequences always had items lasting 200 ms, order could not be identified for this sequence, so that knowledge of the order of the other would be of no help in deciding whether the sequences had same or different arrangements. It was concluded that judgments involved a "temporal template" with the maximum extent of permissible duration mismatch shown in the figure.

Sorkin (1987) reported results consistent with the concept of temporal-template matching in sequence recognition. His listeners attempted to determine whether two sequences consisting of high and low tone bursts separated by intertone gaps had the same or different orders of successive frequencies. The temporal envelopes of the sequences were changed by varying the

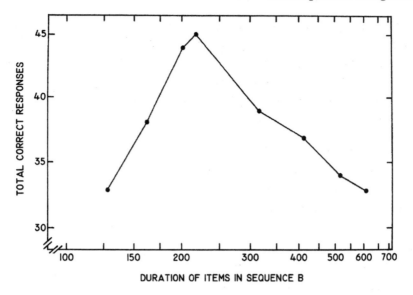

Figure 5.1 Global pattern recognition of sequences with temporal mismatch of item durations. Scores for correct same-or-different judgments are shown for pairs of recycling sequences consisting of the same four sounds arranged in either identical or permuted orders. Sequence A of the pair always had component sounds lasting 200 ms, and the duration of items in sequence B is given by the abscissa. The maximum score for correct responses is 60. Each of the eight data points is based on the mean of the responses made by a separate group of 30 subjects who each made two judgments. (From Warren, 1974b.)

inter-burst intervals and durations of the tones. Two conditions were employed. In the correlated condition, the temporal envelopes varied across trials, but within trials, pairs of sequences used for judgments of identity or difference always had the same temporal envelope. In the uncorrelated condition, temporal envelopes varied both within and across trials. In keeping with observations for same/different judgments described above for sequences with matched and unmatched tone durations (see Figure 5.1), it was found that the use of correlated temporal patterns within trials greatly enhanced the ability of listeners to determine whether or not the same frequency patterns were presented. The quantitative data obtained by Sorkin were used by him to extend a mathematical model for auditory discrimination originally proposed by Durlach and Braida (1969).

The extent of stimulus complexity can have a profound effect upon the training required for detection of differences between extended complex sequences. Watson and his colleagues (Watson, Wroton, Kelly and Benbassat, 1975; Watson, Kelly, and Wroton, 1976; Watson, 1987) have studied the effects of training upon the discrimination of nonrecycling "one-shot" tonal sequences designed to have both temporal complexity and frequency range comparable to those occurring in spoken words. In a typical experiment, "word-length" sequences consisting of ten 40 ms tones were used, and the effects of training were measured for tasks involving detectability of changes in frequency, intensity, or duration of one component within the sequence. Usually, many hours of training were required to reach asymptotic perform-ance with these complex word-length sequences.

Should practiced or unpracticed subjects be used in sequence experiments?

The question of whether to use trained or untrained subjects in perceptual experiments is an important one since it can have profound effects upon the results obtained. Trained subjects can be much more consistent in their responses and make distinctions not possible for untrained subjects. On the other hand, we have seen how subjects can inadvertently be trained to provide correct rote naming of temporal order of sounds lasting only a few milliseconds, even when this information is not provided directly. The report by Divenyi and Hirsh (1974) that highly trained subjects could "identify" the temporal order of nonrecycled three-item tonal sequences at item durations as low as 2 ms, as well as the report by Neisser and Hirst (1974) that one of their highly trained subjects had a threshold for "identification" of order within recycled and nonrecycled four-item sequences of about 30 ms per component could well represent examples of the results of such rote learning. The dangers of misinterpreting results attributable to training procedures are not limited to perception of sequences, and have been discussed earlier in relation to other studies such as time-intensity trading, and loudness judgments.

A comparison of global pattern recognition with identification of the order of components

Results described thus far with recycled sequences have suggested that direct naming of the order of components is a fundamentally different task than the recognition of sequences with particular orders. The nature and extent of these differences was examined directly in a series of experiments by Warren and Ackroff (1976a). Three-item recycled sequences were employed in each experiment, and each of the 795 subjects made either a single judgment involving the order of the items or a single judgment of whether two of these sequences having the three items in identical or permuted orders sounded exactly the same or different in any way.

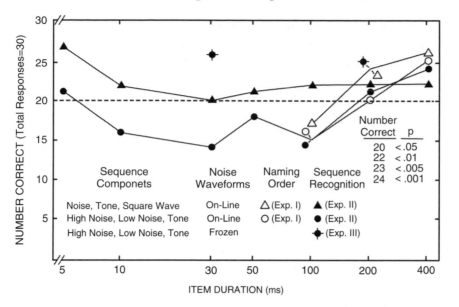

Figure 5.2 The two different ways of distinguishing between sequences having permuted arrangements of the same items: item order identification and recognition of permuted sequence patterns. The hollow symbols show the accuracy of naming the order of components in three-item recycling (looped) sequences having two possible arrangements. The filled symbols show the accuracy of recognizing whether two of these sequences presented successively were identical or different. Each data point represents a separate group of subjects. Random (on-line) generation of noise bursts (having different waveforms for each restatement) was used both in experiment I (naming order) and in experiment II (sequence recognition). "Frozen" or fixed waveform noise bursts (having identical waveforms for each restatement) were used for sequence recognition in experiment III. The dashed horizontal line corresponds to the limit for performance significantly better than chance. For further information, see the text. (From Warren and Ackroff, 1976a.)

There were two sets of sounds used for constructing the three-item sequences and, as we shall see, the choice of particular constituent sounds had a profound effect on same/different judgments, but not upon naming of order. One set consisted of two distinctive periodic sounds (a 2,500 Hz sinusoidal tone and a 1,000 Hz square-wave), as well as a broadband on-line noise. The other set consisted of two distinctive on-line noises (a high frequency noise band and a low frequency noise band), as well as one periodic sound (a 2,000 Hz sinusoidal tone).

Experiment I of this study dealt with the identification of the order of components. After familiarization with the names of the sounds when heard alone, six separate groups of 30 listeners were presented with one of the two possible orders of the recycling three-item isochronous sounds having item durations of 100, 200, or 300 ms, and they attempted to arrange cards with the names of each sound in the order of the item's occurrence. They could listen as long as they wished, and following their single judgment, the subjects were dismissed and served in no further sequence experiments. The results obtained are shown in Figure 5.2. It can be seen that correct identification of the order of the sounds was significantly above the most probable chance total of 15 correct responses for each group at 200 and 400 ms per item, and at chance level for 100 ms per item with both sets of stimuli.

Experiment II used the same two sets of sequences employed in experiment I, but instructions and procedure were changed. Subjects were not required to identify the order of the items. Instead, they listened to a pair of the three-item recycling sequences being played on two separate channels, and were told to report whether the sequences were the same or different. They could switch between the channels at will, and could listen as long as they wished. Both members of each pair had one of the seven item durations shown in Figure 5.2. Half of the 30 subjects in each group received identical and the other half received permuted orders. The results shown in Figure 5.2 indicate that, with sequences consisting of one noise and two periodic sounds (square-wave and sinusoidal tone), accuracy of same/different judgments was significantly above chance at all item durations from 5 through 400 ms. At the shortest item duration of 5 ms, the entire sequence had a period of 15 ms, and a repetition frequency lying in the tonal range (67 Hz), so that the increase in accuracy at this duration might be a consequence of differences in pitch quality or timbre of the two arrangements. The results obtained with repeating sequences consisting of one noise and two periodic sounds demonstrate that listeners without any prior training or practice could discriminate between permuted orders down to 5 ms, as had been reported earlier for highly trained laboratory personnel (Warren, 1974a). But, surprising results with interesting implications were obtained for same/different judgments for the groups receiving the high-band noise, low-band noise, and tone. It can be seen that judgments were at chance level from 10 through 100 ms per item. At 200 and 400 ms per item, judgments were above chance, but since it had been shown in experiment I that subjects could identify order at these longer item durations, same/different judgments could have been mediated by identification of components and their order.

This inability to distinguish between permuted orders with item durations in the range of 10 to 100 ms when only one of the components was a periodic sound suggested that successive noise bursts of the same bandpass characteristics were each treated as a different sound. Although successive bursts of noise derived from the same generators and spectral filters conventionally had been treated as samples of the same sound in earlier experiments dealing with sequence perception (Broadbent and Ladefoged, 1959; Hirsh, 1959; Fay, 1966; Warren, Obusek, Farmer, and Warren, 1969; Neisser and Hirst, 1974), the waveform and short-term running spectra are quite different for separate on-line bursts. Thus, in experiment II, the sequences consisting of high-band noise, low-band noise, and sinusoidal tone contain only a single periodic sound (the tone) surrounded by two ever-changing waveforms. But, when only one of the three items was derived from on-line noise in the sequence consisting of noise, sinusoidal tone, and square-wave, the relative positions of the periodic components consisting of the contiguous sinusoidal tone and the square-wave could permit listeners to discriminate between the fixed patterns corresponding to the permuted orders, even if the noise did not enter into the judgments. This suggested that discrimination between different arrangements of brief sounds is based upon differences in overall waveform, not the ordering of component items. Fortunately, it was possible to test the validity of this conjecture.

Experiment III was undertaken using the three-item sequences consisting of the tone and the high frequency and low frequency on-line noise bands to determine whether stochastic differences in successive restatements of each of the "same" on-line noise bands in experiment II were responsible for the inability to make accurate same/different judgments. New groups of subjects were presented with iterated sequences containing "frozen" or fixed-waveform noise bursts, so that listeners heard sequences having identical frozen noise segments for the high-band noise and for the low-band noise, whether they were within the same or different item orders. The results shown as experiment III in Figure 5.2 indicate that accuracy increased dramatically when frozen noise segments replaced the on-line noise segments. However, frozen waveforms were not required for identifying the order of components at long-item durations; indeed, the score obtained with frozen waveforms was equivalent to that obtained with on-line noise bands for sequences having 200 ms items. In another portion of the study, not shown in Figure 5.2, a separate group of subjects received the same arrangement of components for sequences consisting of the two noise bands and the sinusoidal tone, but different frozen waveforms for each sequence (that is, each of the two sequences to be compared had the same nominal order but independently produced frozen waveforms for both the high-band and the low-band noises). When item durations were 30 ms, it was found that subjects considered the two sequences to be different, despite their having the same nominal order of components.

Perception of tonal sequences and melodies

There are several reasons for considering tonal sequences of interest. Music, of course, employs a special subclass of tonal sequences. But, in addition, tones are valuable research tools for investigating sequence perception since, when sinusoidal tones are used, it is possible to control the extent of frequency differences between successive tones in a continuous manner from near identity (with overlapping loci of stimulation on the basilar membrane), to large differences (involving different loci and different populations of receptors).

Warren and Byrnes (1975) compared holistic pattern recognition with direct identification of components and their orders for four-item recycling sequences of sinusoidal tones using 234 listeners (college students) without special training or any prior experience with such sequences. Among the variables employed were frequency separation of tones (steps ranging from 0.3 to 9 semitones), frequency range (either within the pitch range of orchestral instruments or extending above the approximately 4,500 Hz limit of this range), tonal durations (200 ms or 50 ms), as well as the effect of brief silent intervals. The results are summarized in Figure 5.3. Each data point in the figure represents results from a separate group of subjects, so that each of the listeners performed only one task with one set of stimuli. In experiments 1, 2, and 3, item durations were 200 ms. It can be seen that matching (accomplished by choosing which of six possible arrangements of the four-item sequences matched that of an unknown sequence) was always superior to the naming of order (accomplished by arranging cards – labeled highest, next highest, next lowest, lowest – in the order of occurrence), although both types of judgments had the same chance proportion of correct guessing. Some other results with implications of interest are shown in Figure 5.3. Accuracy of matching did not decrease with increasing frequency separation, as might be anticipated on the basis of experiments with auditory stream segregation of tones (Bregman and Campbell 1971; Bregman, 1990). However, Barsz (1988) suggested that the lack of evidence of streaming might result from differences in stimuli (the streaming study involved the interleaving of tones in two different registers).

Figure 5.3 shows that the correct naming of order was relatively difficult when tones were separated by 0.3 semitones (less than the 1 semitone corresponding to the smallest pitch interval used in most Western music), yet matching accuracy was comparable to that obtained with larger frequency separations. Brief silence between tones did not enhance performance in identification of order, although it has been reported that introduction of equivalent silent gaps facilitated order identification with vowel sequences (Warren and Warren, 1970; Thomas, Cetti, and Chase, 1971). Interestingly,

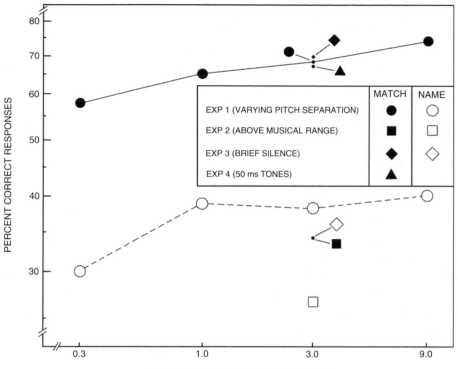

Figure 5.3 Accuracy of matching (filled symbols) and of naming (hollow symbols) the permuted orders of recycled sequences consisting of four sinusoidal tones. Each of the 13 data points is based upon the responses of a separate group of 30 subjects. Item durations were 200 ms except for 50 ms in experiment 4. For further information, see the text. (From Warren and Byrnes, 1975.)

accuracy for both matching and naming decreased dramatically for sequences with separations of 3 semitones when the frequencies were raised from those within the musical range (for which temporal information based on phase-locking to each tonal frequency is available) to those above the musical range (for which phase-locking is lacking). An unexpected finding not shown in Figure 5.3 was that although, as might be expected, the accuracy of matching monotonically increasing or decreasing pitches (glissandi) was higher than the accuracy with non-monotonic pitch changes within the musical range, per-formance matching glissandi was no better than with other arrangements of the same tones above the musical range. (For a discussion of the upper limit of musical pitch, see Semal and Demany, 1990). A duration of 200 ms/tone is within the range of durations of notes in melodies while 50 ms/tone is well below this range, yet Figure 5.3 shows that accuracy in matching was equivalent at both item durations. This equivalency suggests that the lower durational limits employed for notes in melodies of about 150 ms/note (Fraisse, 1963) do not result from an inability to recognize different global properties associated with different arrangements of notes at briefer durations, as has been suggested by some theorists (e.g., Winckel, 1967). As we shall see, subsequent experiments support this suggestion.

Sequences of tones forming melodies are perceived as more than a series of pitches. They have emergent properties, forming recognizable Gestalten or "temporal compounds." If melodies can be considered as temporal compounds, then we would expect to find a temporal template for melody recognition that has both upper and lower durational limits (see Figure 5.1 and associated discussion). An experiment by Warren, Gardner, Brubaker, and Bashford (1991) was undertaken using pure tones to determine whether temporal templates for melodies exist, and if so, the durational limits of the template. The eight melodies used as stimuli are shown in Figure 5.4. These tunes consisting of from seven to nine notes could be recognized by each of the subjects (30 college students) when played at a normal tempo (320 ms/note). None of the subjects had formal musical training, and they could neither name the notes nor transcribe them (the importance of this restriction will be discussed subsequently).

The melodies employed and the durational limits of their temporal templates are shown in Figure 5.4. Presentation of the repeated sequences of notes always started with the third or fourth note of the melodic phrase. Subjects could listen for as long as they wished before attempting to identify the melody. For determining the upper boundary of the recognition template, note durations started well above the range normally employed for melodies (3.6 s/note), and were decreased systematically in steps that varied by a factor of $\sqrt{2}$ (so that two steps halved the duration) until either recognition was achieved, or the notes were 320 ms in duration. The importance of starting the repeated melodic phrase in the middle for long-duration notes was determined in preliminary experiments – if presentation started at the beginning of the phrase, identification was often possible after the first two or three notes, with listeners extrapolating from this limited information and identifying the rest of the melody even if it was not played. When the melody started in the middle of the phrase and was repeated without pauses, such extrapolation was minimized. However, when listeners who could read and transcribe music were presented with the same stimuli consisting of long-duration notes, most of them could recognize the melodies regardless of starting position, apparently through notational coding of the musical intervals. Nevertheless, their ability to use notational coding for melodies did not enable these listeners to recognize melodies played at rapid rates. To return to the formal experiment, the overall grand median for the upper limits of melodic recognition shown in Figure 5.4 was 1,280 ms/note.

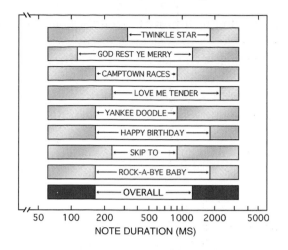

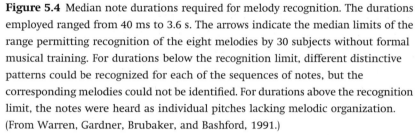

Figure 5.4 Median note durations required for melody recognition. The durations employed ranged from 40 ms to 3.6 s. The arrows indicate the median limits of the range permitting recognition of the eight melodies by 30 subjects without formal musical training. For durations below the recognition limit, different distinctive patterns could be recognized for each of the sequences of notes, but the corresponding melodies could not be identified. For durations above the recognition limit, the notes were heard as individual pitches lacking melodic organization. (From Warren, Gardner, Brubaker, and Bashford, 1991.)

When determining the lower limit for melody recognition, the recycled sequences were first presented at durations much too brief to permit recognitaion (40 ms/note), and durations were increased systematically in steps that varied by a factor of $\sqrt{2}$ until either recognition was accomplished or note durations reached 320 ms/note. The overall median for the lower limit of melody recognition shown in Figure 5.4 was 193 ms/note. The range of durations permitting melody recognition determined in this study is somewhat higher than the values of roughly 150 to 900 ms/note cited by Fraisse (1963) as the range of durations normally used for melodies. However, when played normally, the notes of the melodies are not isochronous, as they were in this experiment.

Although the tunes could not be recognized when played at 40 ms/note, the patterns of notes appeared to be distinctive for each of the melodies. There was no equivalence of different temporal orders or "metathesis" of notes as Winckel (1967) had described for rapid playing. The ability to form nonmelodic temporal compounds for rapidly played melodies is consistent with the earlier report by Warren and Byrnes (1975) that the six possible arrangements of iterated sequences of four 50 ms sinusoidal tones were each distinguishable from the others (see Figure 5.3). It has also been reported that minimal differences in complex tonal patterns can be discriminated – Warren and

Bashford (1993) found that a group of listeners could discriminate between iterated sequences of ten 40 ms tones in which the order of only two contiguous items had been interchanged. In that study, the group accuracy was 94 percent using an ABX procedure (that is, asking whether sequence X was the same as sequence A or B) when subjects were free to switch at will between the three sequences.

Acoustic sequences as unresolved "temporal compounds"

It might be thought that the ability of listeners to distinguish between the different arrangements of the ten 40 ms tones in the 1993 study of Warren and Bashford described above required segmentation into an ordered sequence of discrete components at some level of processing. However, a second experiment in this study using the same listeners and procedure indicated that patterns consisting of brief elements form "temporal compounds" that can be recognized and distinguished from other arrangements even when analysis into distinctive constituent elements is not possible. Ten different 40 ms segments excised from on-line broadband noise were substituted for the ten 40 ms tones. The sequence consisting of the ten concatenated frozen noise segments formed a single 400 ms frozen noise pattern rather than a succession of individual discriminable sounds. Yet when the pattern was iterated, listeners could discriminate between the 400 ms frozen noises that were identical except for the interchanging of orders for two 40 ms frozen noise components (group accuracy of 91 percent). Hence, acoustic sequences of concatenated brief sounds need not be processed as perceptual sequences (that is, segmented into an ordered series of components). This concept has implications for speech-processing models, as illustrated in the following section.

Linguistic temporal compounds formed by repeating sequences of brief steady-state vowels

As discussed earlier in this chapter, a number of studies have found that the threshold for identifying the order for repeating sequences of isochronous steady-state vowels was about 100 ms/vowel, a value above the average duration of phonemes in normal conversational discourse. Several rather interesting phenomena occur when the durations of vowels are decreased to values below the threshold for order identification. Warren, Bashford, and Gardner (1990) reported that the vowel sequences form temporal compounds consisting of illusory syllables and words when the vowels have durations ranging from 30 to 100 ms (corresponding to the durations of phonemes in normal speech). Different arrangements of the same vowels produce different verbal forms. The characteristics of these temporal compounds have provided novel information concerning the perceptual organization of speech sounds, as will be discussed in some detail in Chapter 7. However, at this point it should be noted that the stimulus vowels in these sequences cannot be identified and are perceived as other phonemes (including consonants), even though they are readily discriminated and identified when presented in isolation at the same item durations.

Identification of components and their orders and global pattern recognition for dichotomous patterns

Garner and his associates (Garner and Gottwald, 1967, 1968; Royer and Garner, 1970; Preusser, 1972) used extended complex patterns consisting of various arrangements of two elements (for example, a high tone and a low tone) in which successive presentations of the same item could occur. They observed that: (1) the nature of perceptual organization used by subjects changed with item durations; (2) that a recognition task gave different results than an identification task; and (3) some sequences were perceived globally, without direct identification of the component items. Despite the differences in the extended dichotomous sequences and recycling sequences consisting of three or more sounds, the observations and conclusions derived from experiments with these two types of patterns are similar.

Global pattern recognition in animals other than humans

Although other animals can distinguish between permuted arrangements of brief sounds, true identification of components and their order seems to be possible only for humans since only we appear to have the requisite ability to code, store, and retrieve the symbols representing individual sounds. The inability of monkeys to achieve performance characteristic of human identification of sounds and their orders is demonstrated by an experiment by Dewson and Cowey (1969). After considerable training, their three monkeys were able to discriminate accurately between two-item sequences in which each of the items could be either a tone or a noise (there were four possible patterns consisting of tone-tone, noise-noise, tone-noise, and noise-tone) if, and only if, item durations were briefer than approximately 1.5 s. When durations were increased to more than 3 s, the monkeys could not master the discrimination, apparently being unable to recall the first item after termination of the second (responses could not be made until termination of the entire sequence). Humans can, of course, easily discriminate between such sequences consisting of 3 s items (or, indeed, much longer item durations). But for us, as for monkeys, the actual memory trace of the first sound has probably faded into oblivion within a few seconds, so that the representation of the sound itself is not available for discrimination. It is, rather, the name of the first sound which we retain, and that, together with the name of the second sound, provides the basis for discrimination.

It might be reasoned that monkeys are creatures relying primarily on vision, so that auditory tasks are difficult for these animals. However, this argument would not apply to dolphins. These creatures are readily trainable and rely upon hearing to a great extent for feeding and for social interaction. Nevertheless, an upper limit for sequence discrimination for the dolphin was reported by Thompson (1976) matching that reported earlier for the monkey. Thompson employed four sounds, which can be called, A, B, C, and D. Two-item sequences were created in which the first item could be either A or B, and the second item could be either C or D. The dolphin was trained to press one paddle for either sequence AC or BD and a different paddle for either sequence AD or BC, so that neither the initial sound nor the terminal sound alone provided information that could identify the paddle producing a reward. The animal was not allowed to respond until the sequence was completed. The task was accomplished with ease for brief delays separating the two sounds, but Thompson stated that increasing the delay interval beyond two to three seconds resulted in an abrupt loss in the ability to discriminate between sequences. After using a variety of testing procedures, he concluded that " ... it can be ... argued that the 2- to 3-s ISI (interstimulus interval) delay limit represents a perceptual threshold beyond which the 'wholeness' or gestalt of the configure (sic) is no longer perceived, the animal now hearing two discrete sounds" (p. 116). Colavita, Szeligo, and Zimmer (1974) trained cats to discriminate between sequences consisting of tonal-intensity changes (loud-soft-loud versus soft-loud-soft), each intensity level lasting 900 ms with 100 ms between levels. As a result of the nature of changes in performance and the ability to relearn following bilateral insular-temporal lesions, these investigators concluded that the cats' original sequence discrimination was global, and not based upon pairwise discrimination of the order of individual intensities. Subsequent neurophysiological evidence has supported their conclusion.

Weinberger and McKenna (1988) and McKenna, Weinberger, and Diamond (1989) conducted a series of electrophysiological measurements involving responses of single neurons in the primary (AI) and secondary (AII) auditory cortex of waking cats. These measurements have provided evidence demonstrating the global processing of tone sequences. The investigators used sequences of five iso-intensity sinusoidal tones that either increased or decreased in frequency in a monotonic fashion, or had a non-monotonic frequency pattern. It was found that the vast majority of neurons in both auditory fields responded to the tonal patterns in a global fashion, so that the response to an individual tone was changed by the presence and relative positions of the other tones. McKenna *et al.* concluded that the concept of global pattern recognition "may be related to the present results because neurons in AI and AII can encode permutations of tone sequences as discharge patterns which are not simply a concatenation of the responses to the individual tones."

Conclusions

It has been assumed for some time that the ability to distinguish between different arrangements of the same sounds requires that listeners be able to identify the order of components. However, recent evidence indicates that permuted orders of speech sounds or tones, and permuted orders of unrelated sounds (such as hisses, tones, and buzzes) can be distinguished without the ability to identify the orders within the sequences (or even the component sounds themselves).

It is suggested that we employ two quite different processes for distinguishing between permuted orders of sounds within extended sequences: (1) direct identification of components and their orders; and (2) global pattern recognition. When items are too brief to permit direct order identification, different arrangements of items can still be discriminated through recognition of the overall pattern formed by the components. Following global pattern recognition of familiar sequences, listeners may be able to recite by rote the names of components in their order of occurrence – however, this process should not be confused with the direct identification of components and their order. As will be discussed in Chapter 7, speech perception appears to be based on a global recognition of phonetic patterns without the need to resolve the patterns into an ordered series of speech sounds.

Suggestions for further reading

Plomp, R. 2002. *The Intelligent Ear*. Mahwah, NJ: Erlbaum (see Chapter 3 for a discussion on sequence perception).

Watson, C. S. 1987. Uncertainty, informational masking, and the capacity of immediate memory. In *Auditory Processing of Complex Sounds*, W. A. Yost and C. S. Watson (eds.). Hillsdale, NJ: Erlbaum, 267–277 (a summary of some of Watson's studies using "word length" sequences of nonverbal sounds).

6

Perceptual restoration of missing sounds

The world is a noisy place, and signals of importance are often accompanied by louder irrelevant sounds. Hearing would lose much of its usefulness could we discern only whichever sound was at the highest level. However, there are mechanisms permitting us to attend to sounds that are fainter. In addition, we can, under certain circumstances, perceptually restore sounds that have been completely obliterated.

Some of the mechanisms enhancing the perception of signals in the presence of interfering sounds have been discussed in Chapter 2. One of these mechanisms squelches or reduces the interference produced by echoes and reverberation through the isolation of the early-arriving components that reach the listener directly from the source. Another mechanism is associated with localization, and reduces the threshold for a sound originating at one place when subject to interference by a sound originating at another position. It is also pointed out in Chapter 2 that contralateral induction can restore monaurally masked signals, and prevent mislocalization of a source.

Nevertheless, signals of importance can still be completely masked and obliterated. But when masking is intermittent, snatches of the signal occurring before and after the obliterated segment can furnish information concerning the missing segments. When this occurs, a perceptual synthesis can allow listeners to perceive the missing sounds as clearly as those actually present. As we shall see, this "temporal induction" of missing fragments can not only result in illusory continuity of steady-state sounds such as tones, but it can also restore contextually appropriate segments of time-varying signals such as speech, melodies, and tone glides. Temporal induction depends upon the masking potential of the extraneous sound: that is, restoration requires that the interfering sound have the intensity and spectral characteristics necessary to mask the restored sound. The extraneous sound participates actively in the process of restoration: an appropriate portion of its neural representation is subtracted and used for perceptual synthesis of the obliterated fragment, leaving a diminished residue. On occasion, an extraneous sound may mask some, but not all, frequency regions of a signal. Under these conditions, a "spectral restoration" may occur based upon the concurrent frequencies that have not been masked.

These rather sophisticated mechanisms and strategies allow listeners to repair degraded signals, and can lead them to believe that they are perceiving an intact auditory pattern, rather than fragments joined together with patches they themselves had synthesized.

Temporal induction

Homophonic continuity

The simplest form of temporal induction has been called "homophonic continuity" by Warren, Obusek, and Ackroff (1972). This effect was heard originally when, as part of a study dealing with the perception of temporal order (see Chapter 5), the first author was listening through headphones to a recycling sequence of three successive intensity levels (60, 70, 80 dB) of a one-octave band of noise centered at 2,000 Hz, with each intensity level lasting for 300 ms. The relative order of the three levels could not be perceived directly for an unexpected reason: when this sequence was repeated without pause, the 60 dB level appeared to be on all of the time. Subsequently, it was determined that all listeners, whether psychoacoustically sophisticated or naive, heard the faintest level clearly coexisting with each of the louder levels of the same sound. However, the introduction of silent gaps of 50 ms between successive intensity levels destroyed the apparent continuity of the faintest sound, and each of the three sounds was heard as a separate burst.

Homophonic continuity does not require that the repeated sequence consist of three levels: it was found that alternation of 300 ms bursts of the 2,000 Hz noise band at 70 and 80 dB resulted in the apparent continuity of the fainter sound. Alternating levels of the same sound, whether noise bands having other center frequencies, broadband noise, or sinusoidal tones also produced illusory continuity of the fainter level (Warren *et al.*, 1972).

Illusory continuity is not restricted to sounds differing only in intensity, since a "heterophonic" continuity can occur in which the restored sound differs in spectral composition from the louder sound. Further, restoration of sounds is not limited to production of illusory continuity of a steady sound at a steady level: sounds differing from the preceding and following sounds can be restored under appropriate conditions, as will be discussed below. However, homophonic continuity represents an especially simple type of restoration for which the louder and fainter sounds differ only in intensity. As will be discussed later, the alternation of two levels of the same sound allows us to examine basic differences used for the coding of amplitude of tones and of noise.

Heterophonic continuity

The illusory continuation of one sound when replaced by a different, louder sound has been discovered independently by several investigators. Miller and Licklider (1950) seem to have been the first to report this type of temporal induction. They found that, if a tone was alternated with a louder broadband noise (each sound lasting 50 ms), the tone appeared to be on all of the time. Similar observations were made when they used word lists rather than tones: the voice appeared to be on continuously. However, missing phonemes were not restored, and intelligibility of the lists of monosyllabic words was no better than when the words were interrupted by silent gaps. Miller and Licklider used a visual analogy, stating that this illusory continuity was much like seeing a landscape through a picket fence when "the pickets interrupt the view at regular intervals, but the landscape is perceived as continuing behind the pickets."

Vicario (1960) discovered this type of illusory continuity independently. He called the illusion the "acoustic tunnel effect," again in analogy to vision. In the visual tunnel effect, which had been described by Gestalt psychologists, an object moving behind another appears to continue to exist behind (or within) the blocking object until it emerges on the other side.

Thurlow (1957) also rediscovered heterophonic continuity. He used two alternating tones differing in both intensity and frequency and reported that the fainter tone could be heard to continue through 60 ms bursts of the louder tone. Thurlow described the phenomenon as "an auditory figure-ground effect" using the static model of Gestalt psychology's visual figure-ground effect, in which the background is assumed by viewers to extend behind a superimposed figure. Thurlow's work led to a series of studies on illusory continuity spanning gaps ranging from under 10 ms through 100 ms when these interruptions were filled with a louder sound (Thurlow and Elfner, 1959; Thurlow and Marten, 1962; Elfner and Caskey, 1965; Elfner and Homick, 1966, 1967a, 1967b; Elfner, 1969, 1971). Thurlow and Erchul (1978), on the basis of these studies as well as additional work, indicated their belief in the validity of the suggestion first made by Thurlow and Elfner (1959) that illusory continuity was a consequence of facilitation by the louder sound of a continued firing of the neural units corresponding to the fainter sound. It should be noted that this facilitation model does not require that the louder sound itself be capable of stimulating directly the units responding to or masking the fainter sound. Thus, Thurlow and Elfner reported that a louder pure tone was capable of inducing continuity of an alternating broadband fainter noise. However, the durations used in their studies involved continuity through gaps from 10 to 100 ms, and at these brief durations, spectral splatter or broadening could obscure the role played by potential masking when illusory continuities are longer than 100 ms.

Houtgast (1972) used conditions producing somewhat longer duration heterophonic continuity of tones (125 ms) than the earlier studies, and proposed a rather different basis for this illusion than did earlier investigators. He considered that there was a close relation between illusory continuity and masking, and suggested the following rule: "When a tone and a stimulus S are alternated (alternation cycle about 4 Hz), the tone is perceived as being continuous when the transition from S to tone causes no (perceptible) increase of nervous activity in any frequency region." He called the intensity at which perception of the tone changed from continuous to discontinuous the "pulsation threshold," and went on to say, "The pulsation threshold, thus, is the highest level of the tone at which this condition still holds." With the aid of some assumptions, Houtgast (1972, 1973, 1974b, 1974c) employed this illusory continuity to investigate cochlear spectral analysis. A basic premise underlying Houtgast's investigations was that lateral suppression takes place on the basilar membrane as suggested by Békésy (1959). It was considered that lateral suppression, which reduced the extent of neural responses at the edges of stimulated regions, could not be studied directly by masking experiments (as had been tried by other investigators), since both the masker and the probe would be subject to the same suppression process. However, Houtgast stated that the use of alternating stimuli as used in illusory-continuity experiments permitted an indirect measurement of the magnitude of lateral suppression.

At the same time as the initial report of Houtgast (1972), experiments involving heterophonic continuity were also reported by Warren, Obusek, and Ackroff (1972), along with the experiments involving homophonic induction described earlier. Our experiments involved somewhat longer durations of illusory continuity than did Houtgast's (i.e., 300 ms rather than 125 ms), and we concluded, as did Houtgast, that illusory continuity of the fainter of two alternating sounds required that the louder sound be a potential masker of the fainter. However, we were influenced by earlier work dealing with phonemic restoration. Warren (1970b) had reported that, when a phoneme or group of phonemes in a sentence was replaced by a louder noise, listeners restored the missing phoneme(s) and could not distinguish between the actual and perceptually synthesized speech sounds. Since phonemic restoration had demonstrated that the perceptual synthesis of missing fragments was not restricted to continuity of a steady-state sound, Warren, Obusek, and Ackroff (1972) suggested that temporal induction of continuity could occur when the conditions of the following rule were met: "If there is contextual evidence that a sound may be present at a given time, and if the peripheral units stimulated by a louder sound include those which would be stimulated by the anticipated fainter sound, then the fainter sound may be heard as present." This rule considers that with sufficient contextual support, missing portions of auditory patterns may be perceptually synthesized when replaced by a potential masker. This restoration can lead not only to apparent continuity of a steady tone, as in Houtgast's rule, but to phonemic restorations, continuity of tonal glides, completion of musical phrases, etc.

In order to study the quantitative relation between masking potential and perceptual restoration, four experiments were undertaken by Warren *et al.* (1972). The first of these experiments involved illusory continuity of sinusoidal tones. The inducing sound in the study was always a 1,000 Hz tone at 80 dB SPL which alternated with a fainter tone having the frequencies shown in Figure 6.1. Each tone was on for 300 ms and off for 300 ms, and the six subjects were instructed to adjust the intensity of the fainter tone to the highest level at which it seemed to be on continuously. Listening was through diotically wired matched headphones. The triangular data points in the figure show the highest level permitting continuity at each frequency, this level being expressed as

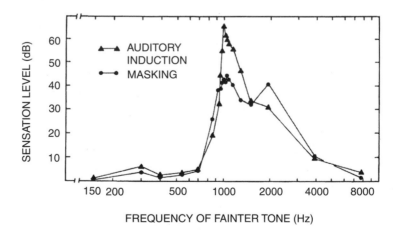

Figure 6.1 Temporal induction (illusory continuity) and masking for tones ranging from 150 Hz to 8,000 Hz in the presence of a louder 1,000 Hz tone presented at 80 dB SPL. (Adapted from Warren, Obusek, and Ackroff, 1972.)

sensation level (dB above a subject's threshold). It can be seen that virtually no continuity occurred until the frequency of the fainter tone was above 700 Hz, so that for these lower frequencies, as long as the tone was loud enough to be heard clearly, it was perceived to be pulsing.

When the weaker tone was 1,000 Hz (the same frequency as the stronger tone), homophonic continuity took place. Most of the subjects chose a 3 dB difference in level between the 1,000 Hz tones as the upper limit of homophonic continuity (rather interesting unexpected phenomena occurring at and near this upper limit will be discussed subsequently). Although the extent of temporal induction increased sharply from 700 through 1,000 Hz, there was a relatively gradual decrease as the frequency of the fainter tone was increased above 1,000 Hz, an asymmetry characteristic of masking functions (see Chapter 3).

The second part of this study measured simultaneous masking using the same subjects and the same frequencies used for determining continuity limits. But rather than alternating the louder and fainter tones, the louder 1,000 Hz tone was kept on continuously at 80 dB SPL, and the threshold was measured for detection of pulsed superimposed tones that were on for 300 ms and off for 300 ms. The data points shown by circles in Figure 6.1 give the simultaneous masking thresholds measured as decibels above the detection threshold for fainter tones having various frequencies when alternated with the louder fixed frequency tone. The figure shows that the simultaneous masking and temporal induction functions were quite similar except for frequencies at or near that of the 1,000 Hz tone and its octave. At identical inducer and inducee frequencies, as indicated earlier, temporal induction became homophonic, and the threshold for masking was equivalent to a jnd in intensity of the 1,000 Hz tone. The masking function is also influenced by the fluctuation in loudness produced by beats when the concurrent louder and fainter tones differ but lie within the same critical band. The functions for apparent continuity and masking were equivalent at 1,500 Hz and above, except for one frequency: there was a separation in the two functions at 2,000 Hz due to an increase in the masked threshold. The increase in masking one and two octaves above the frequency of a tonal masker has been known for some time (Wegel and Lane, 1924), as was described and discussed in Chapter 3. It can be seen in the figure that a change in slope also occurs in the temporal induction curve at 2,000 Hz; the reason for this slight change, while interesting, seems obscure at this time.

The third and fourth experiments provided additional evidence for the close relation between temporal induction and masking. The third experiment used a 1/3-octave band of noise centered on 1,000 Hz as the inducing sound, and found that the upper intensity limit for illusory continuity of tones was highest tonal frequency corresponding to the center frequency of the noise ...d. As with the tonal inducer shown in Figure 6.1, the curve describing the ...ntensity limits for temporal induction of the tone by the noise band was asymmetrical, with steeper slopes at the low frequency end. In the fourth and final experiment, a broadband noise with a frequency notch (that is, a rejected frequency band) centered on 1,000 Hz served as the inducer. In keeping with the hypothesized relation between masking and temporal induction, the upper intensity limit for apparent continuity was lowest for tones at the center frequency of this rejected noise band.

The roll effect as tonal restoration

Van Noorden (1975, 1977) discovered that, when faint 40 ms tone bursts were alternated with louder 40 ms tone bursts with short silent gaps separating the successive bursts, it was possible for listeners to hear the fainter tone burst not only when it actually was present, but also when the louder burst occurred. The gap was also heard, so that there was a discontinuity, and an apparent doubling of the actual rate of the fainter bursts. This "roll effect" required intensity and spectral relations between fainter and louder tones resembling those leading to illusory continuity of the fainter of two alternating temporally continuous tones. As van Noorden pointed out, it was as if the discrete restorations of the fainter tonal bursts leading to the roll effect required that the louder bursts could function as potential maskers. The duration of the silent gap played a critical role in this illusion: if shorter, the gap would not be detected and a continuous homophonic induction would take place, and if longer the percept of the fainter tone could not jump over the silent gap and reappear along with the higher amplitude tone.

Durational limits for illusory continuity

Studies of the illusory continuity of tones have not used interruption times greater than 300 ms, since tonal continuity cannot be maintained for longer periods. (See Verschuure, 1978, for a discussion of temporal limits for the continuity of tones.) Much longer continuity was reported by Warren, Obusek, and Ackroff (1972) for a 1/3-octave band of noise centered on 1,000 Hz when alternated with a louder 500 to 2,000 Hz band of noise of equal duration. All of our 15 subjects heard the fainter noise band continue for several seconds, eight heard illusory continuity for at least 20 s, and six still were hearing the absent noise band continue 50 s after it was replaced by the broadband noise.

Reciprocal changes in inducer and inducee

The upper duration limit for illusory continuity, or pulsation threshold, appears as a fairly sharp break, enabling reproducible measures to be made of this transition (Houtgast, 1972; Warren, 1972; Verschuure, Rodenburg, and Maas, 1974; Fastl, 1975; Schreiner, Gottlob, and Mellert, 1977). Laboratory studies dealing with this topic have concentrated on the conditions needed to produce apparent continuity of a fainter inducee, and have generally ignored possible concurrent changes occurring in the louder inducer. However, Warren (1984) described informal observations suggesting that a portion of the inducer's neural representation was subtracted and used for the perceptual synthesis of the inducee. Subsequent formal experiments have provided quantitative evidence that this reallocation of the neural response from inducer to inducee does indeed occur (Warren, Bashford, and Healy, 1992; Warren, Bashford, Healy, and Brubaker, 1994). In addition, these studies described a number of previously unreported phenomena.

Figure 6.2 shows the reduction in apparent level of a 1,000 Hz sinusoidal inducer when alternated every 200 ms with inducees that were sinusoidal tones of the same or slightly different frequencies. The level of the inducer was fixed at 70 dB, and the inducees were presented at one of three different levels. In keeping with the reallocation hypothesis, the apparent amplitude (loudness) of the inducer decreased with increasing inducee amplitude under eight of the nine conditions, reflecting a greater reallocation of the inducer's auditory

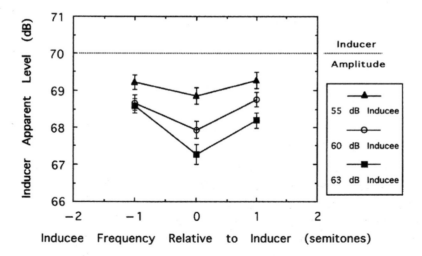

Figure 6.2 Temporal induction: loudness reduction of inducer produced by inducees. Means and standard errors are shown for changes produced in apparent level (loudness) of a 200 ms, 1,000 Hz inducer at 70 dB alternating with 200 ms inducees having three different frequencies, each presented at three different amplitudes. Inducee frequencies are given as the difference in semitones from the inducer frequency (each semitone is 1/12-octave). For further details, see the text. (From Warren, Bashford, Healy, and Brubaker, 1994.)

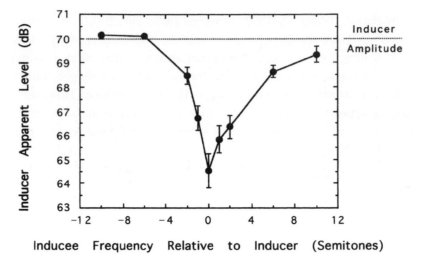

Figure 6.3 Temporal induction: loudness reduction of inducer produced by inducees. Means and standard errors are shown for changes in the apparent level (loudness) of a 200 ms, 1,000 Hz inducer at 70 dB alternating with 200 ms 66 dB inducees having nine different frequencies. Inducee frequencies are given as the difference in semitones from the inducer frequency (each semitone is 1/12-octave). (From Warren, Bashford, Healy, and Brubaker, 1994.)

representation for perceptual synthesis of the inducee. It can be seen that for a given inducee amplitude, the reduction was greatest for homophonic conditions.

Figure 6.3 shows the results of an experiment examining the effect of inducee frequencies covering a range of 22 semitones upon the loudness of a fixed-frequency inducer. As can be seen, a drop in loudness occurred for inducee frequencies within the range extending from 2 semitones below (891 Hz) to 10 semitones above (1,782 Hz) the frequency of the 1,000 Hz inducer. The decrease in the inducer's apparent amplitude occurred even though the inducee appeared to be discontinuous over most of this range. This drop in loudness in the absence of inducee continuity suggested that if reallocation theory was valid, then incomplete induction took place. One possibility is that a portion of the inducer's neural representation was used to increase the apparent duration of the inducee to some extent, but not enough to completely close the gaps. There had been an earlier report by Wrightson and Warren (1981) that a measurable late offset and early onset of a tone alternated with noise can occur when the tone does not appear to be continuous.

An additional experiment by Warren, Bashford, Healy, and Brubaker (1994) provided confirmation that the restoration of obliterated segments is not an all-or-none phenomenon, but rather the end point of a continuum of illusory lengthening. The same stimuli were employed as in the experiment

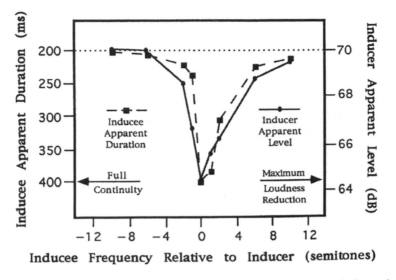

Figure 6.4 Temporal induction: relation of changes in apparent inducee duration to changes in apparent inducer amplitude. The inducer was a 200 ms 1 kHz tone at 70 dB, and the inducees were 200 ms 66 dB tones having various frequencies expressed as semitone separations from the inducer frequency (each semitone is 1/12-octave). The horizontal dotted line represents the actual value of inducee duration (left ordinate) as well as the actual value of inducer amplitude (right ordinate). Data are standardized so that the maximum reduction in apparent inducer amplitude (5.5 dB) matches the ceiling value for inducee apparent duration (full continuity). See the text for further information. (From Warren, Bashford, Healy, and Brubaker, 1994.)

represented in Figure 6.3, but rather than matching the apparent *amplitude* of the inducer, listeners matched the apparent *duration* of the inducee. The changes in apparent duration of inducees are shown in Figure 6.4, along with the corresponding changes in the apparent amplitude of the inducer derived from Figure 6.3. The close relation of the two functions is apparent.

Alternating levels of the same sound: some anomalous effects observed for the higher level sound in the homophonic induction of tones

Figure 6.3 shows that under homophonic conditions (0 semitone separation between the 70 dB 1,000 Hz tonal inducer and the 66 dB tonal inducee), the apparent level of the inducer dropped by 5.5 dB, a decrease in intensity considerably greater than the 2.2 dB change corresponding to a physical subtraction of the inducee level. When the inducee level is raised to about 67 or 68 dB (depending on the listener) continuity of the fainter sound ceases, and the two levels of the pure tones are heard to alternate. When the inducee level was within 1 or 2 dB below the alternation threshold, the inducer no longer seemed tonal, but was heard as an intermittent harsh and discordant sound that was superimposed upon the apparently continuous level of the 66 dB pure tone. It appears that the residue remaining after reallocation does not correspond to the entire neural representation of a tone, but rather it consists of that portion of the inducer's neural representation that normally signals an increase in level above that of the inducee.

There are several changes in the representation of a tone at the level of the auditory nerve that accompany an increase in stimulus amplitude, and any or all of these could serve as a basis for signaling an increase in loudness. These changes include the crossing of the response threshold of less sensitive fibers having the same characteristic frequency as the tone, an increase in the firing rate of fibers responding to the lower level, the asymmetrical further spread of excitation to fibers differing in characteristic frequency from that of the stimulus, and also complex changes associated with phase locking to the stimulus waveform (for a discussion of the possible neural cues employed for the coding of stimulus amplitude, see Javel, 1986; Relkin and Ducet, 1997; Smith, 1988). Although the relative importance of each of these potential cues signaling a loudness increase is not known, homophonic induction appears to shear off those components of the inducer's neural representation that correspond to the lower-level inducee, allowing listeners to hear only those atonal-sounding components that signal the increment in level above that corresponding to the inducee. When the inducer and inducee levels differed by more than 5 or 6 dB the inducer seemed completely tonal despite reallocation. Figures 6.2, 6.3, and 6.4 make it clear that the loudness reduction produced by reallocation cannot be derived from the principles governing the addition and subtraction of sound in physical acoustics.

Differences in the homophonic induction of tone and noise

Warren, Bashford, Healy, and Brubaker (1994) found that the homophonic induction of a broadband noise differed from that of a tone in several respects, indicating that there are basic differences in the neural encoding of amplitude changes for these two types of sounds. It was found that: (1) the reduction in loudness of the inducing noise when the alternating levels are close in amplitude is not accompanied by appreciable change in timbre or quality of the inducer, as is the case with tones; (2) the decrease in inducer loudness is less than that observed for tonal induction involving equivalent amplitudes of inducer and inducee; and (3) there is no transition from homophonic continuity to the perception of alternating amplitudes as heard with tones when the two levels of broadband noise are brought close together. Even when the difference in levels is as little as 0.5 dB (the just noticeable difference in intensity of broadband noise reported by G. A. Miller, 1947), the acoustically lower noise level appears to be continuous, and is heard along with a very faint pulsed additional noise corresponding to the diminished inducer.

These differences in homophonic induction of sinusoidal tones and broadband noise appear to be attributable to the nature of their neural representation: tones are delivered at a fixed amplitude to narrow cochlear regions; noises stimulate broad spectral regions, with individual critical bands receiving different fluctuating amplitude patterns. In order to evaluate the level of a broadband noise with a precision of 0.5 dB, it would seem necessary to combine the input from many loci over some appropriate integration time.

Binaural release from temporal induction

Although temporal induction can occur when the signal (inducee) and the interrupting sound (inducer) are presented monaurally or diotically, and hence appear to originate at the same location, what would happen if the inducer and the inducee appear to originate at different locations? As discussed in Chapter 2, when two sounds occur simultaneously, the ability of one to mask the other is decreased appreciably when interaural phase differences associated with each sound cause them to appear to be located at different azimuths. Kashino and Warren (1996) reported that when interaural phase relations differed for the inducer and inducee, temporal induction was inhibited, as measured both by the upper amplitude limit for inducee continuity, and by loudness reduction of the inducer. This "binaural release from temporal induction" is consistent with the hypothesis that the perceptual synthesis of a missing fragment depends upon the masking potential of an interpolated sound.

Temporal induction of dynamic signals

Temporal induction is not limited to the restoration of continuity of sounds such as tones and noises for which the restored segment resembles the preceding and following segments. Temporal induction can also restore obliterated portions of time-varying signals, such as segments of tonal frequency glides, phonemes of speech, and notes of familiar melodies.

Temporal induction of tonal frequency glides

Dannenbring (1976) studied the illusory continuity of tonal glides interrupted by noise. An example of the stimuli used is shown in Figure 6.5. The difference in frequency between the upper and lower limits of the frequency range transversed by the glides was varied from 100 through 1,000 Hz

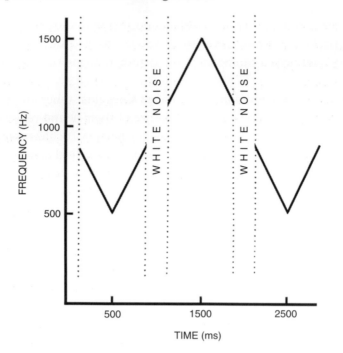

Figure 6.5 Example of conditions used to study illusory continuity (temporal induction) of tonal glides interrupted by louder broadband noise. (Adapted from Dannenbring, 1976.)

(the center frequency of the glide range was always 1,000 Hz), and the duration of the glide from frequency peak to trough was varied from 250 through 2,000 ms. The duration of white noise bursts centered at the middle of each glide was adjusted by the subjects to the maximum duration that permitted the glide to appear continuous. The stimuli were presented diotically, with the noise burst at 90 dB and the tonal glide at 75 dB. Illusory continuity of somewhat longer duration was found as ΔF (the range of the frequency glide) increased. For the longest duration glide (2 s from peak to trough), the tonal glide was heard to continue smoothly through noise durations between 400 and 500 ms (mean of adjustments for the 20 subjects) for each value of ΔF.

Temporal induction of speech: phonemic restoration

It has been reported that listeners cannot tell that a phoneme is missing after it has been excised from a recorded sentence and replaced by an extraneous sound such as a cough or a noise burst (Warren, 1970b; Warren and Warren, 1970). Even when the listeners were told in advance that a particular speech sound (that was not identified) had been removed completely and replaced by another sound and the recording was replayed several times, the sentence still appeared intact, and it was not possible for listeners to distinguish between the perceptually synthesized sound and those physically present (Warren and Obusek, 1971). It might be thought that listeners could identify the position of the extraneous sound in the sentence, and thus locate the missing segment. However, the extraneous sound could not be localized accurately: when subjects attempted to report its position, errors corresponding to a few hundred milliseconds were made. But, when a silent gap was present rather than an extraneous sound, restoration did not occur, and the location of the missing speech sound could be identified with accuracy.

Context provided by both prior and subsequent words can be used to identify an obliterated phoneme in a sentence (Warren and Warren, 1970; Sherman, 1971). However, information provided by the immediately preceding and following speech sounds can be surprisingly ineffective. Thus, when a phoneme in a sentence was deliberately mispronounced before deletion, for example the substitution of /t/ for /n/ in "commu/t/ication," phonemic restoration of the contextually appropriate /n/ occurred despite the inappropriate coarticulation cues present in the intact neighboring phonemes (Warren and Sherman, 1974). Even when listeners were told that a speech sound had been replaced by a noise, the presence of lexically inconsistent coarticulation cues still did not permit them to identify the missing phoneme.

Without sentential context, phonemic restoration does not normally occur. However, when a gap in an isolated word is replaced by speech-modulated noise (as employed by Samuel, 1987, and others) rather than by stochastic noise, then the additional bottom-up cue provided by the amplitude contour of the missing phoneme can permit restoration of the appropriate phoneme (see Bashford, Warren, and Brown, 1996).

Phonemic restorations in Japanese sentences were reported by Sasaki (1980), who reasoned that there might be a melodic restoration effect similar to phonemic restoration. He did indeed find such an effect: when one or two notes were replaced by noise in familiar melodies played on a piano, listeners heard the missing note(s), and mislocalized the noise burst when required to report its location.

The inability to locate extraneous sounds in sentences and in melodies is consistent with reports of a general inability to detect order directly in sequences of nonverbal sounds with equivalent item durations (see Chapter 5). Although the phonemes forming sentences and the notes in musical passages may occur too rapidly to permit direct naming of order, verbal and tonal groupings can be recognized globally and distinguished from groupings of the same brief items in different orders. Following recognition of the overall pattern, the identity and order of components forming these sequences can be inferred if they had been learned previously. This indirect mechanism for naming orders at rates too rapid for direct identification of sounds and their orders is not available for locating the position of extraneous sounds such as a cough replacing or masking a phoneme in a sentence, or a brief click occurring within an otherwise intact sentence.

Both phonemic and melodic restorations can be considered as specialized forms of temporal induction, with the identity of the induced sound determined by the special rules governing these familiar sequences. In keeping with the general principle found to govern temporal induction, there is evidence that restoration of a phoneme is enhanced when the extraneous sound in a sentence is capable of masking the restored speech sound (Layton, 1975; Bashford and Warren, 1987b).

Apparent continuity of speech produced by insertion of noise into multiple gaps

Miller and Licklider (1950) reported that, when recordings of phonetically balanced (PB) lists of monosyllabic words were interrupted regularly by silent gaps at rates from 10 to 15 times a second (50 percent duty cycle, so that on-time and off-time were equal), the silent intervals caused the voice to sound rough and harsh, and the intelligibility dropped. When the silent gaps were filled with a broadband noise that was louder than the speech, Miller and Licklider found that the word lists sounded more "natural" (their "picket fence effect"), but intelligibility was no better than it was with silence. Bashford and Warren (1987b) extended this study of the effects of filling silent gaps with noise, using three types of recorded verbal stimuli: (1) PB word lists of the type employed by Miller and Licklider; (2) an article from a popular news magazine read backwards (the individual words were pronounced normally, but they were read in reverse order with an attempt to preserve normal phrasing contours); (3) the same magazine article read in a normal fashion. The rate at which syllables occurred was matched for all three stimuli, which were presented at peak intensity levels of 70 dB. Twenty listeners adjusted the interruption rate of the verbal stimuli (50 percent duty cycle, rise/fall time of 10 ms) to their threshold for detecting deletions in the speech. Under one condition the gaps were unfilled, and under the other condition the gaps were filled with broadband noise at 80 dB. Table 6.1 lists the deletion detection thresholds obtained in this study.

When each of the types of speech shown in Table 6.1 was interrupted by silent gaps having durations below the deletion detection threshold, they sounded rough or "bubbly," but perceptually discrete gaps were not heard. When the silent gaps were filled with noise, for durations below the deletion

Table 6.1 *Mean deletion detection thresholds (ms) for multiple interruptions of broadband verbal stimuli by broadband noise or silence*

Interrupter	Normal discourse	Discourse read backwards	Word lists
Noise	304	148	161
Silence	52	50	61

From Bashford and Warren (1987b).

detection threshold, listeners reported that the signals sounded like fully continuous speech, with the noise bursts appearing to be superimposed (in keeping with the observations of Miller and Licklider with word lists). It can be seen that detection thresholds for silent gaps were similar for all three types of verbal signals. However, filling gaps with noise caused a considerable increase in the threshold value for recognition of discontinuities in the speech for all conditions. The highest discontinuity threshold (304 ms) was obtained for normal discourse, and corresponded to the average word duration. A subsequent study by Bashford, Myers, Brubaker, and Warren (1988) was undertaken to determine whether this correspondence was fortuitous. A different speaker and a different passage of connected discourse was employed. The recorded speech was played to three groups of listeners, each group hearing the recording at one of the following playback speeds: normal (original speaking rate), 15 percent faster, and 15 percent slower. At each playback rate, the upper limit for apparent speech continuity through noise filled gaps approximated the average word duration regardless of the increase or decrease in word duration, indicating that the limits for illusory continuity for discourse corresponded to a linguistic unit (the word) and not a fixed temporal value.

In order to test whether the restoration of continuity produced by filling gaps in speech with noise follows the rules governing restoration of continuity of nonverbal sounds, an experiment was conducted to determine if speech exhibits the spectral dependency demonstrated for induction with nonverbal stimuli (i.e., if the noise inducing continuity needs to be capable of masking the missing speech fragments if they were really present). Bashford and Warren (1987b) filtered the recording of connected speech (the magazine article described above) to produce a 1/3-octave band centered on 1,500 Hz. This filtered speech was presented at peak levels of 70 dB and alternated with 1/3-octave bands of noise at 80 dB, having the center frequencies shown in Table 6.2. The deletion-detection thresholds were determined using the procedure described above for broadband speech alternated with broadband noise. It was found that the greatest enhancement of continuity occurred with spectral congruence of noise and speech, in keeping with induction studies

Table 6.2 *Mean deletion detection thresholds (ms) for multiple interruptions of narrow-band normal discourse (filter slopes of 48 dB/octave intersecting at 1,500 Hz) when interrupted by the 1/3-octave noise bands with center frequencies listed below*

Noise band (Hz)	375	750	1500	3000	6000
Threshold (ms)	136	221	304	129	128

The threshold off-time with silence substituted for the interpolated noise bands was 79 ms. From Bashford and Warren (1987b).

using nonverbal sounds. Although the deletion detection followed the spectral requirements for nonverbal induction, Bregman (1990) did not accept the contention that restoration involving speech is a linguistic form of temporal induction. He proposed instead that phonemic restoration represents a "schema-driven stream segregation" following Gestalt principles for auditory organization. In keeping with these principles, Bregman hypothesized that reallocation of a portion of the auditory representation of the extraneous noise over to speech does not occur, although he considered that such a reallocation or subtraction does occur with nonverbal induction. Repp (1992) attempted to resolve this dispute by replacing the speech sound "s" in a word with a broadband noise. He had listeners judge whether they could detect a change in the "brightness" or timbre of the interpolated noise when it was used to restore the "s". In two of the five experiments, Repp reported that the subjects' responses indicated a change in the timbre of the noise, which was considered to be consistent with the application of temporal induction rules to phonemic restoration. However, the other three experiments in this study did not indicate a change. In order to test for reallocation directly, Warren, Bashford, Healy, and Brubaker (1994) determined whether or not the illusory continuity of speech reduced the apparent amplitude of an inducing noise. We alternated a narrow-band sentence having a fixed center frequency with the series of louder narrow-band noises as shown in Figure 6.6. It can be seen that the decrease in the amplitude of the noise was greatest when it matched the center frequency of the speech, in keeping with reallocation. The asymmetry of the two limbs reflects the asymmetrical upward spread of masking (and inducing potential) of the noise, as can also be seen in Figure 6.4 for the heterophonic induction of one pure tone by another.

> *Increase in intelligibility produced by insertion of noise into multiple temporal gaps*

As mentioned earlier, Miller and Licklider (1950) found that, although their recorded word lists sounded more natural when interruptions were filled with louder noise rather than being silent, no increase in intelligibility

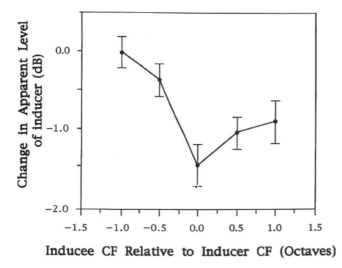

Figure 6.6 Temporal induction of speech (phonemic restorations): changes in the apparent level (loudness) of bandpass noises alternating every 125 ms with a bandpass sentence. The sentence was fully intelligible, and consisted of a 1/3-octave band at a center frequency (CF) of 1.5 kHz, slopes of 48 dB/octave, and a peak level of 70 dB. The inducers were five 1/3-octave noise bands at 70 dB having slopes of 48 dB/octave, and CFs differing from the speech CF by −1.0, −0.5, 0.0, +0.5 and +1.0 octaves. Plotted values are means and standard errors for four listeners. See the text for implications. (Adapted from Warren, Bashford, Healy, and Brubaker, 1994.)

occurred with the introduction of noise. However, later investigators, who used meaningful discourse rather than word lists, did find that an increase in intelligibility was produced by insertion of noise into multiple gaps in speech. Cherry and Wiley (1967) appear to be the first to report such an increase in intelligibility. They passed only the strongly voiced components of speech, and reported that the resultant staccato sequence of high energy voiced speech sounds had an "extremely low intelligibility." But when broadband noise of appropriate intensity was added to the silent gaps, intelligibility increased considerably (from 20 percent to 70 percent). These basic findings were confirmed by Holloway (1970). Wiley (1968) reversed the procedure employed by Cherry and Wiley and by Holloway, and removed the strongly voiced components of running speech, leaving only the low energy speech sounds, and found again that intelligibility was increased when noise was added to the silent gaps. Wiley also deleted the entire speech spectrum at regular intervals, and reported that once more intelligibility was increased by the addition of noise to gaps. Powers and Wilcox (1977) were not aware of Wiley's unpublished dissertation, and discovered independently that addition of noise to silent gaps in regularly interrupted speech increased intelligibility.

The enhancement of intelligibility produced by filling silent gaps in interrupted discourse with noise has given rise to a number of hypotheses concerning its basis. Cherry and Wiley (1967) suggested that noise prevents some disruptive effect of silence upon the natural rhythm of speech which is needed for comprehension. Powers and Wilcox (1977) concluded that their results were consistent with the rhythm hypothesis of Cherry and Wiley. In addition, they mentioned as another possible basis for enhanced intelligibility a suggestion made by Huggins (1964) that noise might serve to mask misleading transitions to silence that could produce illusory consonants. This suggestion, however, is weakened by the observation that although Öhman (1966) verified that illusory consonants are produced by the introduction of silent gaps in isolated monosyllables, no improvement in the identification of disrupted syllables occurs when noise is inserted into gaps in monosyllables (Miller and Licklider, 1950; Dirks and Bower, 1970).

In the study by Warren and Obusek (1971) of a single phonemic restoration in a sentence (which was fully intelligible even without the addition of an extraneous noise in the gap), it was hypothesized that sentences disrupted by multiple gaps could have their missing segments restored by introduction of noise into the gaps, with the restoration of the missing fragments based upon linguistic information provided by the intact segments. As discussed previously, the illusory continuity of both sentences and word lists having multiple interruptions by noise follows the rules governing the temporal induction of nonverbal sounds. An experiment by Bashford, Riener, and Warren (1992) was undertaken to determine whether the restoration of the intelligibility of sentences by adding noise to multiple gaps is also governed by the rules of temporal induction (recall that although filling gaps in broadband word lists with broadband noise produced illusory continuity, intelligibility was not increased). Bashford *et al.* instructed a group of 20 listeners to repeat 100 standardized "everyday speech" sentences developed at the Central Institute for the Deaf (Silverman and Hirsh, 1955). These recorded sentences, containing 500 keywords used for scoring, were bandpass filtered (slopes of 48 dB/octave intersecting at 1,500 Hz) and were interrupted (on/off times of 175 ms) by silence or by one of five 1/3-octave bands of noise (48 dB per octave slopes) with center frequencies as shown in Figure 6.7. The results of the intelligibility test are shown in the figure. It can be seen that intelligibility was greatest when the noise band and speech band were spectrally matched, as would be expected from temporal induction theory.

Taken together, the available evidence indicates that phonemic restoration involves two stages. The first stage (that can be observed when monosyllabic word lists are interrupted by noise) follows the rules for temporal induction of

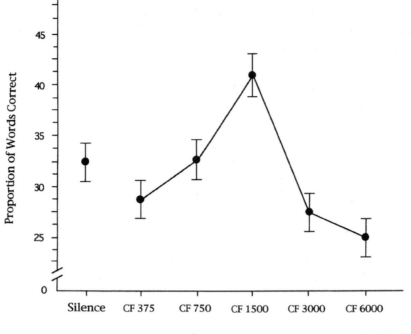

Figure 6.7 Percent repetition accuracy and standard errors for narrow-band (1,500 Hz center frequency) "everyday speech" sentences interrupted by silence or by noise bands of various center frequencies. See the text for further information. (From Bashford, Riener, and Warren, 1992.)

illusory continuity of nonverbal sounds, but does not enhance intelligibility; the second stage can occur when sufficient linguistic context is available, and can result in phonemic restoration, word recognition, and enhanced sentence intelligibility.

Temporal induction in cats and monkeys

Sugita (1997) trained cats to discriminate between an intact tonal glide and a tonal glide with a gap. When noise at different levels was added to the gap, it was found that discrimination between the intact and interrupted glide could be accomplished very well when the noise had a lower level than the tone, but when the noise had a higher level than the missing segment, the ability to discriminate between the intact and interrupted glide dropped considerably. The same stimuli were then presented to humans, and he stated that "very similar and comparable" results were obtained (that is, the noise level required for apparent continuity of the glide through the gap was about the same for cats and humans). Sugita next isolated individual cells in the cat primary auditory cortex that responded to tonal frequency glides. He reported that when a portion of the sweep was replaced by silence, the response was weakened considerably, but was restored when a noise of higher amplitude replaced the missing segment of the glide. Since these cells did not respond well to either the tone with a gap or to the noise when presented separately, Sugita concluded that he had demonstrated a neuronal correlate of temporal induction. Petkov, O'Connor, and Sutter (2003) initially trained their macaque monkeys to discriminate between auditory stimuli with and without silent gaps. The sounds were a 2 kHz tone, a tone glide, and a macaque "coo" sound. Subsequently, when broadband noise was added to each of the three sounds, the stimuli were treated as continuous; but the 2 kHz tone was treated as discontinuous when the noise had a 1-octave wide gap centered on 2 kHz. These observations and others led the authors to state that "primates may share a general mechanism to perceptually complete missing sounds."

Spectral restoration

There have been reports that noise can induce the restoration of absent spectral components of familiar nonverbal sounds. Houtgast (1976) reported that the addition of broadband noise at a level slightly below the masked threshold of a pure tone resulted in perception of the lower pitch of a missing fundamental that had been heard previously along with that tone. Plomp and Larkin (cited in Plomp, 1981) showed that adjacent harmonics could be deleted from a complex tone without affecting its timbre if listeners had been primed with the intact complex tone and if a narrow-band noise replaced the missing region at a level that could have masked the harmonics.

There is also evidence that adding noise to spectral gaps in speech can increase intelligibility. Bashford and Warren (1987a) suggested that a "spectral completion effect" may have contributed to the enhanced intelligibility they observed when complementary filtered noise was added to alternating high-pass and low-pass segments of sentences. However, it was pointed out that the experimental design, which was chosen for other purposes, permitted alternative interpretations of this enhancement of intelligibility. Subsequently, support for spectral restoration of single speech sounds was provided by Shriberg (1992). She found that listeners had difficulty discriminating between vowels when isolated exemplars were low-pass filtered, but identification by her subjects became more accurate when noise replaced the missing spectral portions of the vowels.

Warren, Hainsworth, Brubaker, *et al.* (1997) demonstrated that an increase in intelligibility can indeed occur when noise is added to a spectral gap in speech. We used a list of monosyllabic words and three lists of sentences. The sentence lists varied in the amount of contextual information that could facilitate the identification of the keywords used for scoring intelligibility. The intelligibility of all speech stimuli was reduced by limiting frequencies to two extremely narrow bands that each consisted of high-pass and low-pass slopes of 115 dB/octave that met at 370 Hz (for the low frequency band) and 6,000 Hz (for the high frequency band). These were presented at matched moderate levels that peaked at a combined level at about 70 dB. Scores for the correct identification of the words used for scoring intelligibility for the four types of dual-band speech stimuli in the absence of added noise are shown in Figure 6.8 by the open circles. When noise at 60 dB was added to the spectral gap separating the two speech bands, intelligibility as shown by the filled circles in the figure, was increased by 50 percent or more for each of the speech stimuli. Additional experiments in this study determined the effect of the amplitude and bandwidth of the interpolated noise on intelligibility.

Of course, the presence of noise in the spectral gap provides no additional linguistic information – it merely facilitates the integration of information present in the widely separated spectral regions. A broad spectral gap does not occur normally in speech, and any resulting tendency to treat the individual speech bands as issuing from separate sources could inhibit maximal utilization of the available information. Perhaps stimulation of the auditory lacuna

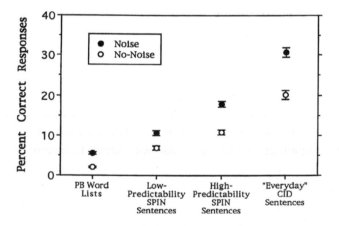

Figure 6.8 Spectral restoration: effects of adding noise at a fixed level and bandwidth to the spectral gap separating two very narrow bands located at opposite extremes of the speech spectrum (center frequencies of 370 Hz and 6,000 Hz). The four types of speech stimuli varied in the extent of linguistic information available for lexical identification. Separate groups of 20 or 24 subjects were used for each stimulus condition. Mean percent accuracy scores and their standard errors are shown. (From Warren, Hainsworth, Brubaker, *et al.*, 1997.)

with noise could reduce this inhibition. Additional experiments in the same study demonstrated that noise levels even 30 dB below the peak speech levels enhanced intelligibility. Maximum intelligibility occurred with a noise 10 dB below the peak level of the speech; higher noise levels decreased intelligibility despite the prior adjustment of the noise bandwidth to compensate for the increased spectral spread of peripheral masking. It appears that when the amplitude of concurrent noise approached that of the speech, an interference with the processing of speech occurred at a central level. This central interference associated with extraneous auditory activity may be a factor contributing to the difficulty of comprehending speech in noisy environments.

Masking and unmasking

Although masking seems to be an apt term for describing the perceptual obliteration of one sound by another, considering temporal induction or spectral restoration as the unmasking of portions of a signal can be misleading. Unmasking suggests drawing aside a curtain of noise to reveal the presence of an intact signal. But the truly masked signal is no more, and any restoration should be considered a recreation or perceptual synthesis of the contextually appropriate sound involving the central nervous system. There have been a few attempts to examine the neurological bases for human temporal induction. Husain, Lozito, Ulloa, and Horwitz (2005) proposed a neurological model for temporal induction involving the auditory cortex which was in agreement with behavioral data, and Micheyl, Carlyon, Shtyrov, Hauk, *et al.* (2003) employed the mismatch negativity component of auditory event-related potentials and obtained results indicating that the illusion of continuity can occur outside the focus of attention.

This chapter has demonstrated that restoration of speech fragments follows rules governing the restoration of portions of nonverbal signals. In Chapter 5, we have seen that sequences consisting solely of phonemes, tones, and arbitrarily selected unrelated sounds follow common rules, and the next chapter on speech will attempt to show how linguistic skills are superimposed upon general auditory principles.

Suggestions for further reading

For additional studies on the heterophonic induction of dynamic signals,
see: Ciocca, V., and Bregman, A. S. 1987. Perceived continuity of gliding and steady-state tones through interrupting noise. *Perception and Psychophysics*, **42**, 476–484.

Dannenbring, G. L. 1976. Perceived auditory continuity with alternately rising and falling frequency transitions. *Canadian Journal of Psychology*, **30**, 99–114.

Sasaki, T. 1980. Sound restoration and temporal localization of noise in speech and music sounds. *Tohuku Pschologica Folia*, **39**, 79–88.

7

Speech

Earlier chapters dealing with nonlinguistic auditory perception treated humans as receivers and processors of acoustic information. But when dealing with speech perception, it is necessary also to consider humans as generators of acoustic signals. The two topics of speech production and speech perception are closely linked, as we shall see.

We shall deal first with the generation of speech sounds and the nature of the acoustic signals. The topic of speech perception will then be described in relation to general principles, which are applicable to nonspeech sounds as well as to speech. Finally, the topic of special characteristics and mechanisms employed for the perception of speech will be examined.

Speech production

The structures used for producing speech have evolved from organs that served other functions in our prelinguistic ancestors and still perform nonlinguistic functions in humans.

It is convenient to divide the system for production of speech into three regions (see Figure 7.1). The subglottal system delivers air under pressure to the larynx (located within the Adam's apple) which contains a pair of vocal folds (also called vocal cords). The opening between the vocal folds is called the glottis, and the rapid opening and closing of the glottal slit interrupts the air flow, resulting in a buzz-like sound. The buzz is then spectrally shaped to form speech sounds or phonemes by the supralaryngeal vocal tract having the larynx at one end and the lips and the nostrils at the other. In addition to modifying the laryngeal buzz, the vocal tract is also used to produce noises and plosive sounds with phonetic significance.

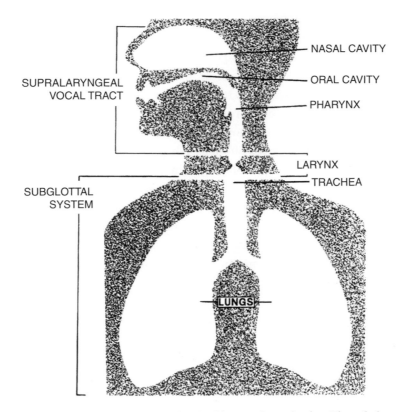

Figure 7.1 Anatomical structures involved in speech production. The subglottal system delivers air under pressure to the larynx. The vocal folds in the larynx are capable of generating broadband sounds. The supraglottal system can spectrally shape the sound produced in the larynx by altering dimensions along the vocal tract, and by opening or closing access to the nasal passages. The supraglottal system is also capable of adding some hisses and pops of its own.

The subglottal system

The glottis remains open during normal breathing without phonation. Inhalation is accomplished through expansion of the chest cavity, largely through contraction of the diaphragm and the external intercostal muscles. Exhalation is accomplished mainly through elastic recoil when the contraction of the muscles used for inhalation ceases. However, during more active breathing, including that accompanying speaking, the passive compression of air in the lungs following active inhalation is supplemented by contraction of the internal intercostal and abdominal muscles. The air passes from the lungs through the windpipe or trachea up to the larynx. During speaking, the subglottal pressure is traditionally described as equivalent to about 5 to 10 cm of water (that is, equal to the force per unit area exerted by a water column of this height), although during very loud shouting it can rise to the equivalent of 60 cm of water. The average flow rates of air while speaking are roughly 150 to 200 cm^3/s, and since the average inhalation during speech is about 500 to 800 cm^3, about 3 to 5 s of speech or about 10 to 15 words are produced by a single breath in normal speech. Delicate muscular control of the subglottal pressure and flow rate appropriate to particular articulatory gestures is essential for generating the normal amplitude patterns of speech.

Production of all English phonemes is powered by subglottal compression of air. However, there are languages in which some of the phonemes are produced by different means. A rapid downward movement of the closed glottis is used to create implosive phonemes in some American Indian and African languages, and an upward movement of the closed glottis can be used to produce "ejective" pops and hisses with phonetic significance. Movements of the tongue to suck air into the mouth are used to produce clicks in several languages of southern Africa.

The larynx

The larynx is homologous with a valve that protects the lungs of the lungfish from flooding, and is used generally for phonation or sound production by terrestrial vertebrates (Negus, 1949). The human larynx is at the top of the trachea and houses vocal folds consisting of two strips of ligaments and muscles attached to a firm cartilagenous support. During swallowing, the epiglottis moves down to seal off the larynx as solid and liquid material is moved into the esophagus. During normal breathing without phonation, the glottal opening between the vocal folds remains in a half-open position, although it can be opened more fully during rapid intake of breath. During voicing or phonation, the vocal folds open and close rhythmically to produce puffs of air. These puffs correspond to a buzz-like periodic sound which furnishes the raw acoustic substrate from which vowels and voiced consonants are shaped. The harmonic components of the buzz decrease in amplitude with increasing frequency, so that there is roughly equal power per octave. During whispering, the vocal folds are kept in a nearly closed position, creating turbulence that produces a hiss-like sound, which is shaped by the supraglottal region in the same manner as the glottal buzz of voiced sounds. Whispered speech also can be produced by other constrictions leading to hisses at positions near the laryngeal end of the vocal tract.

The opening and closing of the vocal folds are not synchronous with muscle twitches, as once thought by some investigators but, rather, follow from the effects of rapid air flow through the glottis. During normal phonation, prevoicing changes in muscle tension cause the vocal folds to move close together.

The increase in the velocity of air moving through this constricted passage produces a drop in air pressure, and Bernoulli's principle (that is, an increase in a fluid's velocity causes a decrease in its pressure) causes the vocal folds to be drawn together, and to close. The closure results in a build-up of subglottal pressure, forcing the vocal folds open, releasing a puff of air which causes the cycle to repeat for as long as phonation is maintained.

Much information about the operation of the vocal folds has been obtained by direct observation. By placing a mirror at the appropriate angle at the back of the throat, it is possible both to illuminate and to view glottal configurations. Since movements are rapid during phonation, a succession of pictures taken at high speed has been useful in studying the cycle of opening and closing during voicing.

The rate at which the glottis opens and closes is the voice's fundamental frequency, and determines the pitch. The rate of glottal vibration is under the control of several sets of muscles which can raise the pitch by stretching and hence increasing the tension of the vocal folds. The intensity of the voice can be controlled by changing both the subglottal pressure and the portion of the glottal period during which the vocal cords are open. Decreasing the portion of the cycle during which the vocal folds are open results in a louder sound as well as a change in quality associated with a greater vocal effort.

The fundamental frequency of the voice is about 120 Hz for an adult male and about 250 Hz for an adult female. Children may have fundamental frequencies as high as 400 Hz. The low frequency in adult males is associated with thickening and lengthening of the vocal folds resulting from hormonal changes occurring at puberty. The range of frequencies employed in speech by male and female adults is usually a little more than one octave, with a modal frequency about 1/3-octave above the lower limit of this range.

The trained voice of a singer exhibits exceptionally fine control of pitch, loudness, and quality of phonation. There are three sets of intrinsic laryngeal muscles, which are "synergistic" in terms of fundamental frequency and intensity (Hirano, Ohala, and Vennard, 1969); while untrained people often change intensity when they change their fundamental frequency, trained singers can alter intensity and frequency independently. Singers deliberately introduce an instability or periodic fluctuation in pitch called the vibrato, which is centered upon the frequency corresponding to the sung note. (The usual rate of this fluctuation is about six or seven per second, and the frequency excursion as large as one semitone.) Interestingly, the pitch extracted by a listener from this rapid succession of glissandi involves not a moment-by-moment evaluation but, rather, an averaging over time (in keeping with the obligatory perceptual integration of events during this time period, as described in Chapter 3). The almost universal use of the vibrato in singing is a fairly recent development in our culture: as late as the nineteenth century, the ability to sing notes with a fixed pitch was an admired ability of trained singers. Vibrato is not the only vocal ornamentation used by operatic singers: they occasionally use tremolo which consists of an irregular amplitude modulation superimposed upon the frequency modulation of the vibrato to convey particular emotional moods.

Trained singers usually are capable of producing a range of pitches well beyond that used in speech. In order to cover this range, they employ a number of different production modes, each corresponding to a different "register." Thus, the falsetto register (used by male singers in reaching their highest notes) involves a tensing of the vocal folds so that only a portion of the edges vibrate. The "laryngeal whistle" register (used by female singers in reaching their highest notes) does not involve vibration of the vocal folds, but instead, a whistle is produced by air passing through a small opening in the otherwise closed vocal folds. One of the goals of voice training is to permit transitions between different registers to be made smoothly and, ideally, without the listener being able to detect a discontinuity in the passage from one production mode to another. A trained soprano may be able to cover the range of fundamental frequencies from 130 through 2,000 Hz by employing the so-called "chest register" below 300 Hz, the "head voice" from about 300 to 1,000 Hz, the "little register" from about 1,000 to 1,500 Hz, and the "whistle register" above 1,500 Hz. (For a discussion of the various registers and theories concerning their production see Deinse, 1981.)

Although people are quite unaware of the mechanisms employed for changing pitch in speaking, it might be thought that singers would have insight into their methods for pitch change, since so much time and effort is devoted to studying and practicing pitch control. Yet, only a rather vague and ambiguous vocabulary is available for describing the registers and qualities of the singing voice. The location of the muscles employed and their exquisitely delicate control through acoustic, tactile, and proprioceptive (muscular) feedback is accomplished with little or no direct knowledge on the part of the performer, providing an example of what Polanyi (1958, 1968) has called "tacit knowledge." However, the ability to describe and to respond to instructions concerning the positions and movements of the articulatory organs increases as we move upward along the airstream from the larynx to the tongue tip and lips. The basis for this increasing awareness will be discussed later when we deal with the perceptual status of the phoneme.

The vocal tract and articulation of speech sounds

The buzz produced by the larynx becomes speech only after being modified by its passage through the vocal tract. During this trip, phonemes are formed by the spectral shaping of the laryngeal buzz, and by obstructing the airflow. A highly simplified model of the vocal tract considers it to be a tube, like an organ pipe, which is open at one end. In a male, the length of this tube is about 17.5 cm. As an initial simplifying approximation, this tube can be considered to have a uniform cross-section. The lowest resonant frequency of such a tube has a wavelength four times the tube length, corresponding to about 500 Hz for a male. Those spectral components of the broadband laryngeal source having frequencies of about 500 Hz are increased in intensity by this resonance to produce the first formant band. Additional resonances occur in the tube at odd-numbered integral multiples of the first formant, so that the second formant is at 1,500 Hz, and the third formant at 2,500 Hz. The vocal tracts of women are somewhat shorter, and the wavelengths associated with their corresponding formants are on the average about 80 to 85 percent of the male's. Formants are associated with standing waves (which correspond to fixed regions of high and low pressure), with all formants having one pressure maximum at the glottis and one pressure minimum at the lips. The first formant has only this one maximum and minimum, the second formant one additional maximum and minimum, and the third formant two additional maxima and minima, each spaced regularly along the uniform tube in this simplified model of the vocal tract.

Of course, the vocal tract is not a uniform tube. The length of the tube can be changed by movement of portions of the tract and, in addition, cavities and constrictions can be created at the back of the throat and within the mouth. A decrease in cross-sectional area at a region of a formant's pressure-amplitude minimum lowers the formant's frequency, whereas an increase in area at this region raises its frequency. Corresponding cross-sectional changes at places of pressure maxima have the opposite effect in changing the formant's frequency.

Vowels differ in the frequencies and relative intensities of their formants. Figure 7.2 shows the complex positional adjustments of the highly flexible tongue that must be learned in order to produce the vowels that are shown. The procedure of preceding the vowel by /h/ and following it by /d/ minimizes the influence of adjacent phonemes by coarticulation, and produces vowels much like those produced in isolation. Table 7.1 gives the formant frequencies for the vowels shown in Figure 7.2 as measured by Peterson and Barney (1952) for men, women, and children. The words used in speaking the vowels are given above their phonetic symbols. The single vowels shown are sometimes called monophthongs to distinguish them from diphthongs consisting of a pair such as /iu/ occurring in the word "few."

Several cycles of a periodic sound such as a vowel are necessary to establish the fundamental and the line spectrum (see Figure 1.3.1), and so it might be

Table 7.1 *Averages of fundamental and formant frequencies and formant amplitudes of vowels by 33 men, 28 women, and 15 children*

		heed i	hid ɪ	head ɛ	had æ	hod ɑ	hawed ɔ	hood ʊ	who'd u
Fundamental frequencies (Hz)									
	M	136	135	130	127	124	129	137	141
	W	235	232	223	210	212	216	232	231
	Ch	272	269	260	251	256	263	276	274
Formant frequencies (Hz)									
F_1	M	270	390	530	660	730	570	440	300
	W	310	430	610	860	850	590	470	370
	Ch	370	530	690	1010	1030	680	560	430
F_2	M	2290	1990	1840	1720	1090	840	1020	870
	W	2790	2480	2330	2050	1220	920	1160	950
	Ch	3200	2730	2610	2320	1370	1060	1410	1170
F_3	M	3010	2550	2480	2410	2440	2410	2240	2240
	W	3310	3070	2990	2850	2810	2710	2680	2670
	Ch	3730	3600	3570	3320	3170	3180	3310	3260
Formant amplitudes (dB)									
L_1		-4	-3	-2	-1	-1	0	-1	-3
L_2		-24	-23	-17	-12	-5	-7	-12	-19
L_3		-28	-27	-24	-22	-28	-34	-34	-43

From Peterson and Barney, 1952.

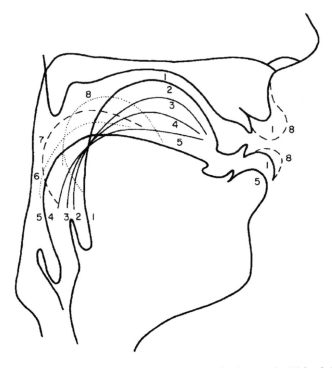

Figure 7.2 Tongue positions for vowels in the words: (1) *heed*, (2) *hid*, (3) *head*, (4) *had*, (5) *hod*, (6) *hawed*, (7) *hood*, (8) *who'd*. (From MacNeilage and Ladefoged, 1976.)

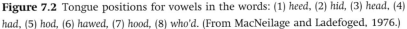

thought that a vowel could not be identified from a single glottal pulse. However, there have been reports that single glottal pulses, and even segments excised from single pulses, can be used to identify vowels with accuracy not much below that found for extended statements (Gray, 1942; Moore and Mundie, 1971). Vowel recognition from a single pulse (or portions of that pulse) probably is based upon the distribution of spectral power in bands corresponding to the formants of extended vowel statements. Observations in our laboratory have indicated that conditions resembling those producing temporal induction (see Chapter 6) can enhance the vowel-like characteristics of a single glottal pulse and facilitate its recognition. The procedure works well when the glottal pulse is preceded and followed by 1 second bursts of pink noise (that is, noise with equal power per octave) separated from the glottal pulse by no more than 5 ms of silence, and presented at a level about 10 dB above that corresponding to the extended statement of the vowel from which the single pulse was excised.

Table 7.2 lists the English consonants by place and manner of articulation. All consonants involve some type of obstruction of the vocal tract. When accompanied by glottal vibration, they are voiced; otherwise they are

Table 7.2 *Classification of English consonants by place and manner of articulation*

Place of articulation	Stops		Fricatives		Nasals		Glides and laterals	
	Voiceless	Voiced	Voiceless	Voiced	Voiceless	Voiced	Voiceless	Voiced
Labial	[p] (p̱in)	[b] (ḇin)				[m] (sum̱)	[hw] (w̱hat)	[w] (w̱ill)
Labiodental			[f] (f̱ine)	[v] (v̱ine)				
Dental			[θ] (ṯẖigh)	[ð] (ṯẖy)				
Alveolar	[t] (ṯin)	[d] (ḏin)	[s] (s̱ip)	[z] (ẕip)		[n] (suṉ)		[l] (ḻess)
Palatal	[tʃ] (c̱ẖar)	[dʒ] (j̱ar)	[ʃ] (s̱ẖip)	[ʒ] (aẕure)				[r] (ṟim)
								[j] (y̱es)
Velar	[k] (ḵilt)	[g] (g̱ilt)				[ŋ] (suṉg̱)		
Glottal			[h] (ẖill)					

Based on Zemlin, 1998.

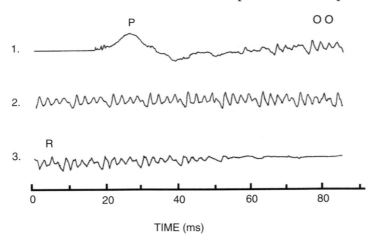

Figure 7.3 Waveform of the word "poor." Three successive 85 ms segments are shown. (From Fletcher, 1953.)

unvoiced. Places of articulation are the lips (labial), teeth (dental), gums (alveolar), hard palate (palatal), soft palate or velum (velar), and vocal folds or glottis (glottal). Stop consonants involve complete closure of the vocal tract. When the closure is followed by an audible release of air it is sometimes called a stop plosive or, simply, plosive. The length of time between the hiss-like release of air and the onset of voicing (the "voice-onset time") can determine whether a stop consonant is considered voiceless or voiced. Incomplete closure results in a fricative. When a stop is followed by a fricative, an affricative is produced (such as /tʃ/ in "choice" and /dʒ/ in "judge"). The glides /r/, /w/, /j/, and /l/ are produced by rapid articulatory movements and have characteristics in some ways intermediate between those of consonants and vowels. The nasal consonants are generated by blocking the passage of air through the mouth at the places characteristic of the consonant (see Table 7.2), while lowering the velum to permit release of air through the nasal passages.

Visual representation of speech sounds

The most direct way of representing the acoustic nature of speech is through its waveform. The waveform describes pressure changes over time. By construction of devices that record these changes in some mechanical, magnetic, or digital fashion, we can use this record to recreate a more or less perfect copy of the original sound. Figure 7.3 shows the waveform corresponding to the word "poor."

Although visual representations of waveforms can accurately depict the acoustic signal, they are of little use in identifying speech sounds. One reason is that the waveforms do not reveal the component harmonics or formants in any recognizable fashion. Waveforms of complex sounds do not correspond to the pattern of stimulation at any receptor site, since stimulation takes place only after segregation of spectral components. It is possible to give an approximate description of the pattern of acoustic stimulation at individual receptor sites along the organ of Corti using multiple tracings corresponding to the output of a bank of bandpass filters representing successive critical bands. Such tracings have some use in studying the perception of periodic sounds, as was discussed in Chapter 3 and illustrated in Figures 3.9, 3.11, 3.13, and 3.18. However, such a depiction of speech would be quite cumbersome, and would represent only a rough approximation of local stimulus patterns. A more convenient and conventional depiction (but one that does not take into account critical bandwidths), is produced by a sound spectrograph.

The sound spectrograph was developed at Bell Telephone Laboratories during the early 1940s. The device consists of a series of narrow-band filters that are used successively to scan repetitions of a recorded speech sample. A sound spectrogram shows three variables: time is shown along the horizontal axis, frequency along the vertical axis, and intensity by the darkness of the tracing. Figure 7.4(a) shows a spectrogram of the phrase "to catch pink salmon." The formants of vowels are seen as dark horizontal bars. The silences of the stop consonants are shown as the vertical blank areas, and the fricative consonants correspond to the dark regions lacking discrete bars.

A group of workers at Haskins Laboratory developed a "pattern playback" which can optically scan a sound spectrogram and recreate the original sounds. Using this device, one can hand paint patterns on a transparent base and play back the optical pattern to produce intelligible speech. Hand-painted versions shown in Figure 7.4(b) were produced by first drawing the most obvious features of the original and then modifying the patterns while listening to the results until, usually by trial and error, the simplified drawn spectrograms were fairly intelligible. In the example shown in Figure 7.4, both the original and the hand-painted versions could be used with the pattern playback to produce an understandable acoustic rendition of "to catch pink salmon." Pattern playback not only permits editing of sound spectrograms to determine which components are necessary for intelligibility, but also permits synthesis of acoustic patterns with desired characteristics. Although this device has provided useful information and is of value in illustrating the acoustic features of importance to speech perception, today computer software allows us to synthesize and analyze speech with considerably greater ease and flexibility.

In the early years of the sound spectrogram's use, it was hoped that it would provide a "visual speech" permitting deaf individuals to see and comprehend

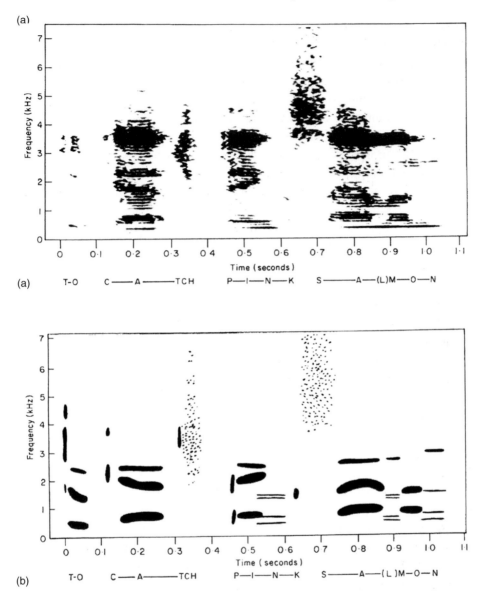

(a)

(a)   T-O   C——A———TCH   P—I—N—K   S———A—(L)M—O—N

(b)   T-O   C——A———TCH   P—I—N—K   S———A—(L)M—O—N

Figure 7.4 (a) Sound spectrogram of a phrase; (b) simplified version of the same phrase, painted by hand. Both of these versions were intelligible after conversion to sound by the "pattern-playback" device. (From Liberman, Delattre, and Cooper, 1952.)

spoken words as much as they can written words (see Potter, Kopp, and Kopp, 1947). However, sound spectrograms have proved disappointingly difficult to read as a succession of identifiable phonemes interpretable as words, even with considerable training. One reason for this difficulty appears to be the interaction of phonemes in normal speech. The statement has been made by an investigator having a great deal of experience using spectrograms that "as a matter of fact I have not met one single speech researcher who has claimed he could read speech spectrograms fluently, and I am no exception myself" (Fant, 1962). Samples of single vowels produced in isolation or by careful choice of neighboring sounds in monosyllables (such as /h*d/, where * represents the vowel) can be characterized and identified relatively easily using spectrograms; but, in running speech, the boundaries between phonemes are often lost, and the acoustic nature of a speech sound is found to be influenced greatly by the nature of the neighboring sounds. The coarticulation effect of one speech sound upon another can extend not only to the neighboring speech sounds, but for a few phonemes before and after its occurrence. It has been suggested that such context-sensitive allophones (acoustic variants of the same phoneme) may enhance identification of the brief phonemic components of speech by providing information concerning more than one phoneme simultaneously (Wickelgren, 1969). However, as will be discussed subsequently, there is the possibility that phonemic segmentation is not required for the identification of syllables and words.

It is evident that coarticulation does not interfere with either comprehension of speech or the identification of constituent phonemes by listeners. Why then does coarticulation appear to make the reading of sound spectrograms so difficult? One possible explanation is that we have had many thousands of hours practice listening to speech, and a tremendous amount of practice in reading spectrograms may be required before we could achieve comprehension comparable to that of speech that is heard. In support of this explanation, fairly good performance (although still not matching auditory perception of speech) has been reported for an individual having an estimated 2,000 to 2,500 hours practice reading sound spectrograms (Cole, Rudnicky, Zue, and Reddy, 1980). However, it also is possible that acoustic cues playing important roles in the auditory perception of speech are not apparent in the visual display provided by sound spectrograms.

Intelligibility of sentences heard through narrow spectral slits

In an experiment by Bashford, Riener, and Warren (1992) dealing with the intelligibility of bandpassed sentences interrupted by bandpassed noise, it was noted that one of the control conditions employing intact narrow-band speech had a surprisingly high intelligibility. These bandpassed sentences had high-pass and low-pass slopes (48 dB/octave) intersecting at 1,500 Hz, yet despite the extremely limited frequency range and the spectral tilts of the intersecting filter slopes, over 95 percent of the keywords could be identified. A search of the literature indicated that no systematic study of intelligibility of bandpass sentences heard in the clear (that is, without interfering noise) had been reported. We decided that it would be of interest to determine the extent of spectral information needed to understand everyday speech.

In our first detailed study of the intelligibility of narrow-band sentences, Warren, Riener, Bashford, and Brubaker (1995) employed Central Institute of the Deaf (CID) "everyday speech" sentences (Silverman and Hirsh, 1955) and determined their intelligibility when heard through narrow spectral slits. Steep filter slopes were employed (roughly 100 dB/octave) with two band-widths (1/3-octave and 1/20-octave). Separate groups of 20 subjects (each presented with the same 100 CID sentences containing a total of 500 keywords) were used for the nine center frequencies employed with each bandwidth. The results are shown in Figure 7.5. It can be seen that very little spectral information is required to identify the keywords in the "everyday speech" sentences. Close to perfect intelligibility was obtained for 1/3-octave bands with center frequencies in the vicinity of 1,500 Hz. Even with bands having a nominal bandwidth of 1/20-octave (produced by filter slopes of 115 dB/octave meeting at the center frequency), a score of better than 75 percent was achieved for a center frequency of 1,500 Hz. This relatively high intelligibility occurred on the basis of information present along the filter slopes, despite their severe spectral tilt, and the absence of spectral information necessary for discriminating between speech sounds and individual words when heard in

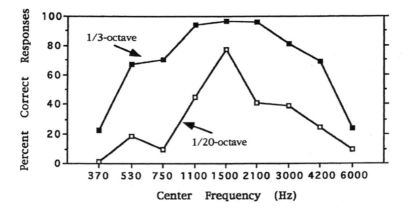

Figure 7.5 Effect of bandwidth on intelligibility: percentage of keywords reported correctly for "everyday speech" sentences presented as nominal 1/3-octave bands (transition-band slopes 96 dB/octave) and as nominal 1/20-octave bands (transition-band slopes 115 dB/octave). (From Warren, Riener, Bashford, and Brubaker, 1995.)

188   Speech

isolation. It appears that "top-down" information remaining in the spectrally impoverished sentences permitted identification of lexical components that could not be recognized on their own.

As can be seen in Figure 7.5, the 1/20-octave bands centered at 370 Hz and 6,000 Hz had very low intelligibilities. However, when Warren *et al.* presented both of these bands together, the intelligibility rose to more than double the sum of the intelligibility of each of the bands when presented alone, indicating that information in the two bands was being integrated in a super-additive fashion despite the wide frequency separation.

The high intelligibility obtained with a triangular band consisting solely of slopes of approximately 100 dB/octave demonstrated that transition band slopes steeper than those achievable with analog filters would be needed to separate the contributions made by passbands and transition bands. By using digital FIR (finite impulse response) filtering it is possible to produce extremely steep slopes while leaving the passband intact. Warren and Bashford (1999) used FIR filtering to produce high-pass and low-pass slopes averaging 1,000 dB/octave that were used to isolate the passband and transition bands of one of the 1/3-octave bands shown in Figure 7.5. The original band was centered on 1,500 Hz, and had transition-band slopes of approximately 100 dB/octave. When

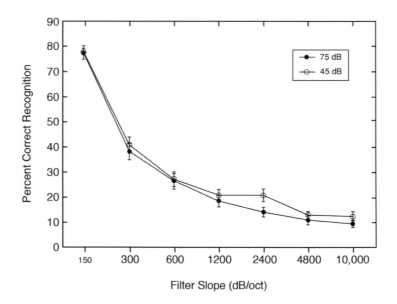

Figure 7.6 Effect of filter-band slopes upon intelligibility. Means and standard errors for intelligibilities of 1/3-octave bands of "everyday" sentences centered on 1,500 Hz and having transition-band slopes adjusted to values ranging from 150 to 10,000 dB/octave. Sentences were presented to two separate groups of 35 listeners at slow rms peak levels of either 45 or 75 dB. (From Warren, Bashford, and Lenz, 2004.)

intact, the 1/3-octave band had an intelligibility of over 95 percent, and following separation, the 1/3-octave passband with slopes averaging 1,000 dB/octave had an intelligibility of only 24 percent, and the two transition bands separated by a 1/3-octave gap had the much higher intelligibility of 82 percent. However, there was no assurance that the slopes of 1,000 dB/octave flanking the passband were steep enough to remove all transition band contributions.

An experiment by Warren, Bashford, and Lenz (2004) used FIR filtering and systematically increased the slopes until asymptotic intelligibility was reached for the nominal 1/3-octave band used by Warren and Bashford (1999). As shown in Figure 7.6, matched high-pass and low-pass slopes of 4,800 dB/octave were needed to produce effectively rectangular passbands having an intelligibility of 12 percent. Even with slopes of 1,200 dB/octave the score was 20 percent, well above that of rectangular bands.

Intelligibilities of passbands heard singly and together

The relative contributions to speech perception made by different regions of the spectrum have been of major interest for a long time, both for theory and for practical concerns (e.g., telephony, computer speech recognition, hearing aids, cochlear implants, and architectural acoustics). In the early and mid twentieth century, researchers at Bell Telephone Laboratories became involved in studying the relative intelligibilities of passbands spanning the speech spectrum. An obvious reason for this interest was its use in telephony, but their interest went far beyond that. As part of their research, they wished to be able to determine the intelligibility of 1/3-octave and 1-octave bands of speech heard singly and in combination. However, there was a major impediment to achieving this goal at that time. It was recognized that intelligibility of a particular band was determined not only by center frequency and bandwidth, but also by information in the flanking transition bands (filter slopes) produced by filtering. (In 1960, Kryter estimated that frequencies as far as 30 dB down the filter slopes might contribute to intelligibility.) Since the analog audio filters available at that time could not produce slopes steep enough to eliminate transition band contributions without introducing unacceptable passband distortion, an ingenious procedure was developed that could lead to estimates of passband intelligibilities spanning the speech spectrum by canceling out the contributions of slopes. This was accomplished by combining intelligibility scores of high-pass and low-pass speech having graded cut-offs that covered the range of frequencies contributing to intelligibility. Ceiling intelligibilities were avoided by partially masking the speech by the addition of noise. Computations were rather complex, and worksheets for calculating relative importance values of passbands spanning the speech spectrum were published as the Articulation Index (AI) by the American National Standards Institute (ANSI, 1969/1986). These importance values represented the proportion of the total broadband information contained within a given band. The importance values of adjacent bands can be combined, and by application of an appropriate transfer function, the intelligibility of single passbands and multiple contiguous (but not separated) passbands can be estimated. Subsequently, the AI was updated (ANSI S3.5, 1997/ 2007) and renamed the Speech Intelligibility Index (SII). The basic AI/SII procedure has been used by the Speech Transmission Index (Steeneken and Houtgast, 1980, 2002) with modified calculations to compensate for distortions such as reverberation. The Speech Recognition Sensitivity Model (Müsch and Buus, 2001a, 2001b) also used modified AI/SII calculations to compensate for estimates of intelligibility scores of bands that were either too high or too low based upon slopes and the bands' relative positions.

The basic AI/SII procedure for estimating passband intelligibilities has been accepted as a standard and used widely over the years. However, the ability to eliminate contributions from transition bands (see Figure 7.6) led to a study demonstrating that direct measurement could provide an alternative to the AI/ SII procedure for estimating passband intelligibilities. Warren, Bashford, and Lenz (2005) employed a "low-predictability" list of sentences, and used FIR filtering to produce six 1-octave rectangular passbands that covered the range of frequencies making appreciable contributions to speech intelligibility (center frequencies of 0.25, 0.5, 1, 2, 4, and 8 kHz). The slopes employed were 3.2 dB/Hz which were sufficient to remove contributions from transition bands (increasing slopes to 8.0 dB/Hz produced no significant change in any of the passband intelligibilities). Table 7.3 provides the results obtained for measurements of the intelligibilities of these individual bands along with the intelligibility scores obtained for each of their 15 possible pairings. The extents of synergy or redundancy are also shown for the pairs, whether they were contiguous or separated. The synergy/redundancy scores were based on the assumption that the error probabilities (one minus proportion correct) for the two bands were independent and multiplicative. All dual bands were found to exhibit synergy.

The protean phoneme

As we have seen, a phoneme can assume different forms that are determined, to a great degree, by the identity of the neighboring speech sounds. This has led to what Klatt (1979) has called the "acoustic-phonetic non-invariance problem." If phonemes have a perceptual reality, they might be

Table 7.3 *Intelligibilities of individual rectangular 1-octave passbands spanning the speech spectrum and their synergistic or redundant interactions when paired*
The dark diagonal boxes show the intelligibility scores and standard errors for the six 1-octave rectangular passbands when heard alone. The boxes to the left of the diagonal show the dual-band intelligibility scores and standard errors (in parentheses) for all 15 possible pairings of the six bands. The boxes to the right of the diagonal show the percentage difference (Δ%) between the dual-band scores and the predicted scores based on the scores of the two component bands when heard alone; $+\Delta$% values indicate synergy, $-\Delta$% values (none found) would indicate redundancy, for further details see text.

	0.25 kHz	0.5 kHz	1 kHz	2 kHz	4 kHz	8 kHz
8 kHz	9.2% (1.0)	40.7% (2.5)	68.1% (2.2)	71.2% (2.3)	23.5% (1.3)	6.8% (1.7)
4 kHz	17.9% (1.3)	66.8% (1.5)	82.5% (1.5)	75.6% (2.3)	16.8.6% (1.5)	$\Delta+5$%
2 kHz	65.6% (2.4)	89.9% (1.0)	90.0% (1.1)	54.8% (3.3)	$\Delta+21$%	$\Delta+23$%
1 kHz	50.8% (1.4)	71.3% (1.3)	38.8% (2.5)	$\Delta+24$%	$\Delta+69$%	$\Delta+59$%
0.5 kHz	18.5% (1.3)	16.8% (1.5)	$\Delta+45$%	$\Delta+44$%	$\Delta+122$%	$\Delta+81$%
0.25 kHz	0.0% (0.0)	$\Delta+10$%	$\Delta+31$%	$\Delta+20$%	$\Delta+1$%	$\Delta+35$%

Based on Warren, Bashford, and Lenz, 2005.

expected to possess some acoustic characteristics, or cluster of characteristics, that serve to differentiate one phoneme from another. However, despite careful searches for such phonetic invariance, it has not been possible to find convincing evidence of its existence for all phonemes.

Individual plosive consonants are especially difficult to characterize in terms of acoustically invariant properties. They cannot be produced in isolation, and when articulated with a vowel to form a consonant-vowel syllable, sound spectrograms indicate that their acoustic forms are determined by adjacent vowels. Figure 7.7 shows spectrogram patterns which can be played back to produce syllables corresponding to /di/ and /du/. It can be seen that in /di/, the second formant rises from about 2,200 to 2,600 Hz, while in /du/ it falls from about 1,200 to 700 Hz. When the formant transitions are heard in isolation without the subsequent portion corresponding to the vowels, the frequency glides of the plosives resemble whistles or glissandos rather than speech sounds.

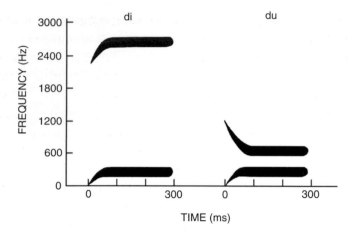

Figure 7.7 Spectrographic patterns sufficient for the perception of /d/ before /i/ and before /u/ when converted to sound. Note that the frequency transitions of the stop consonants (which have durations less than 100 ms) are not perceived as such, but can be heard as chirps when separated from the rest of the diphones. (From Liberman, Cooper, Shankweiler, and Studdert-Kennedy, 1967.)

In the 1960s, there were attempts to save the acoustically elusive phoneme by considering it to be closely related to speech production. According to the motor theory of speech perception (Liberman, Cooper, Shankweiler, and Studdert-Kennedy, 1967) as revised by Liberman and Mattingly (1985), phonetic analysis is accomplished by a specialized "module" that interprets the afferent auditory signal in terms of the efferent motor commands necessary to produce the phonemes. Since, as shown in Figure 7.7, acoustic invariance is not a necessary concomitant of motor invariance, the theory appears to handle the perceptual equivalence of acoustically different allophones. However, MacNeilage (1970) has presented evidence that as a result of coarticulation, electromyographic (muscle) recordings made during the production of phonemes in different contexts have indicated that the articulatory gestures corresponding to particular phonemes lack motor invariance. This complication was met by Liberman and Mattingly (1985) by considering that it is "the intended gestures of the speaker that are the basis for phonetic categories" rather than "the peripheral realization of the gestures."

Analysis-by-synthesis (Stevens, 1960; Stevens and Halle, 1967; Halle and Stevens, 1972) also posits that there is a close relation between speech perception and production. It is considered that the auditory signal is subject to analysis in terms of distinctive features possessed by phonemes, such as those hypothesized in the feature systems of Chomsky and Halle (1968) or of Jakobson, Fant, and Halle (1963). This analysis permits generation of rules used for production of the sound. Hypotheses are then constructed based on these generative rules, and these hypotheses are used to construct an internal auditory pattern consisting of phonetic segments. This internal pattern is compared with the pattern produced by the acoustic input, and recognition results if the match is close. If the match is not close, new hypotheses and new internal patterns are generated for comparison with the patterns produced by the stimulus.

Although both analysis-by-synthesis and the motor theory of speech perception accept the existence of phonemes as perceptual entities, they do not require them to have an acoustic invariance. However, starting in the 1970s there have been several attempts to describe phonemes in terms of invariant aspects. A number of investigators have suggested that although many acoustic characteristics of phonemes vary with context, certain cues (not always apparent when looking at waveforms or spectrograms) are invariant and are used for phonemic identification (Stevens, 1971; Cole and Scott, 1974; Searle, Jacobson, and Rayment, 1979; Jusczyk, Smith, and Murphy, 1981; Stevens and Blumstein, 1981). Although it appears that some acoustic characteristics are invariant for some phonemes, it seems that definitive evidence for acoustic invariance of other phonemes, particularly the plosive consonants, is not available at present. Diehl (1981) has gone so far as to suggest that some evidence cited as supporting an acoustic invariance model actually provides evidence against this model.

A different type of invariance has been proposed for phonemic identification, based upon integrated responses from specialized neural analyzers operating as subphonemic feature detectors (Eimas and Corbit, 1973; Cooper, 1974). The difficulties encountered in specifying particular acoustic characteristics defining individual phonemes are met by considering identification of a phoneme to be based upon a set of characteristics analyzed by a set of hypothetical linguistic feature detectors. Claims of experimental support for this approach are based upon studies using "feature detector adaptation" in which listeners report apparent changes in a test stimulus occurring after repeated presentation of an adapting stimulus (for reviews of this work, see Eimas and Miller, 1978; Simon and Studdert-Kennedy, 1978; Cooper, 1979). The general rule found was that repetition caused category boundaries, such as the voice-onset time boundary (i.e., the duration of a noise burst preceding voicing) that separates perception of /t/ from /d/ to shift in the direction of the voice onset time of the repeated stimulus. These changes were attributed to the adaptation of linguistic feature detectors. However, several investigators have suggested that the effects of repetition are the consequence of general effects of auditory adaptation and fatigue applicable to both speech and nonspeech, so that there is no need to postulate the existence of specifically linguistic feature detectors (see Simon and Studdert-Kennedy, 1978; Elman, 1979; Rosen, 1979; Sawusch and Nusbaum, 1979; Diehl, 1981). It has also been suggested that changes in category boundaries need not be the consequence of adaptation or fatigue of any type of feature detector, but can reflect a general "criterion shift rule" that is applicable across sensory modalities (see Chapter 8). The rule has been expressed as follows: "If we are exposed to a stimulus having a particular level along a continuum of possible values, then the internal standards or criteria used for subsequent evaluations of other stimuli within this continuum are shifted in the direction of the exposure level" (Warren, 1985). In hearing, this simple principle applies to shifts in auditory medial plane localization (as described in Chapter 2), and to the pitch of sinusoidal tones (Cathcart and Dawson, 1928–1929; Christman, 1954). Criterion shifts, unlike adaptation or fatigue, may require the presence of contingent conditions. Thus Ganong (1976) reported amplitude-contingent category boundary shifts that required matching the amplitudes of "adaptor" and test syllables, indicating that separate linguistic feature detectors would be needed for the same syllable at different levels. Hall and Blumstein (1978) reported that it was not sufficient to have the same phonetic and syllabic structure for the "adaptor" and the test syllable – when other syllables were also present in the stimulus, the same arrangement of syllables was required for the effects attributed to detector adaptation of the test syllable to occur.

Before proceeding further with mechanisms for speech perception, it is necessary to look more deeply into the role of the phoneme as a perceptual unit. There can be little doubt that phonemes are extremely useful (and perhaps indispensable) constructs for the study of speech production and for linguistic analysis. However, as we have seen, perceptual models based on the recovery of phonemes from speech have run into difficulties, leading to questions concerning the role of phonemes in the perceptual organization of speech.

Are phonemes perceptual units?

The alphabet and the phoneme

The concept that speech can be analyzed into a sequence of phonemes can be traced back to alphabetic writing. Unlike other forms of writing, the alphabet appears to have been invented only once when it was used to transcribe the Semitic language spoken in northern Palestine and Syria about 3,700 years ago, and then used to construct the Phoenician, Hebrew, and Arabic alphabets. These early alphabets had systematic symbolic representation only for the consonants, but as these languages had many consonants and only a few vowels, this did not present a problem. Indeed, modern Hebrew and Arabic are usually written without symbols for vowels (although optional diacritic markings can be used for vowels). The Phoenician alphabet was used as a model by the Greeks about 3,000 years ago. The Greek language is richer in vowels, and vowel symbols were added to create the first complete alphabet. The alphabets used in Western languages are derived from the Greek.

In addition to requiring only a few graphemic symbols (26 in English compared to thousands in logographic systems such as Chinese), alphabetic writing is a how-to-produce description. Of course, modern English spelling differs considerably from modern English pronunciation, but it is still possible to pronounce an unfamiliar word from inspection of its written form with a fair chance of success.

Alphabetic writing has traditionally been considered as a phonological system, with each symbol representing a distinct sound. Thus, Bishop Berkeley (1732/ 1948) stated " … it is requisite that each word contain in it so many distinct characters as there are variations in the sound it stands for. Thus the single letter *a* is proper to mark one simple uniform sound; and the word *adultery* is accommodated to represent the sound annexed to it in the formation whereof there being eight different collisions or modifications of the air by the organs of speech, each of which produces a difference of sound, it was fit the word representing it should consist of as many distinct characters thereby to mark each particular difference or part of the whole sound." However, it is more accurate to consider the alphabetic symbols as representing articulatory gestures rather than sounds. The same gesture can produce different sounds (consider the different acoustic forms corresponding to the single acoustic gesture symbolized by "d" as represented in Figure 7.7). As we shall see, the confounding of graphemic symbols, speech sounds, articulatory gestures, and perceptual units employed in the perception of speech has resulted in much confusion.

One school of thought considers that the alphabetic system for segmenting speech is the recognition of a fact of nature, and that phonemes corresponding to this system are units employed by listeners for the comprehension of speech. Thus, Miller and Jusczyk (1989) stated "We take as the goal of a theory of speech perception an account of how the listener recovers the phonetic structure of an utterance from the acoustic signal during the course of language processing." However, there is a growing body of experimental evidence indicating that phonetic segmentation is not required for speech comprehension.

Illiterate adults cannot segment phonetically

Morais, Cary, Alegria, and Bertelson (1979) tested adults of "peasant origin" living in a poor agricultural region of Portugal. Half of these adults were illiterate (Group I), and the other half had some familiarity with reading following attendance in special classes for illiterates (Group R). Both groups were required either to add the sounds /m/, /p/ or /ʃ /, or to delete these sounds from utterances produced by the experimenter. It was found that Group I could neither delete nor add the designated speech sounds at the beginning of a nonsense word, while Group R had little difficulty with this task. Morais and his colleagues concluded that their results "clearly indicate that the ability to deal explicitly with the phonetic units of speech is not acquired spontaneously. Learning to read, whether in childhood or as an adult, evidently allows the ability to manifest itself." Subsequent studies have demonstrated that this link between literacy and the ability to identify and manipulate phonemes occurs in other languages using alphabetic writing systems. However, literacy in a nonalphabetic system does not help listeners' performance in tasks requiring phonetic segmentation. Thus, Chinese adults literate only in Chinese characters could not add or delete individual consonants in spoken Chinese words (Read, Zhang, Nie, and Ding, 1986).

Ability to segment phonetically and reading ability are related in children

Before learning to read, children can identify the number of syllables in a short utterance much better than they can the presence of an equal number of phonemes. Liberman, Shankweiler, Fischer, and Carter (1974) tested three groups of children in nursery school, kindergarten, and first grade (4-, 5-, and 6-year-olds) who listened to utterances containing one to three units (either syllables or phonemes depending on the "game") and then indicated by the number of taps on a table how many units were present. Each age group performed much better at syllabic segmentation than phonetic segmentation. Only the children five and six years of age had been receiving instruction in reading; and it was found that while no children could segment phonetically at four years of age, 17 percent could segment at age five, and 48 percent at age six.

A considerable number of studies demonstrate that the ability to associate letters with speech sounds is of great importance in achieving adequate reading skills (for reviews of this literature, see Goswami and Bryant, 1990; Brady and Shankweiler, 1991). Interestingly, Rozin, Poritsky, and Sotsky (1971) found that children in the second grade with reading disabilities made rapid progress in learning to read when ideographic characters representing entire English words were used rather than alphabetic writing. Other investigators working with children demonstrating reading difficulties have noted that these children also encounter problems when presented with other tasks requiring phonetic segmentation. Thus, children with reading disabilities have difficulties in finding syllables that rhyme, and in learning to speak Pig Latin (which involves shifting the initial consonant cluster of a word to its end and adding the diphthong /ei/ (see Monroe, 1932; Savin, 1972)).

Cues for identifying phonemes and characterizing letters

If there is no obvious acoustic invariance for a stop consonant such as /p/, but rather a number of acoustic patterns that depend upon the neighboring phonemes, why are these different sounds designated by the same alphabetic symbol and considered as the same phoneme? The answer appears to be that they are all produced in the same fashion, so that all tokens of the phoneme /p/ involve stopping and releasing the flow of air at the lips. Additional information concerning voicing permits discrimination between /p/ and /b/, and characterizes the phoneme unambiguously. Phonemes defined by articulatory position are not subject to the acoustic-phonetic noninvariance problem; thus, variations in formant transitions when /p/ is followed by different vowels become irrelevant. Also, MacNeilage's (1970) observation that there is no invariance in muscle activity associated with production of individual stop consonants is not a problem, since the articulatory invariance represents the end point of muscle activity (lip closure), not the muscular activity needed to achieve this position.

However, not all articulatory positions corresponding to phoneme produc-tion are available for analysis. As pointed out by Helmholtz (Warren and Warren, 1968, p. 234),

> we have no idea at all of the form and the movements of such exquisitely sensitive parts as our soft palate, our epiglottis and our larynx because we cannot see them without optical instruments and cannot easily touch them ... . The extraordinarily varied and minute movements of the larynx teach us also, regarding relation between the act of volition and its effect, that what we are able to produce first and directly is not the innervation of a certain nerve or muscle, nor is it always a certain position of the movable parts of our bodies, but it is the first observable external effect. As far as we can ascertain by eye and hand the position of the parts of our bodies, this is the first observable effect with which the conscious intent in the act of volition is concerned. Whenever we cannot do this, as in the larynx and in the posterior parts of the mouth, the different modifications of voice, breathing, swallowing, etc., are these first effects.

Helmholtz's comments would lead us to expect that, when people profoundly deaf from an early age are taught to produce intelligible speech, they have the greatest difficulty in exercising control over their larynx and articulatory positions at the back of the mouth. In keeping with these expectations, Peterson (1946) has observed that the three major problems associated with quality of speech by the deaf are pitch variations (under laryngeal control), breathiness (under laryngeal control), and nasality (under velar, or soft palate, control).

Vowels are usually more difficult to characterize in terms of articulatory position than consonants. This difficulty may explain why children acquiring reading skills find it harder to deal with vowels than consonants, and make a larger number of errors with the letters corresponding to vowels (Shankweiler and Liberman, 1972).

Phonemes in speech are not perceived, but are inferred

There are three lines of experimental evidence indicating that listeners do not, and indeed cannot, perceive phonemes in running speech directly, but that their presence is inferred following prior identification of larger units: (1) an inability to distinguish between speech sounds that are "heard" when replaced by noise (the phonemic restoration effect) and those physically present; (2) the need to identify syllabic organization before identifying constituent phonemes; and (3) the inability to identify brief phonetic components (steady-state vowels) when chained together into a sequence, even though they are readily recognizable when presented singly. Evidence supporting these three statements is given below.

"Restored" and "real" phonemes are perceptually equivalent

It has been reported that listeners cannot detect which speech sound is missing after listening to a recorded sentence in which a phoneme has been deleted and replaced by a cough or noise burst (Warren, 1970b; Warren and Warren, 1970; Warren and Sherman, 1974). The restoration of obliterated phonemes was dealt with in some detail in Chapter 6, and we will return to the phonemic restoration effect later when discussing skilled storage and delayed perceptual organization of speech. The point of special interest here is that the restored phonemes are indistinguishable from those phonemes that are actually present as acoustic components of the stimulus. Evidence presented in the following sections indicates that "restored" phonemes and "real" phonemes are both inferred entities based upon a prior recognition of acoustic patterns representing syllables or words.

Identification of syllables and words precedes identification of constituent phonemes

The task of "phoneme monitoring" was introduced by Foss (1969) and Foss and Lynch (1969) who studied the effect of lexical item difficulty and position in a sentence upon the time required to identify the occurrence of a target phoneme. This procedure was modified by Savin and Bever (1970) and used to compare the times required to identify a syllable and a phoneme within that syllable. Their listeners were instructed to press a key as soon as they detected a given target in a sequence of nonsense syllables. The targets consisted of an initial consonant, the vowel following the consonant, or the entire syllable. It was found that the time required to respond to the syllable target was less than for the phonemes within the syllable. They concluded that access to the syllable occurred first, and that identification of the phonemes followed the recognition of the syllable.

The experimental results reported by Savin and Bever were confirmed in an independent study by Warren (1971) that was completed shortly before their work was published. Besides employing stimuli consisting of nonsense syllables, as did Savin and Bever, lexical syllables were also studied under various conditions. The four types of monosyllabic stimuli used were: (1) a nonsense syllable list, (2) a word list, (3) sentences with the target word having a low contextual probability, and (4) sentences with the target word having a high contextual probability. For each type, the identification time for a phoneme was always greater than the identification time for the syllable containing that phoneme. The identification times for syllables (and the longer identification times for phonemes within the syllables) were about the same for types 1, 2, and 3. When prior context made a target word's occurrence more probable with stimulus type 4, identification time for the word decreased appreciably, as would be expected. In addition, identification times for a phoneme within that word changed correspondingly, indicating that the phoneme identification was derived from a prior higher-level organization. The observations reported by Foss (1969), by Savin and Bever (1970), and by Warren (1971) have been confirmed and elaborated by a number of subsequent studies (see Connine and Titone, 1996).

Obligatory transformation of brief steady-state phonemes into syllables and words: the vowel-sequence illusion

Perhaps the most direct evidence that phoneme identification is a consequence that follows and does not precede linguistic organization is provided by observations made using sequences of brief steady-state vowels.

As described in Chapter 5, different arrangements of sounds other than those of speech can be discriminated readily when items are presented too rapidly to permit identification of order. Experiments with repeating sequences of tones and sequences of different arbitrarily selected sounds have shown that when the constituent sounds have durations below the threshold for order identification, they coalesce to form distinctive "temporal compounds" that permit listeners to discriminate easily between different arrangements of the same sounds, even if the constituent elements of the compounds cannot be identified. Sequences of steady-state speech sounds also form temporal compounds: these have rather interesting characteristics.

Warren, Bashford, and Gardner (1990) employed repeating sequences of three to ten contiguous steady-state vowels presented loudly and clearly at isochronous item durations that were below the lower limit of 100 ms/item required for identification of the vowels and their orders. It was found that at durations between 30 and 100 ms/vowel, the vowel sequences were transformed into syllables and words having illusory consonants and illusory vowels having an apparently smooth succession of speech sounds lacking the actual abrupt acoustic changes. These linguistic organizations permitted listeners to distinguish readily between different arrangements of the same items. When the listeners were monolingual English speakers, there was considerable inter-subject agreement on the verbal forms reported for particular sequences (Warren, Healy, and Chalikia, 1996). Listeners' linguistic organizations not only conformed to phonotactic rules for grouping of consonants and vowels, but they typically were syllables occurring in English. The illusory phonemes seemed quite real, and Chalikia and Warren (1991) were able to map their perceptual boundaries relative to the acoustic boundaries of the steady-state stimulus vowels for individual listeners using the mapping procedure described by Warren and Sherman (1974). These boundaries were quite stable, and differed from the boundaries of the stimulus vowels. These observations are consistent with the hypothesis that sequences of brief speech sounds form linguistic temporal compounds consisting of syllables and words, and that analysis into an ordered sequence of phonemes follows an initial linguistic organization.

There was an additional, rather surprising characteristic of the verbal organization of brief vowel sequences: listeners usually reported hearing two concurrent voices having different timbres, each voice saying something different (Warren, Bashford, and Gardner 1990). A subsequent study by Chalikia and Warren (1994) found that different spectral ranges were employed for each of the simultaneous voices. When listeners were instructed to adjust the cut-off frequencies of a bandpass filter to the narrowest range required for the perception of each of the verbal forms, the median limits were 300–1,200 Hz for the low voice and 1,500–3,500 Hz for the high voice. This spectral fissioning of broadband vowel sequences into two verbal forms corresponding to low and high frequency regions suggests the existence of a powerful organizational principle capable of overcoming the strong acoustic cues indicating a common source for all spectral components of the acoustic phones. These cues indicating a single source for a vowel sequence include the abrupt simultaneous onset and offset of components across the spectrum, the harmonic relations of all spectral voicing components to a common 100 Hz fundamental, and the spacing of the formants within each vowel indicating a single phone produced by a single vocal tract. Nevertheless, the tendency to match these phonetic sequences to separate frequency-limited templates for syllables and words was sufficient to overcome these forces of fusion.

The spectral splitting of vowel sequences occurred in the vicinity of the "cross-over frequency" of approximately 1,500 Hz that divides normal broadband speech into high and low spectral regions contributing equally to intelligibility. Sentences consisting of normal speech limited to either of these two frequency regions can be understood. Chalikia and Warren (1994) pointed out that the ability to comprehend speech on only one side of the crossover frequency could allow listeners to process broadband speech independently in each of these ranges. Such independent concurrent processing could be useful when the spoken message is unclear. Normally, the linguistic information obtained in each of the two ranges would be consistent, so that they could be integrated and fused into a single broadband auditory image. However, the concurrent linguistic organizations achieved with vowel sequences are incompatible, integration is not possible, and listeners hear two voices with different timbres, each saying something different.

When nonsense words are reported for vowel sequences, as they often are, they almost always consist of syllables that occur in polysyllabic English words for monolingual English speakers, suggesting the existence of a stored syllabary. The accessing of this syllabary could be an initial stage in the normal processing of sentences and discourse: it would, of course provide direct access to monosyllabic lexical items, and in addition could allow the accessing of polysyllabic words by the chaining together of appropriate units. This perceptual syllabary may be linked to a syllabary employed for speech production.

It has been suggested that the pre-planning required for speaking is accomplished with the assistance of a production syllabary consisting of listings of the sequence of motor commands needed to produce the syllables occurring in English. Crompton (1982) argued that the construction of articulatory programs involves the accessing of this library of articulatory routines, and that these routines correspond to syllables. It was claimed that confirmatory evidence for the existence of a production syllabary is provided by errors associated with "slips of the tongue." Crompton considered that such speech errors are due to the faulty operation of the mechanism for accessing these various syllable routines. This notion of a pre-existing production syllabary was elaborated by Levelt (1992) and Levelt and Wheeldon (1994). They used this concept to sketch a framework for planning the construction of motor programs that a speaker implements to generate the syllables in connected speech. Experimental evidence for the existence of a production syllabary was reported for Dutch (Wheeldon and Levelt, 1995), French (Ferrand, Segui, and Grainger, 1996), and English (Ferrand, Segui, and Humphreys, 1997).

Implications of the vowel-sequence illusion for theories of aphasia

Since discriminating between different arrangements of phonemes is required for lexical recognition (e.g., "pets" versus "pest"), a number of investigators have concluded that speech comprehension requires initial segmentation into an ordered series of discrete phonemes at some stage of perceptual processing (Joos, 1948; Efron, 1963; Jones, 1978; Morais and Kolinsky, 1994). If recovering an ordered string of rapid phonemes is required for comprehension of speech, then aphasias could be due in part to a general inability to achieve temporal resolution of brief sounds. A number of studies have tested this hypothesis, comparing the performance of individuals with aphasia and nonaphasic listeners in ordering tasks involving sequences of nonverbal sounds such as tones, clicks, and noises (Efron, 1963; Carmon and Nachshon, 1971; Brookshire, 1972; Tallal and Piercy, 1973; Bond, 1976). These studies found that listeners with aphasia indeed did not perform as well as the nonaphasic listeners in identifying the order of components. However, it has been pointed out that aphasias are associated with a broad pattern of deficits, and it may be inappropriate to conclude that deficits in ordering auditory stimuli are either the same as, or the cause of, this disorder (Swisher and Hirsh, 1972).

The vowel sequence illusion, together with other evidence, demonstrates that segmentation of speech into an ordered sequence of brief component sounds is not required for verbal organization. If this is indeed the case, then individuals with aphasia may be able to discriminate between the patterns formed by different arrangements of phonemes as brief or briefer than those occurring in speech, but their disorder may result from an inability to utilize these discriminable temporal compounds linguistically. Warren and Gardner (1995) tested this hypothesis using adults with aphasia who had suffered cerebral accidents at least one year prior to testing and were judged to be neurologically stabilized. It was predicted that they would be able to perform at significantly above chance levels in discriminating between sequences consisting of different arrangements of the same brief vowels having durations comparable to phonemes in speech, as long as the task did not require them to name the components in their proper order. In addition, it was predicted that they would no longer be able to discriminate between different arrangements if the durations of items were increased to 2 s or more since, as discussed in Chapter 5, this task requires linguistic skills that include labeling, storage, and comparison of one ordered string of verbal labels with another.

The listeners in our experiment were sixteen adult subjects with receptive aphasia who had normal hearing as determined by audiometric testing. They had diverse etiologies of brain damage: three had both left and right hemisphere lesions, ten had only left hemisphere lesions, and three undetermined sites of brain damage. All were neurologically stabilized, with the trauma responsible for aphasia occurring at least one year prior to testing. They were tested within three months of participation in the experiment with the Western Aphasia Battery, resulting in a classification of twelve subjects with anomia, three with Broca's aphasia, and one with Wernicke's aphasia. In the experiment, they were presented with repeating sequences of three steady-state isochronous vowels at seven item durations ranging from 12 ms/vowel up to 5 s/vowel. Each trial consisted of a succession of sequences separated by brief silences, with successive sequences either being identical, or alternating in the arrangement of the vowels. The subject indicated whether successive sequences in a trial were the same or different using a nonverbal response procedure.

As hypothesized, the listeners with aphasia were generally able to distinguish between the different orders down to 12 ms/vowel, but they could not determine whether the arrangements were the same or different when the vowels were each 3 s or more in length (a task that the nonaphasic control groups accomplished with great ease). These results indicate that their difficulty in comprehending speech was not the consequence of an inability to distinguish between different arrangements of brief phonemes: the difficulty seems to involve a diminished ability to process phonetic temporal compounds of syllabic duration linguistically. An impaired ability to achieve linguistic organization above the level of the syllable has been noted in the production of speech by individuals suffering from jargon aphasia. G. A. Miller (1991, p. 83) stated:

> The rules forming admissible syllables ... seem to be learned at an extremely deep level. Even when injuries to the brain result in 'jargon aphasia,' a condition in which the victim can speak fluently but is largely unintelligible because the speech is dense with nonwords, nearly all the neologisms that are generated still conform to the conventional rules of syllable formation.

Perceptual changes occurring during repetition of syllables and words

Verbal and visual satiation

When a word is repeated over and over to oneself, a lapse in meaning occurs which has been called verbal satiation, semantic satiation, and adaptation. Titchener (1915, pp. 26–27) described the effect as follows: "Repeat aloud some word – the first that occurs to you; house, for instance – over and over again; presently the sound of the word becomes meaningless and blank; you are puzzled and a morsel frightened as you hear it." Many studies have been reported on this topic, with some authors claiming that occasionally alternate meanings for the word may be introduced (see Amster, 1964).

The loss of meaning of words with continued stimulation is not unique for hearing, and occurs with viewing of printed words (Severance and Washburn, 1907; Don and Weld, 1924). Another type of perceptual change also occurs in vision. When a pattern is viewed which has two or more plausible interpretations that are mutually incompatible (that is, it is physically impossible for more than one of the forms represented by the figure to be present simultaneously), then continued inspection can lead to an apparent change from one of the forms to another without conscious volition. Many of these ambiguous figures involve reversible perspective. Since Necker (1832) called attention to this phenomenon, a large number of reversible figures have been reported in the literature. Perhaps the best known of these is the "Necker cube" (although Necker actually described a parallelopiped). Necker pointed out that reversible geometric figures appear in Euclid's solid geometry, and he reasoned that the ancient Greeks and others must have noticed the illusory shifts in perspective which are so obvious to us. Evidence that Necker's assumption is correct has been provided by a series of photographs of reversible designs used for floor mosaics, some dating back to the temple of Apollo at Pompeii and the Roman Emperor Hadrian's Villa near Rome. Photographs of these mosaics were taken in the 1950s and subsequently published in a paper on perceptual transformations (Warren, 1981b). Among these photographs are beautiful and ingenious floor designs found on the floors of the fifth century Great Saint Mary's Basilica in Rome and the eleventh to fourteenth century Saint Mark's Cathedral in Venice – some of these mosaic figures have three or four plausible perspective interpretations.

The phenomena observed with ambiguous visual configurations suggested that it would be of interest to study the perception of ambiguous auditory configurations such as the syllable "ace," which when repeated without pause might alternate with perception of "say," or repetition of a more complex syllable such as "rest" that might produce three plausible lexical interpretations ("rest," "tress," and "stress") (Warren and Gregory, 1958). Realizing that the neuromuscular effects of self-repetition might inhibit illusory changes as well as introducing other complicating factors associated with self-production, it was decided to employ passive listening to a recorded word repeated on a tape loop. Listeners did hear some changes of the sort we expected, but it was also observed that other words were reported that involved phonetic distortion of the stimulus. However, our preconceived bias was such that these distortions were attributed to mechanical instabilities in the playback of our small tape loops, and we entitled our paper "An auditory analogue of the visual reversible figure" (Warren and Gregory, 1958). However, further work, using improved procedures ensuring that repetitions were identical, demonstrated that the phonetic distortions were not the result of changes in the stimulus. This disruption of veridical perceptual organization has revealed aspects of verbal organization that are not otherwise readily accessible for study.

Verbal transformations

When listening to a recording of any repeating word, phrase, or short sentence, a succession of illusory changes are heard that have been called "verbal transformations." The first detailed study of verbal transformations (Warren, 1961a) employed young adults (British naval ratings), who heard illusory changes while listening to recordings of repeated monosyllabic words and nonwords, polysyllabic words, and short sentences. Illusory changes were heard with all stimuli. When presented with a monosyllable repeated twice a second for 3 minutes, the average young adult heard about 30 transitions (or changes in what was heard) usually involving about six different illusory syllables, with transitions not only involving forms reported for the first time, but sometimes returning to those heard previously. An example of the illusory changes heard by a subject in this study listening to the monosyllabic word "right" follows: "ripe, right, white, white-light, right, right-light, ripe, right, ripe, bright-light, right, ripe, bright-light, right, bright-light." Changes in the stimulus level had no effect on the rate of illusory changes as long as clarity was unimpaired, but when the words were made indistinct by the addition of on-line noise, the rate of changes dropped to less than half.

Profound age differences have been found for verbal transformations. Warren (1961b) reported that the elderly (62–86 years) heard less than one-fifth the number of transitions from one form to another than did young adults (18–25 years) listening to the same repeating syllables for the same 3 minute time period. The study was then extended to four groups of children that were 5, 6, 8, and 10 years of age (Warren and Warren, 1966), using the same stimuli employed in the earlier study with adults. It was found that almost no verbal transformations occurred for nursery school children at the age of 5 years. At 6 years, half of the children heard verbal transformations; appearance was all-or-none, so that the 6 year olds heard either no changes at all, or heard them occurring at a rate corresponding to that of older children and young adults. By the age of 8, all subjects heard verbal transformations. The rate of illusory changes remained approximately constant from 8 years of age through young adulthood, and declined markedly for the elderly group of subjects. The number of different forms reported during 3 minutes of listening behaved somewhat differently, and declined regularly with age. Children often heard extensive changes involving several phonemes in going from one form to the next. A sample of all forms reported by an 8 year old child listening to the nonsense syllable "flime" repeated twice a second for 3 minutes follows: "flime, crime, clime, like, oink, clime, flime, haw, flying, flime, crime, fly-um, flime, flyed, oink, flyed, fly-in, Clyde, fly-in, oink, wink, fly-in, I'm flying, flying, Clyde, flying, oink, flyed, I'm flying, flyed, I wink, flyed, aw-wenk-ah" (Warren and Warren, 1966). In addition to age differences in the number of phoneme changes in going from one perceptual form to the next, there were differences in the nature of the words reported, suggesting that processing units change with age. G. A. Miller (1962) has pointed out that " ... language must contain some natural coding units of finite length. But what these coding units are for an articulate human being still remains something of a mystery." Verbal transformations do not solve this mystery, but do offer some clues indicating that the size of the "coding units" used for linguistic grouping changes consistently with age.

From ages 6 to 10, nonsense words were reported frequently with phonemes occurring in orders not permitted in English: for example, starting a word with the cluster "sr" as in "sreb." Organization of young adults appeared to be limited strictly by the rules governing phoneme clustering. That is, they reported nonsense words fairly frequently; but, with no exceptions, the phonemes were clustered according to the rules of English for monolingual speakers of that language. In addition, these nonsense words almost invariably consisted of syllables occurring in English in polysyllabic words. The group of elderly listeners generally employed meaningful English words as their units of organization. When presented with the repeated nonsense syllable "flime," the elderly heard it as a meaningful word (an interesting exception is an incorrect past participle "flyed," reported more frequently than the actual nonsense stimulus by the aged). These restrictions concerning forms reported by adults applied only to monolingual English speakers – those familiar with a second language could report forms corresponding to rules governing that language while listening to a repeating English word.

Warren (1968c) suggested that the transformation of repeated words may be related to mechanisms employed for the reorganization of connected discourse employed when an initial linguistic organization is not confirmed by subsequent context. If verbal transformations reflect skilled reorganizational processes, they should not appear in children until their language skills have attained a certain level. The requisite level does not seem to have been reached at age 5, but seems to be reached normally by the age of 6 or 7. The decrease in the nature and rate of verbal transformations in the aged may be attributable to adaptive changes in processing strategy. It is well established that considerable difficulty is encountered by the aged with tasks involving the use of recently stored information following intervening activity (Welford, 1958). In view of this difficulty, the optimal strategy for the aged might be to organize speech directly into English words, with very little use of reorganization based on subsequent information and, hence, very few verbal transformations.

We maintain a mastery of linguistic skills over the greater part of our life span. It appears that this proficiency may be maintained, not through preserving a fixed repertoire of processing mechanisms, but rather through adaptive changes. A sort of perceptual homeostasis might be achieved through the use of mechanisms appropriate to changes in functional capacity. (See Chapter 8 for a discussion of evidence that the rules and criteria governing perceptual interpretation of sensory input are labile and are continually being evaluated for accuracy, and are revised when appropriate.) If this view concerning adaptive changes is correct, then accuracy in speech perception can be achieved through a variety of perceptual strategies, and it could be a grave error to assume a similarity in perceptual mechanisms used for achieving accuracy from a similarity in performance.

It seemed that the verbal transformation effect and the phonemic restoration effect may be linked, each being related to skilled mechanisms employed normally for the resolution of ambiguities and correction of errors (Warren and Warren, 1970). Acting on this possibility, Obusek and Warren (1973) combined these two illusions by presenting a repeated word ("magistrate") to college students with a portion deleted and replaced by noise. If illusory changes are indeed corrective, they would be expected to be directed to the phonemically restored segment. When the /s/ of "magistrate" was removed and replaced by a louder noise, 42 percent of the illusory changes involved the position corresponding to the deleted /s/, compared to 5 percent when a different group of subjects heard the intact word as the repeated stimulus. When the /s/ was deleted and replaced by silence rather than noise (so that phonemic restorations were inhibited), the lability of phonemes heard in this position was greater than with the intact word, but much less than that associated with the presence of noise: only 18 percent of changes involved the position of the silent gap. When the noise was present, it was not possible for a listener to detect which phoneme corresponded to the noise bursts any more than with phonemic restorations of nonrepeated sentences (Warren, 1970b). Yet, it appears that, at some level of processing, the distinction between speech-based and noise-based organization was maintained, and the perceptual reorganization was directed to the portion lacking direct acoustic justification.

Identifying lexical neighbors using verbal transformations

Verbal transformations appear to result from the concurrent operation of two effects produced by continued exposure to an unchanging stimulus: (1) the decay of any particular verbal organization, and (2) the emergence of a new verbal form, which is followed by (1) and then (2), etc. The first stage has already been discussed in this section under the topic of verbal satiation (which can also be considered a repetition-induced decrease of activation of the perceived verbal organization). The second stage can be considered as a repetition-induced increased activation of the listener's most salient alternative organization, and it can be used to explore the lexical neighborhood of any repeating word.

As mentioned previously, when listening to a repeated word for a period of 3 minutes, an average of about six different verbal forms are heard by young adults. The forms reported towards the end of the stimulation period can be quite different phonetically from the stimulus, and are often more closely related to one of the previously heard forms. But the very first change heard has a special status; it is free from the influence of prior illusory forms, typically differs from the stimulus by only a single phoneme, and may represent the listener's most salient surrogate or competitor for that word. Hence, the listener's first transform may identify that individual's closest neighbor for any word chosen by the experimenter.

There are a number of models that consider that the identification of a spoken word results from a competition among structurally similar words (McClelland and Elman, 1986; Norris, 1994; Luce and Pisoni, 1998; Luce, Goldinger, Auer, and Vitevitch, 2000; Norris, McQueen, and Cutler, 2000). It is generally considered that these competitors form a lexical neighborhood consisting of words differing from the stimulus by a single phoneme (see Luce, Pisoni, and Goldinger, 1990). This single-phoneme-difference rule for defining neighbors has been supported by a number of experimental studies, for example reports that prior exposure to one word reduces the reaction time to a subsequent word if the words are neighbors, and also that words having many neighbors with a high frequency of occurrence are usually accessed more slowly and with less accuracy than those words having only a few, low frequency neighbors (see Goldinger, Luce, and Pisoni, 1989; Luce and Pisoni, 1998).

A study by Bashford, Warren, and Lenz (2006) was designed to use the verbal transformation illusion to identify the effectively competing neighbors of a selection of monosyllabic words and nonwords. A brief silence separated the restatements of the stimulus word to prevent resegmentation (for example, preventing contiguous restatements of "say" from being heard as "ace").

Although the results obtained provide general support for the one-phoneme-distance rule for neighbors, there were also conditions under which an effective neighbor having a high frequency of usage differed by more than one phoneme. This "verbal-transform procedure" makes it possible to use the first illusory forms reported by a group of listeners to construct a frequency-weighted list of the most salient neighbors of any desired word (or nonword) among the population of listeners being polled.

Dichotic verbal transformations

Verbal transformations of dichotic stimuli have been used to study the nature of neural analyzers used for speech perception (Warren and Ackroff, 1976b; Warren, 1977b). In one of the conditions described in these papers, the stimulus word "tress" with a repetition period of 492 ms was passed through a digital delay line with two delay taps, and the delay between the taps was adjusted so that the asynchrony of the outputs was exactly half the repetition period (246 ms). Listening was through a pair of headphones wired separately so that temporally dichotic but otherwise identical stimuli were heard in each ear. Neither ear could be considered as leading with the half-cycle delay, and there was a lateral symmetry in the nature of simultaneous contralateral input. Since the interaural asynchrony was a few hundred milliseconds, there was no possibility of binaural fusion (see Chapter 2); and all listeners initially identified the stimulus accurately on each side. The question of interest to theory was whether or not the same illusory changes would be heard simultaneously on the right and left. If the changes were identical and simultaneous, it would indicate that there was a sharing of a single set of neural linguistic analyzers. If independent changes were to occur at each ear, then it would indicate that two sets of functionally separate analyzers were used for the acoustically identical verbal stimuli.

It was found that for each of 20 subjects, the times at which changes occurred were uncorrelated at each ear. Also, the forms heard at the two sides were independent, so that while the word "dress" might be perceived at one ear, a word as far removed phonetically from the repeating stimulus "tress" as "commence" might be heard at the other after a few minutes and several previous changes.

Continuous monitoring of changes occurring on each side is demanding and tiring, and can lead to confusions and omissions. A procedure of reporting what is heard on each side only when cued by a brief light signal has been used in recent studies by Peter Lenz in our laboratory. One of the findings using this improved method has been that the rate of illusory changes differs dramatically with the nature of dichotic competition: it is highest when the same monosyllabic word is delivered asynchronously to each ear and tends to decrease with the extent of phonetic mismatch of the two signals. It has been suggested that the increased complexity of the combined input to a shared prelexical auditory/phonetic processor determines the rate of change, and that the output from this initial stage is then employed by independent higher-level syllabic/lexical processors identified with separate azimuths. Although it is tempting to attribute the independent syllabic organization of the dichotic signals to the bilateral anatomical and functional organization of the auditory system, this approach is weakened by the reports that independent changes of the same word were not limited to only two competing versions (Warren and Ackroff, 1976b; Warren, 1977b). Listeners were presented with three asynchronous versions of a single repeated word, each separated from the other two by exactly one-third of the word's duration. Two versions were delivered monaurally (one on the right, and one on the left), and one was diotic with its apparent location lying in the medial plane. Each of the five listeners heard the three versions of the word (right, left, and center) change independently. These observations demonstrate a rather impressive feat of parallel processing – not only can three sets of linguistic analyzers be employed for verbal organization of the same stimulus, but independent shifts in the criteria for other verbal forms can also occur concurrently at each of the three spatial locations.

Recent unpublished observations by Bashford and Warren using dichotic verbal transformations have indicated that the mechanisms involved in producing resegmentation changes of "reversible" repeating words may be quite different from the mechanisms resulting in the phonetic changes of verbal transformations. When the reversible repeating stimulus that could be heard as "ace" or "say" was presented to each ear with an interaural asynchrony of one-half the repetition period, then if "ace" was heard at one ear, "say" was always heard at the other. Changes occurred at the same time, and consisted of a reversal of the ears hearing each form. Similarly, when bisyllabic "welfare" was repeated at each ear with a half-period interaural delay, it was obligatory that initially one ear heard "welfare" and the other "farewell" with reversals in syllabic order occurring synchronously at the two ears. This inability to hear the same organization at each ear at the same time along with the temporal linkage of resegmentation changes at each side are quite different from the independent changes occurring when the resegmentation of the stimulus to form different words is not possible. However, with continued listening to reversible words, phonetic changes do occur, and then independent asynchronous changes can be heard at each side. This shift from synchronous to asynchronous changes provides further evidence that resegmentation and verbal transformations occur at different levels of processing.

The relation between production and perception of speech: organization above the lexical level

Since humans function as both producers and receivers (perceivers) of speech, it has been tempting, and to some extent useful, to look for similarities and interdependence of these two modes of linguistic behavior. Certainly, when operating as speaker or listener we use the same lexicon and linguistic conventions. However, there are basic differences between the goals and strategies employed for production and perception. A major distinction is that the course of temporal organization is reversed for producing and for perceiving speech.

When producing speech, knowledge of what is to be said precedes (or should precede) vocalization. In extended discourse, the general plan of what is to be communicated may be formulated by the speaker several sentences in advance; and, by the time a particular sentence is started, its structure must be well organized if speech is to maintain fluency and intelligibility. When listening rather than speaking, the temporal nature of the task is quite different: processing obviously does not precede but rather follows reception. The message as received may be subject to perceptual errors and confusions resulting from environmental noises, unfamiliarity with the speaker's pronunciation and style, false expectations of the speaker's intent, unintentional ambiguities in what the speaker is saying, etc. It is not always possible or desirable to ask the speaker to repeat or clarify statements, and misunderstandings are not uncommon, as we all know. There is evidence that one important technique for minimizing errors in comprehension of speech involves delaying the perceptual organization of a word until several subsequent words have been received.

Skilled storage and delayed perceptual organization of speech

Several investigators have noted that speech must be stored and perceptual decisions deferred if errors are to be minimized. Chistovich (1962) reported that many errors were made when her subjects were instructed to repeat speech heard through headphones as quickly as possible. She suggested that these mistakes reflected the temporal course of speech identification, with an appreciable delay in response time being needed for more accurate performance. Both Miller (1962) and Lieberman (1963) have emphasized that successful speech perception cannot proceed as a Markovian process, with perception occurring first on lower and then higher levels of organization, with no feedback from higher to lower levels. Markovian processing of this nature does not benefit fully from the redundancy of the message and does not permit the correction of mistakes. Without the possibility of correction, an error would continue to provide incorrect prior context, producing still more errors until comprehension became blocked. This is the sort of difficulty which can be encountered by someone with less than complete mastery of a foreign language.

Bryan and Harter (1897, 1899) reported evidence concerning the importance of skilled storage in linguistic comprehension. They worked with expert telegraphers who they claimed had learned a "telegraphic language" similar to other languages. Complete mastery required several years of continual use, perhaps ten years to achieve the speed and accuracy required for a press dispatcher. Skill in sending messages was achieved relatively quickly; it was the receiving of messages which was considerably more difficult. When mastery in receiving was achieved, the receiver could work automatically with little conscious effort, often transcribing complex messages while thinking about something quite different. The story has been told that a telegrapher who had transcribed the message that Lincoln had just been shot exhibited surprise when he overheard this news some time later.

An expert telegrapher usually delayed several words before transcribing the ongoing text in normal messages. When receiving messages transmitted in cipher or when receiving stock quotations, the lack of hierarchical organization and redundancy made the task much harder for experts. In recognition of this difficulty, the sender slowed down transmittal rate, and the receiver decreased the number of items held in storage by following the text more closely in time. Thus, long storage was used only when the context permitted useful interactions between information received at different times.

Skilled storage similar to that reported for telegraphy has been observed for typewriting (Book, 1925), for reading aloud (Huey, 1968), and for tactile reading by the blind (Love, cited by Bryan and Harter, 1899; M. W. Moore and Bliss, 1975). It appears that storage with continuing processing and revision is employed quite generally for comprehension of linguistic input. Lashley (1951) gave a classic demonstration of the use of storage to correct errors in speech perception made evident by subsequent context. He first spoke of the process of *rapid writing* to an audience. Several sentences after creating a set for the word "writing," Lashley spoke the sentence: "Rapid righting with his uninjured hand saved from loss the contents of the capsized canoe." He then noted that the context required for the proper interpretation of the sounds corresponding to "righting" was not activated for some 3 to 5 s after hearing the word.

Phonemic restorations provide a technique for studying prelinguistic storage of auditory information until lexical identity can be established. The original studies dealing with phonemic restoration (Warren, 1970b; Warren and Obusek, 1971) employed the stimulus sentence: "The state governors met with their respective legi*latures convening in the capitol city" (* designates an extraneous sound, such as a cough or noise burst, replacing the phoneme). All the information necessary to identify the missing sound as /s/ is present before the end of "legislatures," with no need for storage of subsequent acoustic information. However, other observations have indicated that listeners can defer the restoration of an ambiguous word fragment for several words until context is provided which resolves the ambiguity (Warren and Warren, 1970). Since the 1970s, numerous studies have investigated the storage capacity of this "working memory" that can permit listeners to retain acoustic information until subsequent context permits appropriate interpretation (see Daneman and Merikle, 1996, for review). The integration of degraded or reduced acoustic information permits comprehension of sentences when many of the cues necessary to identify a word heard in isolation (or in a list of unrelated words) are lacking. An example of sentence intelligibility based on reduced cues is furnished by the intelligibility of "sine-wave sentences" in which listeners heard only sinusoidal tones that tracked the frequency and amplitude fluctuations of formants. Remez, Rubin, Berns, *et al.* (1994) reported that listeners could identify as many as 70 percent of the syllables in sentences when "Three or four sinusoids were used to replicate each sentence, one sinusoid for each of the three lowest frequency formants and a fourth for a fricative formant when necessary." Another example of the robustness of sentence intelligibility is evidenced by a study by Warren, Riener, Bashford, and Brubaker (1995) in which sentences were filtered to produce a wedge shaped band consisting solely of slopes of 115 dB/octave meeting at 1,500 Hz. Despite the limited spectral range and slopes distorting the spectral profile, the intelligibility score was 77 percent.

Speech errors in everyday life

There is an old medical maxim that pathology represents normal function laid bare. Disorders and errors in speech perception may also provide a means of glimpsing the otherwise hidden mechanisms of normal function. This hope of enhancing understanding of normal processes may underlie the continued study of speech errors since the late nineteenth century.

Most collections of naturally occurring speech errors deal with spontaneous errors in production, or "slips of the tongue." These are difficult to gather since they occur relatively infrequently, except from individuals especially prone to make these errors, such as the Reverend Dr. W. A. Spooner, an Oxford don who was Warden of New College, Oxford from 1903 to 1924. His "spoonerisms" include such statements as "you hissed my mystery lecture" for "you missed my history lecture" and "tasted the whole worm" rather than "wasted the whole term." The first comprehensive collection of slips of the tongue was Meringer's compendium published in Vienna (Meringer and Mayer, 1895). Collections of English slips of the tongue have been gathered by Fromkin (1971) and Shattuck (1975). These errors have been used in attempts to understand the planning and execution of phrases and sentences (see Fromkin, 1973, 1980).

In addition to studies of production errors, there have been a few attempts to collect errors in speech perception that have been detected while listening to speech in everyday life (see Browman, 1980; Celce-Murcia, 1980; Garnes and Bond, 1980). Errors in perception are much more common than errors in production, but they are quite difficult to study systematically. Perceptual errors by people with normal hearing can be caused by a variety of factors, including interference by extraneous sounds, anticipatory bias, an unfamiliar accent or dialect, as well as a speaker's poor pronunciation. Often, errors remain undetected and listeners are left with an incorrect interpretation of the message. Despite the difficulties in collecting listeners' errors and evaluating their causes, compendia of errors can provide a measure of the reliability and accuracy of verbal communication under particular conditions, and can point to factors liable to cause difficulties in perceiving speech.

Besides observing and collecting of perceptual errors occurring under normal listening conditions, it is possible to induce errors in the laboratory. The use of repeated verbal stimuli provides a convenient way of initiating misperceptions.

Syllable recognition by nonhuman species

Holistic pattern recognition is not restricted to humans. Evidence discussed in Chapter 5 indicates that monkeys, cats, and dolphins can distinguish between permuted orders of nonverbal sounds, recognizing the overall pattern rather than the individual components and their orders. In addition, a number of laboratories have successfully taught animals to distinguish between different samples of speech, and have reported similarities in discrimination by these animals and by humans. Dewson (1964) taught cats to distinguish between /i/ and /u/ whether spoken by a male or female voice. Warfield, Ruben, and Glackin (1966) taught cats to distinguish between the words "cat" and "bat," and reported that the limits of acoustic alteration of the words permitting discrimination were similar for cats and for humans.

Kuhl and Miller (1978) used synthetic speech and showed that chinchillas can distinguish between /ta/ and /da/, /ka/ and /ga/, and /pa/ and /ba/. In another study using natural speech, Kuhl and Miller (1974) found that, following training, syllables containing /t/ or /d/ could be discriminated by chinchillas, despite variations in talkers, the vowels following the plosives, and the intensities. Work with monkeys by Sinnott, Beecher, Moody, and Stebbins (1976) has shown that they are able to discriminate between acoustic correlates of the place of human articulation with /ba/ and /da/. These studies involving several mammalian species indicate the extent to which the phylogenetic development of speech exploited common perceptual abilities. In addition, Kluender, Diehl, and Killeen (1987) reported that Japanese quail can learn phonetic categories. For further discussion, see Warren, 1976, 1988.

Suggestions for further reading

Greenberg, S., and Ainsworth, W. A. (eds.) 2006. *Listening to Speech: An Auditory Perspective*. Mahwah, NJ: Erlbaum. (Chapters on various topics were assembled to provide "a multi-tier framework" for understanding spoken language.)

Liberman, A. M., and Mattingly, I. G. 1985. The motor theory of speech perception revisited. *Cognition*, **21**, 1–36.

Warren, R. M., 1988. Perceptual basis for the evolution of speech. In *The Genesis of Language: A Different Judgement of Evidence*, M. E. Landsberg (ed.). Berlin: Mouton de Gruyter, 101–110.

8

The relation of hearing to perception in general

Books on perception usually concentrate on a single modality, such as vision or hearing, or a subdivision of a modality, for example, color vision or speech perception. Even when an introductory book on perception deals with several modalities, it is generally subdivided into sections with little overlap. The few books treating the senses together as a single topic generally emphasize philosophy or epistemology (but see Gibson, 1966; Marks, 1978).

Yet the senses are not independent. Events in nature are often multi-dimensional in character and stimulate more than one sensory system. An organism which optimizes its ability to interact appropriately with the environment is one that integrates relevant information across sensory systems. In a book dealing largely with single neurons that respond to more than one modality, Stein and Meredith (1993) stated that "we know of no animal with a nervous system in which the different sensory representations are organized so that they maintain exclusivity from one another."

Multimodal perception

Interaction of vision with senses other than hearing

Depth perception in vision is based on a number of cues, including disparity of the images at the two retinae, and motion parallax. But, in addition to these cues transmitted by the optic nerve, there are proprioceptive ocular cues from the muscles producing accommodation (changes in the curvature of the lens necessary to produce a sharp image) and convergence (adjustment of the ocular axes so that the fixated object is imaged on corresponding points of each fovea). These proprioceptive cues originating in muscles are integrated with the purely optical cues to depth. For a person perceiving an object at a particular distance, these muscle-sense cues are indistinguishable and are as fully visual as those providing information via the optic nerve.

Another example of cross-modal visual integration is afforded by the vestibulo-ocular reflex, which enables the viewer to maintain visual fixation that might otherwise be lost during head movements. Receptors in the semi-circular canals and the utricle and saccule found in the inner ear signal acceleration along any of the three mutually perpendicular planes as well as rotary acceleration of the head, and this information is transmitted by the vestibular branch of the auditory nerve. In addition to neuromuscular reflexes that normally aid in maintaining balance, reflex eye movements are produced by this stimulation in a direction that compensates for the effects of head movements. When the vestibular and ocular systems are operating normally in a coordinated fashion, we are unaware of the contribution of vestibular input to the stability of our visual world.

Graybiel, Kerr, and Bartley (1948) have studied the effect of vestibular information on visual perception in a quantitative fashion using the "oculo-gyral illusion." This illusion can be observed when a person is accelerated in a rotating chair while viewing a dim starlike pattern in an otherwise dark room, with the position of the visual pattern being fixed relative to the head of the subject. At very low acceleration rates which would be imperceptible with the eyes closed ($0.12°/s^2$) the visual target appears to be displaced in the direction of acceleration, so that the only way of detecting acceleration is through the effect of vestibular input on vision.

In the examples of the interaction of vision with other sensory modalities described above, the contributions provided by other senses are not perceived, but influence what is seen. However, this dominance of vision does not occur when vision is pooled with hearing in speech perception.

Interaction of vision and hearing in speech perception

People with normal hearing can use speech-reading (lip-reading) as an aid to comprehension. This usually takes place without awareness – the visual information concerning what is being said seems to be heard rather than seen; that is, it enters into determining what we believe we hear the speaker say.

Comprehension based on speech-reading alone is very difficult, although some deaf individuals can achieve some understanding of what a speaker is saying solely through visual observation. Although lip movements are con-sidered the most important cues, some articulatory information may be fur-nished by movements of the jaw and Adam's apple. In addition, a variety of facial expressions and other gestures are correlated with meaning but not related directly to articulation. Nevertheless, speech-reading, at best, provides incomplete and ambiguous information concerning articulation. Some speech sounds are produced by articulatory movements which cannot be seen (for example, /h/ and /k/), and some sounds with articulatory movements which can be seen have "homophenes" with the same appearance (/m/, /p/, and /b/ involve similar lip movements, so that "may," "pay," and "bay" all look alike).

Experiments have shown not only that speech-reading can function as a rather poor surrogate available to deaf individuals, but also that visual cues to articulation provide a supplementary source of information used by people with normal hearing to enhance intelligibility under noisy environmental conditions (for example, see Dodd, 1977, 1980). Speech-reading can also produce comprehension of speech which would otherwise not be understood. Rosen, Fourcin, and Moore (1981) tested listeners with normal hearing and compared their ability to perceive what a speaker said using speech-reading alone and speech-reading supplemented with acoustic input corresponding to the fundamental frequency pattern of the speaker's voice. While the voice-pitch information by itself was unintelligible, it was found to produce a dramatic increase in the ability to understand what the speaker was saying when used in conjunction with speech-reading.

Perceptual resolution of conflicting visual and auditory information concerning speech

In a dissertation by Cutting (1973, p. 5) it was reported that, when "ba" was delivered to one ear while a synchronous statement of "ga" was presented to the other ear, the listener heard "da" (an example of "dichotic fusion"). Subsequently, McGurk and MacDonald (1976) reported an analogous audio-visual fusion. In a paper entitled "Hearing lips and seeing voices," they used a video recording of a talker producing a consonant-vowel syllable while a sound track simultaneously produced a different consonant-vowel syllable. For example, when the sound of "ba" was dubbed onto a video recording of "ga" which was repeated twice a second, it was reported that 98 percent of adults and 80 percent of preschool children reported hearing "da." It should be noted that there was no awareness of a visual contribution to perception – listeners believed that the illusory "da" was heard and was solely auditory. The illusion occurred even with knowledge of the nature of the visual and auditory input; by closing their eyes, subjects could hear "ba" which reverted to "da" when their eyes were opened. It is as if the modality serving as the source of the information were irrelevant to the perceptual task of determining the nature of the acoustic utterance, and so is not perceived directly. This "McGurk effect" has been studied extensively using a variety of synchronous visual and auditory cues (see Massaro, 1987; Massaro and Cohen, 1995; Green and Norrix, 1997). While these studies have demonstrated that a conflict between vision and hearing in speech perception can lead to the pooling of cues and the "hearing" of visual information, this type of conflict resolution does not take place with other tasks in which vision is pitted against hearing. When visual and auditory cues to the localization of a source are in disagreement, vision tends to dominate, and the sound usually is heard to come from the position determined by vision (for a discussion of this "ventriloquism" effect, see Thurlow and Jack, 1973; Thurlow and Rosenthal, 1976; Bertelson and Radeau, 1981; Bertelson and de Gelder, 2004).

Multimodal sensory control of speech production

The level of our vocal output is monitored not only by hearing but also by nonauditory information, including "vocal effort" as signified by proprioceptive feedback from the muscles involved in controlling subglottal pressure and laryngeal pulsing (see Chapter 7), together with tactile cues indicating the magnitude of vibration along the vocal tract (Borden, 1979). Normally, these cues are in agreement, and each supplements and confirms the information provided by the others. Blocking, or at least partial blocking, of one of the monitoring systems (such as the masking of auditory feedback by noise) does not produce the disruption associated with conflicting cues, since other monitoring systems can be used to maintain normal functioning. However, when a conflict in self-monitoring cues is introduced by recording a speaker's voice and then playing the recording back to the speaker after a delay of a few hundred milliseconds ("delayed auditory feedback"), speech production by the speaker becomes disrupted, and an effect resembling stuttering occurs (Yates, 1963; Zimmerman, Brown, Kelso, *et al.*, 1988; Stuart, Kalinowski, Rastatter, and Lynch, 2002).

Multimodal information concerning the level of our voice alone is insufficient to allow us to speak at an appropriate intensity. It is inappropriate to speak softly to someone far away, and a listener might show annoyance were we to shout in his or her ear. We use visual cues to estimate our distance from a listener and employ this information to adjust our vocal level appropriately. It has been demonstrated experimentally that we are quite familiar with the manner in which sound changes with distance and can make accurate compensatory adjustments in our vocal level (Warren, 1968a; see Chapter 4). In addition, it would be unsuitable to use the same level at a cocktail party that we would use when speaking to someone at the same distance in a quiet room.

The Lombard reflex increases our vocal level with an increase in background noise, and this automatic gain control helps to ensure that we can be understood by our targeted listeners. It is only after both the distance to the listener and the ambient noise level are determined that the level of our voice required for comprehension by the listener can be reckoned and compared with the feedback from the several sensory systems that we use to monitor our voice.

General perceptual rules and modality-specific rules

The close interrelation of sensory systems might lead us to believe that some of the rules governing perception in one modality would apply to others as well. While this is indeed the case, care must be taken in considering how general principles are utilized across modalities and for different tasks within single modalities. Three such general principles will be described briefly along with a few examples of their application.

1.　　*Sensory input is interpreted in terms of familiar causative agents or events, and not in terms of the manner and nature of neural stimulation*

This principle is illustrated in vision when a gentle pressure against the upper right quadrant of the closed eye can be seen as a circle or a ring of light (a "pressure phosphene") located in the lower left quadrant of the visual field. This misidentification of pressure as light and mislocalization of the stimulus is the consequence of the fact that stimulation of the optic nerve is usually produced by light rather than pressure, and receptors at the upper right of the retina usually respond to light at the lower left of the visual field.

Whereas pressure phosphenes represent a correct identification of the stimulated sensory modality but a misinterpretation of the causative agent, this is reversed in "facial vision" of the blind. Obstacles can be detected by some sightless people through sounds reflected from surfaces (a skill more highly developed by bats, cetaceans, and some cave-dwelling birds). Some blind people capable of detecting obstacles need not generate sounds by their cane-tapping or footsteps – spectral changes produced by the reflection of ambient sounds from surfaces can suffice (see Chapter 3). Yet the detection of obstacles is usually not attributed by blind individuals to hearing, but to sensitivity of their face and forehead. Acoustic cues to impending collision when walking are perceived by them as "pressure waves" stimulating their skin, producing a sensation which gets stronger and assumes an unpleasant quality if they continue on the same course (see Supa, Cotzin, and Dallenbach, 1944; Worchel and Dallenbach, 1947). Indeed, if blind individuals do not heed the auditory information indicating their approach to an obstacle, they might suffer actual cutaneous stimulation of an unpleasant nature along with injury to the head. Their inability to appreciate that hearing serves as the basis for their obstacle sense and their false perception of auditory input as cutaneous stimulation seem anomalous only if we consider that people can appreciate directly the nature of sensory input used for perceptual evaluation. However, this misattribution is consistent with the hypothesis that consciousness is directed to events correlated with sensory input rather than sensation per se.

A somewhat different example of the misinterpretation of sensory input was given in Chapter 2. When a sound source changes its location relative to the position of a listener's head, the convolutions of the pinnae produce changes in the spectral composition of sound reaching the auditory receptors. Despite appreciable alteration of the spectral profile, the timbre of the sound seems to be unchanged, and the spectral changes are interpreted in terms of the azimuth and/or elevation of the source.

A final example of the inability to evaluate sensory input per se was discussed in some detail in Chapter 4, in which evidence was presented indicating that attempts to estimate subjective magnitudes for loudness and pitch result in responses based upon estimates of the magnitudes of associated physical correlates. There is also evidence that this physical correlate theory applies to judgments of other sensory magnitudes as well (see Warren, 1958, 1981a; Warren and Warren, 1963).

2.   *Perceptual changes occur during exposure to an unchanging stimulus pattern*

Chapter 7 has discussed the illusory changes that occur while listening to a repeating word. Perceptual instability also occurs when the pattern of visual stimulation does not change. If the continuous small eye movements or tremors (called physiological nystagmus) that are normally present during vision are canceled through optical means, the perception of objects becomes fragmented, and portions of the image disappear. This disappearance is not attributable solely to adaptation or fatigue, since contours and lines corresponding to meaningful symbols and objects tend to be more stable. Also, portions of a frozen retinal image that have disappeared can spontaneously reappear. Even when normal eye movements are occurring, continuing inspection of an ambiguous figure, such as an outline cube, results in changes from one plausible perspective interpretation to another. Instability was the subject of John Locke's musings when he stated more than 300 years ago (Locke, 1690/1894) that, "*the mind cannot fix long on one invariable idea*" (italics his). He concluded (p. 245) that any attempt by an individual to restrict their thoughts to any one concept will fail, and new concepts or modifications of the old " ... will constantly succeed each other in his thoughts, let him be wary as he can."

3.   *Prior stimulation influences perceptual criteria*

While verbal transformations of a repeating word and illusory changes in unchanging visual displays occur *during* a continued exposure to the same stimulus, there are other perceptual changes that occur *after* exposure to a stimulus. These poststimulatory changes follow a rule applying to many types of judgments involving different sensory modalities (Warren, 1985). This "criterion shift rule" states that the criteria used for evaluating stimuli are displaced in the direction of recently experienced values. Following exposure to an exemplar occupying a particular position along a continuum, judgmental boundaries are shifted towards the previously experienced value. Criterion shifts can produce unwanted effects in laboratory studies when stimuli presented earlier in an experiment can influence subsequent judgments (see Chapter 4). These effects have been known for some time, and have been called hysteresis, time-order error, series effects, and central tendency of judgments.

Some examples may clarify the nature and broad applicability of criterion shifts. As discussed in Chapter 7, the time separating the noise produced by the plosive release of air and the onset of voicing can determine whether a syllable is heard as /ta/ or /da/. The voice-onset time corresponding to this category boundary is shifted noticeably after listening to multiple repetitions of either the syllable /ta/ or /da/. Thus, following exposure to exemplars of /ta/, the category boundary moves into what previously was the /ta/ domain, so that some syllables that previously would have been heard as /ta/ can be clearly heard as /da/. It is not necessary to use category boundaries separating phonemes to observe such perceptual shifts. Remez (1979) reported that the perceptual boundary for a vowel in a continuum extending from the vowel to a nonspeech buzz could be changed in an analogous fashion by exposure to an exemplar at one end of the continuum. Similar effects of prior stimulation were described for judgments along a variety of visual continua by Gibson, one such continuum being that of visual curvature. Gibson observed that if a curved line convex to the left was examined for some time, a line presented subsequently had to be curved in the same direction to appear straight, and an objectively straight line appeared convex to the right. Gibson called this phenomenon "adaptation with negative after-effect" and described it in terms of the following general rule: "If a sensory process which has an opposite is made to persist by a constant application of its appropriate stimulus-conditions, the quality will diminish in the direction of becoming neutral, and therewith the quality evoked by any stimulus for the dimension in question will be shifted temporarily toward the opposite or complementary quality" (Gibson, 1937). Gibson's observations are consistent with the after-effect of seen motion described by Aristotle, rediscovered several times in the nineteenth century, and cataloged and classified by Wohlgemuth (1911). These reports indicate that perceptual criteria for movement shift in the direction of previously seen motion. The motions inducing these shifts can be lateral (to the left or right), vertical (up or down), rotary (clockwise or counterclockwise), radial (contraction or expansion of a rotating spiral), or combinations of these types. Thus, after a moving display has been viewed, a new display must move slightly in the manner previously seen in order to appear stationary, so that an objectively stationary display is seen to move in the opposite fashion. Related observations with other perceptual continua were described in 1910 by von Kries (1962, p. 239) who attributed these errors to what he called "the law of contrast." Cathcart and Dawson (1927–1928; 1928–1929) also discovered this rule governing perceptual shifts for color, pitch of sinusoidal tones, visual area, and time intervals; they recognized the rule's very broad applicability, naming it the "diabatic" effect. Helson (1964) tried to quantify this general principle with his "adaptation level theory" for predicting the extent of shifts, but this theory has had rather limited success. There have been attempts to explain perceptual shifts produced by prior stimulation in terms of the adaptation of hypothetical neural feature detectors, but this mechanism, at least applied to phoneme boundary shifts, has come under considerable criticism (see Chapter 7). Of course, the criterion shift rule is, as is perception in general, subserved by neural mechanisms. The value of this rule is that it predicts the existence and the direction of changes. But, it says nothing about the mechanisms producing these changes, as is the case for other rules predicting the nature and direction of changes occurring when dynamic systems are perturbed (i.e., Le Chatelier's principle in chemistry and physics, and Claude Bernard's and W. B. Cannon's homeostasis in biological systems).

The ubiquitous nature of after-effects in perception reflects a relativistic basis for judgments, with the criteria used for perceptual evaluation constructed from past exemplars in such a way that greater weighting is assigned to recent exemplars. It may not be necessary that neural adaptation or fatigue take place for perceptual judgments to change. A shift or recalibration of criteria used for evaluation could be responsible for judgmental shifts.

There is a phenomenon related to criterion shifts: "Sensory Deprivation," the absence of patterned sensory input providing information concerning environmental conditions, can lead to a breakdown in normal perceptual processing (see Vernon, 1963; Schultz, 1965; Riesen, 1975). When subjects see only a featureless white field through translucent goggles and hear only white noise, hallucinations occur in which the unpatterned stimulation is interpreted as an exemplar of some particular ordered pattern. After a few hours of such sensory deprivation, subjects experience after-effects producing errors and distortions in perception when returned to a normal environment.

It appears that there is a continual calibration (i.e., verification or modification) of criteria used for perceptual evaluation of sensory input. Perception is a function that is particularly vital – without homeostatic adjustments to ensure accuracy of perception under changing conditions, our actions would become inappropriate, and our survival would be in jeopardy.

Suggestions for further reading

Marks, L. E. 1978. *The Unity of the Senses: Interrelations Among the Modalities.* New York: Academic Press.

Warren, R. M. 1985. Criterion shift rule and perceptual homeostasis. *Psychological Review*, **92**, 574–584.

References

Abbagnaro, L. A., Bauer, B. B., and Torick, E. L. 1975. Measurements of diffraction and interaural delay of a progressive sound wave caused by the human head II. *Journal of the Acoustical Society of America*, **58**, 693–700.

Adrian, E. D. 1931. The microphone action of the cochlea: An interpretation of Wever and Bray's experiments. *Journal of Physiology*, **71**, 28–29.

American National Standards Institute, 1969 (Reaffirmed, 1986). *Methods for the Calculation of the Articulation Index, S3.5.* New York: American National Standards Institute.

American National Standards Institute, 1976 (Reaffirmed, 1999). *Acoustical Terminology, S1.1.* New York: American National Standards Institute.

American National Standards Institute, 1997 (Reaffirmed, 2007). *Methods for Calculation of the Speech Intelligibility Index, S3.5.* New York: American National Standards Institute.

Amster, H. 1964. Semantic satiation and generation: Learning? Adaptation? *Psychological Bulletin*, **62**, 273–286.

Ashmore, J. F. 1987. A fast motile response in guinea-pig outer hair cells: The cellular basis of the cochlear amplifier. *Journal of Physiology*, **388**, 323–347.

Ayres, T., Aeschbach, S., and Walker, E. L. 1980. Psychoacoustic and experimental determinants of tonal consonance. *Journal of Auditory Research*, **20**, 31–42.

Bachem, A. 1948. Chroma fixation at the ends of the musical frequency scale. *Journal of the Acoustical Society of America*, **20**, 704–705.

Barsz, K. 1988. Auditory pattern perception: The effect of tonal frequency range on the perception of temporal order. *Perception & Psychophysics*, **43**, 293–303.

Bartlett, F. C., and Mark, H. 1922–1923. A note on local fatigue in the auditory system. *British Journal of Psychology*, **13**, 215–218.

Bashford, J. A., Jr., Brubaker, B. S., and Warren, R. M. 1993. Cross-modal enhancement of periodicity detection for very long period recycling frozen noise. *Journal of the Acoustical Society of America*, **93**, 2315 (Abstract).

Bashford, J. A., Jr., Myers, M. D., Brubaker, B. S., and Warren, R. M. 1988. Illusory continuity of interrupted speech: Speech rate determines durational limits. *Journal of the Acoustical Society of America*, **84**, 1635–1638.

Bashford, J. A., Jr., Riener, K. R., and Warren, R. M. 1992. Increasing the intelligibility of speech through multiple phonemic restorations. *Perception & Psychophysics*, **51**, 211–217.

Bashford, J. A., Jr., and Warren, R. M. 1987a. Effects of spectral alternation on the intelligibility of words and sentences. *Perception & Psychophysics*, **42**, 431–438.

Bashford, J. A., Jr., and Warren, R. M. 1987b. Multiple phonemic restorations follow the rules for auditory induction. *Perception & Psychophysics*, **42**, 114–121.

Bashford, J. A., Jr., and Warren, R. M. 1990. The pitch of odd-harmonic tones: Evidence of temporal analysis in the dominance region. *Journal of the Acoustical Society of America*, **88**, S48 (Abstract).

Bashford, J. A., Jr., Warren, R. M., and Brown, C. A. 1996. Use of speech-modulated noise adds strong "bottom-up" cues for phonemic restoration. *Perception & Psychophysics*, **58**, 342–350.

Bashford, J. A., Jr., Warren, R. M., and Lenz, P. W. 2006. Polling the effective neighborhoods of spoken words with the Verbal Transformation Effect. *Journal of the Acoustical Society of America*, **119**, EL55.

Batteau, D. W. 1967. The role of the pinna in human localization. In *Proceedings of the Royal Society (London), Series B*, **168**, 158–180.

Batteau, D. W. 1968. Listening with the naked ear. In *Neuropsychology of Spatially Oriented Behavior*, S. J. Freedman (ed.). Homewood, IL: Dorsey Press, 109–133.

Békésy, G. von 1938. Ueber die Entstehung der Entfernungsempfindung beim Hören, *Akustische Zeitung*, **3**, 21–31.

Békésy, G. von 1959. Similarities between hearing and skin sensation. *Psychological Review*, **66**, 1–22.

Békésy, G. von 1960. *Experiments in Hearing*. New York: McGraw-Hill.

Belin, P., Zatorre, R. J., Hoge, R., Pike, B., and Evans, A. C. 1999. Event-related fMRI of the auditory cortex. *NeuroImage*, **10**, 417–429.

Bergman, M. 1957. Binaural hearing. *Archives of Otolaryngology*, **66**, 572–578.

Berkeley, G. 1948. An essay towards a new theory of vision, Section 143. In *The Works of George Berkeley, Bishop of Cloyne*, vol. 1, A. A. Luce and T. E. Jessop (eds.). London: Thom. Nelson & Sons (First published 1709, text from the 1732 revised edition).

Bertelson, P., and de Gelder, B. 2004. The psychology of multimodal perception. In *Cross Modal Space and Cross Modal Attention*, C. Spence and J. Driver (eds.). Oxford: Oxford University Press, 141–177.

Bertelson, P., and Radeau, M. 1981. Cross-modal bias and perceptual fusion with auditory-visual spatial discordance. *Perception & Psychophysics*, **29**, 578–584.

von Bezold, W. 1890. Urteilstauschungen nach Beseitigung einseitiger Harthörigkeit. *Zeitschrift für Psychologie*, **1**, 486–487.

Bilger, R. C., Matthies, M. L., Hammel, D. R., and Demorest, M. E. 1990. Genetic implications of gender-differences in the prevalence of spontaneous otoacoustic emission. *Journal of Speech and Hearing Research*, **33**, 418–433.

Bilsen, F. A. 1970. Repetition pitch: Its implication for hearing theory and room acoustics. In *Frequency Analysis and Periodicity Detection in Hearing*, R. Plomp and G. F. Smoorenburg (eds.). Leiden: Sijthoff, 291–302.

Bilsen, F. A. 1977. Pitch of noise signals: Evidence for a "central spectrum." *Journal of the Acoustical Society of America*, **61**, 150–161.

Bilsen, F. A., and Goldstein, J. L. 1974. Pitch of dichotically delayed noise and its possible spectral basis. *Journal of the Acoustical Society of America*, **55**, 292–296.

Bilsen, F. A., and Ritsma, R. J. 1969–1970. Repetition pitch and its implication for hearing theory. *Acustica*, **22**, 63–73.

Bilsen, F. A., and Wieman, J. L. 1980. Atonal periodicity sensation for comb filtered noise signals. *Proceedings of the 5th International Symposium in Hearing*. Delft: Delft University Press, 379–383.

Blauert, J. 1969–1970. Sound localization in the median plane. *Acustica*, **22**, 205–213.

Blauert, J. 1997. *Spatial Hearing: The Psychophysics of Human Sound Localization*. Cambridge, MA: MIT Press.

Bloch, E. 1893. Das binaurale Hören. *Zeitschrift für Ohrenheilkunde*, **24**, 25–85.

Blodgett, H. C., Wilbanks, W. A., and Jeffress, L. A. 1956. Effects of large interaural differences upon the judgment of sidedness. *Journal of the Acoustical Society of America*, **28**, 639–643.

de Boer, E. 1956. *On the "Residue" in Hearing*. Unpublished Doctoral Dissertation, University of Amsterdam.

de Boer, E. 1976. On the "residue" and auditory pitch perception. In *Handbook of Sensory Physiology*, vol. V. *Auditory system, Part 3: Clinical and Special Topics*, W. D. Keidel and W. D. Neff (eds.). Berlin: Springer-Verlag, 479–583.

Bond, Z. S. 1976. On the specification of input units in speech perception. *Brain and Language*, **3**, 72–87.

Book, W. F. 1925. *The Psychology of Skill with Special Reference to its Acquisition in Typewriting*. New York: Gregg.

Borden, G. J. 1979. An interpretation of research on feedback interruption. *Brain and Language*, **7**, 307–319.

Boring, E. G. 1942. *Sensation and Perception in the History of Experimental Psychology*. New York: Appleton-Century-Crofts.

Brady, S. A., and Shankweiler, D. P. (eds.). 1991. *Phonological Processes in Literacy*. Hillsdale, NJ: Erlbaum.

Braun, M. 1994. Tuned hair cells for hearing, but tuned basilar membrane for overload protection: Evidence from dolphins, bats, and desert rodents. *Hearing Research*, **78**, 98–114.

Bregman, A. S. 1990. *Auditory Scene Analysis: The Perceptual Organization of Sound*. Cambridge, MA: MIT Press.

Bregman, A. S., and Campbell, J. 1971. Primary auditory stream segregation and perception of order in rapid sequences of tones. *Journal of Experimental Psychology*, **89**, 244–249.

Broadbent, D. E., and Ladefoged, P. 1959. Auditory perception of temporal order. *Journal of the Acoustical Society of America*, **31**, 1539–1540.

Brookshire, R. H. 1972. Visual and auditory sequencing by aphasic subjects. *Journal of Communication Disorders*, **5**, 259–269.

Browman, C. P. 1980. Perceptual processing: Evidence from slips of the ear. In *Errors in Linguistic Performance: Slips of the Tongue, Ear, Pen, and Hand*, V. A. Fromkin (ed.). New York: Academic Press, 213–230.

Brown, E. L., and Deffenbacher, K. 1979. *Perception and the Senses*. New York: Oxford University Press.

Brownell, W. E., Bader, C. R., Bertrand, D., and de Ribaupierre, Y. 1985. Evoked mechanical responses of isolated cochlear outer hair cells. *Science*, **227**, 194–196.

Bryan, W. L., and Harter, N. 1897. Studies in the physiology and psychology of the telegraphic language. *Psychological Review*, **4**, 27–53.

Bryan, W. L., and Harter, N. 1899. Studies on the telegraphic language: The acquisition of a hierarchy of habits. *Psychological Review*, **6**, 345–375.

Bukofzer, M. F. 1947. *Music in the Baroque Era*. New York: Norton.

Burns, E. M., and Viemeister, N. F. 1976. Nonspectral pitch. *Journal of the Acoustical Society of America*, **60**, 863–869.

Butler, R. A. 1969. Monaural and binaural localization of noise bursts vertically in the median sagittal plane. *Journal of Auditory Research*, **3**, 230–235.

Butler, R. A., Levy, E. T., and Neff, W. D. 1980. Apparent distance of sounds recorded in echoic and anechoic chambers. *Journal of Experimental Psychology: Human Perception and Performance*, **6**, 745–750.

Butler, R. A., and Naunton, R. F. 1962. Some effects of unilateral auditory masking upon the localization of sound in space. *Journal of the Acoustical Society of America*, **34**, 1100–1107.

Butler, R. A., and Naunton, R. F. 1964. Role of stimulus frequency and duration in the phenomenon of localization shifts. *Journal of the Acoustical Society of America*, **36**, 917–922.

Buus, S. 1997. Auditory masking. In *Encyclopedia of Acoustics*, vol. 3, M. J. Crocker (ed.). New York: Wiley, 1427–1445.

Carmon, A., and Nachshon, I. 1971. Effect of unilateral brain damage on perception of temporal order. *Cortex*, **7**, 410–418.

Cathcart, E. P., and Dawson, S. 1927–1928. Persistence: A characteristic of remembering. *British Journal of Psychology*, **18**, 262–275.

Cathcart, E. P., and Dawson, S. 1928–1929. Persistence (2). *British Journal of Psychology*, **19**, 343–356.

Caton, R. 1875. The electric currents of the brain. *British Medical Journal*, **2**, 278.

Celce-Murcia, M. 1980. On Meringer's corpus of "slips of the ear." In *Errors in Linguistic Performances: Slips of the Tongue, Ear, Pen, and Hand*, V. A. Fromkin (ed.). New York: Academic Press, 199–211.

Celesia, G. G. 1976. Organization of auditory cortical areas in man. *Brain*, **99**, 403–417.

Chalikia, M. H., and Warren, R. M. 1991. Phonemic transformations: Mapping the illusory organization of steady-state vowel sequences. *Language and Speech*, **34**, 109–143.

Chalikia, M. H., and Warren, R. M. 1994. Spectral fissioning in phonemic transformations. *Perception & Psychophysics*, **55**, 218–226.

Chatterjee, M., and Zwislocki, J. J. 1997. Cochlear mechanisms of frequency and intensity coding. I. The place code for pitch. *Hearing Research*, **111**, 65–75.

Cherry, C. 1953. Some experiments on the recognition of speech, with one and two ears. *Journal of the Acoustical Society of America*, **25**, 975–979.

Cherry, C., and Wiley, R. 1967. Speech communications in very noisy environments. *Nature*, **214**, 1164.

Chistovich, L. A. 1962. Temporal course of speech sound perception. In *Proceedings of the 4th International Commission on Acoustics, (Copenhagen), Article H 18*.

Chocholle, R., and Legouix, J. P. 1957a. On the inadequacy of the method of beats as a measure of aural harmonics. *Journal of the Acoustical Society of America*, **29**, 749–750.

Chocholle, R., and Legouix, J. P. 1957b. About the sensation of beats between two tones whose frequencies are nearly in a simple ratio. *Journal of the Acoustical Society of America*, **29**, 750.

Chomsky, N., and Halle, M. 1968. *The Sound Patterns of English*. New York: Harper & Row.

Christman, R. J. 1954. Shifts in pitch as a function of prolonged stimulation with pure tones. *American Journal of Psychology*, **67**, 484–491.

Ciocca V., and Bregman A. S., 1987. Perceived continuity of gliding and steady-state tones through interrupting noise. *Perception & Psychophysics*, **42**, 476–484.

Colavita, F. B., Szeligo, F. V., and Zimmer, S. D. 1974. Temporal pattern discrimination in cats with insular-temporal lesions. *Brain Research*, **79**, 153–156.

Cole, R. A., Rudnicky, A. I., Zue, V. W., and Reddy, D. R. 1980. Speech as patterns on paper. In *Perception and Production of Fluent Speech*, R. A. Cole (ed.). Hillsdale, NJ: Erlbaum, 3–50.

Cole, R. A., and Scott, B. 1973. Perception of temporal order in speech: The role of vowel transitions. *Canadian Journal of Psychology*, **27**, 441–449.

Cole, R. A., and Scott, B. 1974. The phantom in the phoneme: Invariant cues for stop consonants. *Perception & Psychophysics*, **15**, 101–107.

Coleman, P. D. 1963. An analysis of cues to auditory depth perception in free space. *Psychological Bulletin*, **60**, 302–315.

Collet, L., Kemp, D. T., Veuillet, E., Duclaux, R., Moulin, A., and Morgon, A. 1990. Effect of contralateral auditory stimuli on active cochlear micromechanical properties in human subjects. *Hearing Research*, **43**, 251–262.

Connine, C. M., and Titone, D. 1996. Phoneme monitoring. *Language and Cognitive Processes*, **11**, 635–645.

Cooper, N. P. 1999. An improved heterodyne laser interferometer for use in studies of cochlear mechanics. *Journal of the Neuroscience Methods*, **88**, 93–102.

Cooper, N. P., and Rhode, W. S. 1993. Nonlinear mechanics at the base and apex of the mammalian cochlea; *in vivo* observations using a displacement-sensitive laser interferometer. In *Biophysics of Hair Cell Sensory Systems*, H. Duifhuis, J. W. Horst, P. van Dijk, and S. M. van Netten (eds.). Singapore: World Scientific, 249–257.

Cooper, W. E. 1974. Contingent feature analysis in speech perception. *Perception & Psychophysics*, **16**, 201–204.

Cooper, W. E. 1979. *Speech Perception and Production: Studies in Selective Adaptation.* Norwood, NJ: Ablex.

Cowan, N., Lichty, W., and Grove, T. R. 1990. Properties of memory for unattended spoken syllables. *Journal of Experimental Psychology: Learning, Memory, and Cognition,* **16,** 258–269.

Cramer, E. M., and Huggins, W. H. 1958. Creation of pitch through binaural interaction. *Journal of the Acoustical Society of America,* **30,** 413–417.

Crompton, A. 1982. Syllables and segments in speech production. In *Slips of the Tongue and Language Production,* A. Cutler (ed.). Berlin: Mouton, 109–162.

Cullinan, W. L., Erdos, E., Schaefer, R., and Tekieli, M. E. 1977. Perception of temporal order of vowels and consonant-vowel syllables. *Journal of Speech and Hearing Research,* **20,** 742–751.

Cutting, J. E. 1973. *Levels of Processing in Phonological Fusion.* Doctoral dissertation, Yale University (see p. 7).

Dallos, P. 1973. *The Auditory Periphery: Biophysics and Physiology.* New York: Academic Press.

Dallos, P. 1978. Biophysics of the cochlea. In *Handbook of Perception,* vol. 4, E. C. Carterette and M. P. Freedman (eds.). New York: Academic Press, 125–162.

Dallos, P. 1981. Cochlear physiology. *Annual Review of Psychology,* **32,** 153–190.

Dancer, A. 1992. Experimental look at cochlear mechanics. *Audiology,* **31,** 301–312.

Daneman, M., and Merikle, P. M. 1996. Working memory and language comprehension: A meta-analysis. *Psychonomic Bulletin & Review,* **3,** 422–433.

Dannenbring, G. L. 1976. Perceived auditory continuity with alternately rising and falling frequency transitions. *Canadian Journal of Psychology,* **30,** 99–114.

David, E. E., Guttman, N., and van Bergeijk, W. A. 1958. On the mechanism of binaural fusion. *Journal of the Acoustical Society of America,* **30,** 801–802.

Davis, H. 1961. Some principles of sensory receptor action. *Physiological Review,* **41,** 391–416.

Davis, H. 1965. A model for transducer action in the cochlea. In *Cold Spring Harbor Symposium on Quantitative Biology,* **30,** 181–190.

Davis, H. 1968. Discussion of Batteau's contribution. In *Hearing Mechanisms in Vertebrates, CIBA Foundation Symposium,* A. V. S. de Reuck and J. Knight (eds.). Boston, MA: Little, Brown, 241–242.

Davis, H., Benson, R. W., Covell, W. P., Fernandez, C., Goldstein, R., Katsuki, Y., Legouix, J.-P., McAuliffe, D. R., and Tasaki, I. 1953. Acoustic trauma in the guinea pig. *Journal of the Acoustical Society of America,* **25,** 1180–1189.

Davis, H., Fernandez, C., and McAuliffe, D. R. 1950. The excitatory process in the cochlea. In *Proceedings of the National Academy of Sciences (USA),* **36,** 580–587.

Deinse, J. B. van 1981. Registers. *Folia Phoniatrica,* **33,** 37–50.

Del Castillo, D. M., and Gumenik, W. E. 1972. Sequential memory for familiar and unfamiliar forms. *Journal of Experimental Psychology,* **95,** 90–96.

Deutsch, D. 1974. An auditory illusion. *Nature,* **251,** 307–309.

Deutsch, D. 1975. Two-channel listening to musical scales. *Journal of the Acoustical Society of America,* **57,** 1156–1160.

Deutsch, D. 1981. The octave illusion and auditory perceptual integration. In *Hearing Research and Theory*, vol. 1, J. V. Tobias and E. D. Schubert (eds.). New York: Academic Press, 99–142.

Deutsch, D., and Roll, P. L. 1976. Separate "what" and "where" decision mechanisms in processing a dichotic tonal sequence. *Journal of Experimental Psychology: Human Perception and Performance*, **2**, 23–29.

Dewson, J. H. III 1964. Speech sound discrimination by cats. *Science*, **144**, 555–556.

Dewson, J. H. III 1968. Efferent olivocochlear bundle: Some relationships to stimulus discrimination in noise. *Journal of Neurophysiology*, **31**, 122–130.

Dewson, J. H. III, and Cowey, A. 1969. Discrimination of auditory sequences by monkeys. *Nature*, **222**, 695–697.

Diehl, R. L. 1981. Feature detectors for speech: A critical reappraisal. *Psychological Bulletin*, **89**, 1–18.

Dirks, D. D., and Bower, D. 1970. Effect of forward and backward masking on speech intelligibility. *Journal of the Acoustical Society of America*, **47**, 1003–1008.

Divenyi, P. L., and Hirsh, I. J. 1974. Identification of temporal order in three-tone sequences. *Journal of the Acoustical Society of America*, **56**, 144–151.

Dodd, B. 1977. The role of vision in the perception of speech. *Perception*, **6**, 31–40.

Dodd, B. 1980. Interaction of auditory and visual information in speech perception. *British Journal of Psychology*, **71**, 541–549.

Don, V. J., and Weld, H. P. 1924. Minor studies from the psychological laboratory of Cornell University. LXX. Lapse of meaning with visual fixation. *American Journal of Psychology*, **35**, 446–450.

Dorman, M. F., Cutting, J. E., and Raphael, L. J. 1975. Perception of temporal order in vowel sequences with and without formant transitions. *Journal of Experimental Psychology: Human Perception and Performance*, **104**, 121–129.

Dowling, W. J. 1973. The perception of interleaved melodies. *Cognitive Psychology*, **5**, 322–337.

Durlach, N. I., and Braida, L. D. 1969. Intensity perception. I: Preliminary theory of intensity resolution. *Journal of the Acoustical Society of America*, **46**, 372–383.

Efron, R. 1963. Temporal perception, aphasia, and déjà vu. *Brain*, **86**, 403–424.

Efron, R. 1973. Conservation of temporal information by perceptual systems. *Perception & Psychophysics*, **14**, 518–530.

Efron, R., and Yund, E. W. 1976. Ear dominance and intensity independence in the perception of dichotic chords. *Journal of the Acoustical Society of America*, **59**, 889–898.

Egan, J. P. 1948. The effect of noise in one ear upon the loudness of speech in the other. *Journal of the Acoustical Society of America*, **20**, 58–62.

Egan, J. P., and Hake, H. W. 1950. On the masking pattern of a simple auditory stimulus. *Journal of the Acoustical Society of America*, **20**, 622–630.

Eimas, P. D., and Corbit, J. D. 1973. Selective adaptation of linguistic feature detectors. *Cognitive Psychology*, **4**, 99–109.

Eimas, P. D., and Miller, J. L. 1978. Effects of selective adaptation on the perception of speech and visual patterns: Evidence for feature detectors. In *Perception and Experience*, R. D. Walk and H. L. Pick (eds.). New York: Plenum, 307–345.

Elfner, L. F. 1969. Continuity in alternately sounded tone and noise signals in a free field. *Journal of the Acoustical Society of America*, **46**, 914–917.

Elfner, L. F. 1971. Continuity in alternately sounded tonal signals in a free field. *Journal of the Acoustical Society of America*, **49**, 447–449.

Elfner, L. F., and Caskey, W. E. 1965. Continuity effects with alternately sounded noise and tone signals as a function of manner of presentation. *Journal of the Acoustical Society of America*, **38**, 543–547.

Elfner, L. F., and Homick, J. L. 1966. Some factors affecting the perception of continuity in alternately sounded tone and noise signals. *Journal of the Acoustical Society of America*, **40**, 27–31.

Elfner, L. F., and Homick, J. L. 1967a. Continuity effects with alternately sounding tones under dichotic presentation. *Perception & Psychophysics*, **2**, 34–36.

Elfner, L. F., and Homick, J. L. 1967b. Auditory continuity effects as a function of the duration and temporal location of the interpolated signal. *Journal of the Acoustical Society of America*, **42**, 576–579.

Elman, J. L. 1979. Perceptual origins of the phoneme boundary effect and selective adaptation to speech: A signal detection analysis. *Journal of the Acoustical Society of America*, **65**, 190–207.

Evans, E. F. 1986. Cochlear nerve fiber temporal discharge patterns, cochlear frequency selectivity and the dominant region for pitch. In *Auditory Frequency Selectivity*, B. C. J. Moore and R. D. Patterson (eds.). New York: Plenum, 253–264.

Fant, C. G. M. 1962. Descriptive analysis of the acoustic aspects of speech. *Logos*, **5**, 3–17.

Fastl, H. 1975. Pulsation patterns of sinusoids vs. critical band noise. *Perception & Psychophysics*, **18**, 95–97.

Fay, W. H. 1966. *Temporal Sequence in the Perception of Speech*. The Hague: Mouton.

Fechner, G. T. 1860. *Elemente der Psychophysik*. Leipzig: Breitkopf und Härtel.

Feddersen, W. E., Sandel, T. T., Teas, D. C., and Jeffress, L. A. 1957. Localization of high frequency tones. *Journal of the Acoustical Society of America*, **29**, 988–991.

Ferrand, L., Segui, J., and Grainger, J. 1996. Masked priming of word and picture naming: The role of syllabic units. *Journal of Memory & Language*, **35**, 708–723.

Ferrand, L., Segui, J., and Humphreys, G. W. 1997. The syllable's role in word naming. *Memory & Cognition*, **25**, 458–470.

Fettiplace, R., and Crawford, A. C. 1980. The origin of tuning in turtle cochlear hair cells. *Hearing Research*, **2**, 447–454.

von Fieandt, K. 1951. Loudness invariance in sound perception. *Acta Psychologica Fennica*, **1**, 9–20.

Flanagan, J. L. 1972. *Speech Analysis, Synthesis, and Perception*, 2nd edition. Berlin: Springer-Verlag.

Flanagan, J. L., and Guttman, N. 1960a. On the pitch of periodic pulses. *Journal of the Acoustical Society of America*, **32**, 1308–1319.

Flanagan, J. L., and Guttman, N. 1960b. Pitch of periodic pulses without fundamental component. *Journal of the Acoustical Society of America*, **32**, 1319–1328.

Fletcher, H. 1924. The physical criterion for determining the pitch of a musical tone. *Physical Review*, **23**, 427–437.

Fletcher, H. 1930. A space-time pattern theory of hearing. *Journal of the Acoustical Society of America*, **1**, 311–343.

Fletcher, H. 1940. Auditory patterns. *Review of Modern Physics*, **12**, 47–65.

Fletcher, H. 1953. *Speech and Hearing in Communication*. New York: Van Nostrand.

Flock, A., Flock, B., and Murray, E. 1977. Studies on the sensory hairs of receptor cells in the inner ear. *Acta Oto-Laryngologica*, **83**, 85–91.

Flügel, J. C. 1920–1921. On local fatigue in the auditory system. *British Journal of Psychology*, **11**, 105–134.

Foss, D. J. 1969. Decision processes during sentence comprehension: Effects of lexical item difficulty and position upon decision times. *Journal of Verbal Learning and Verbal Behavior*, **8**, 457–462.

Foss, D. J., and Lynch, R. H., Jr. 1969. Decision processes during sentence comprehension: Effects of surface structure on decision times. *Perception & Psychophysics*, **5**, 145–148.

Foulke, E., and Sticht, T. G. 1969. Review of research on the intelligibility and comprehension of accelerated speech. *Psychological Bulletin*, **72**, 50–62.

Fourcin, A. J. 1965. The pitch of noise with periodic spectral peaks. In *Reports of the 5th International Congress on Acoustics (Liège)*, lA, B42.

Fourcin, A. J. 1970. Central pitch and auditory lateralization. In *Frequency Analysis and Periodicity Detection in Hearing*, R. Plomp and G. F. Smoorenburg (eds.). Leiden: Sijthoff, 319–328.

Fraisse, P. 1963. *The Psychology of Time*, J. Leith, translator. New York: Harper & Row.

Freedman, S. J., and Fisher, H. G. 1968. The role of the pinna in auditory localization. In *Neuropsychology of Spatially Oriented Behavior*, S. J. Freedman (ed.). Homewood, IL: Dorsey Press, 135–152.

Fromkin, V. A. 1971. The non-anomalous nature of anomalous utterances. *Language*, **7**, 27–52.

Fromkin, V. A. 1973. *Speech Errors as Linguistic Evidence*. The Hague: Mouton.

Fromkin, V. A. 1980. Introduction. In *Errors in Linguistic Performance: Slips of the Tongue, Ear, Pen, and Hand*, V. A. Fromkin (ed.). New York: Academic Press, 1–12.

Gacek, R. R. 1972. Neuroanatomy of the auditory system. In *Foundations of Modern Auditory Theory*, vol. 2, J. V. Tobias (ed.). New York: Academic Press, 241–262.

Gamble, E. A. McC. 1909. Minor studies from the psychological laboratory of Wellesley College, I. Intensity as a criterion in estimating the distance of sounds. *Psychological Review*, **16**, 416–426.

Ganong, W. F. III 1976. Amplitude contingent selective adaptation to speech. *Journal of the Acoustical Society of America*, **59**, S26 (Abstract).

Gardner, M. B. 1968. Historical background of the Haas and/or precedence effect. *Journal of the Acoustical Society of America*, **43**, 1243–1248.

Gardner, M. B. 1969. Distance estimation of 0° or apparent 0° oriented speech signals in anechoic space. *Journal of the Acoustical Society of America*, **45**, 47–53.

Gardner, M. B., and Gardner, R. S. 1973. Problem of localization in the median plane: Effect of pinnae cavity occlusion. *Journal of the Acoustical Society of America*, **53**, 400–408.

Garner, W. R. 1951. The accuracy of counting repeated short tones. *Journal of Experimental Psychology*, **41**, 310–316.

Garner, W. R. 1954. Context effects and the validity of loudness scales. *Journal of Experimental Psychology*, **48**, 218–224.

Garner, W. R., and Gottwald, R. L. 1967. Some perceptual factors in the learning of sequential patterns of binary events. *Journal of Verbal Learning and Verbal Behavior*, **6**, 582–589.

Garner, W. R., and Gottwald, R. L. 1968. The perception and learning of temporal patterns. *Quarterly Journal of Experimental Psychology*, **20**, 97–109.

Garnes, S., and Bond, Z. S. 1980. A slip of the ear: A snip of the ear? A slip of the year? In *Errors in Linguistic Performance: Slips of the Tongue, Ear, Pen, and Hand*, V. A. Fromkin (ed.). New York: Academic Press, 231–239.

Gibson, J. J. 1937. Adaptation with negative after-effect. *Psychological Review*, **44**, 222–244.

Gibson, J. J. 1966. *The Senses Considered as Perceptual Systems*. Boston, MA: Houghton Mifflin.

Gilkey, R., and Anderson, T. (eds.) 1997. *Binaural and Spatial Hearing in Real and Virtual Environments*. Hillsdale, NJ: Erlbaum.

Goldinger, S. D., Luce, P. A., and Pisoni, D. B. 1989. Priming lexical neighbors of spoken words: Effects of competition and inhibition. *Journal of Memory and Language*, **28**, 501–518.

Goldstein, J. L. 1973. An optimum processor theory for the central formation of the pitch of complex tones. *Journal of the Acoustical Society of America*, **54**, 1496–1516.

Goldstein, J. L. 1978. Mechanisms of signal analysis and pattern perception in periodicity pitch. *Audiology*, **17**, 421–445.

Goswami, U., and Bryant, P. 1990. *Phonological Skills and Learning to Read*. Hillsdale, NJ: Erlbaum.

Gray, G. W. 1942. Phonemic microtomy: The minimum duration of perceptible speech sounds. *Speech Monographs*, **9**, 75–90.

Graybiel, A., Kerr, W. A., and Bartley, S. H. 1948. Stimulus thresholds of the semicircular canals as a function of angular acceleration. *American Journal of Psychology*, **61**, 21–36.

Green, D. M. 1976. *An Introduction to Hearing*. Hillsdale, NJ: Erlbaum.

Green, D. M., and Yost, W. A. 1975. Binaural analysis. In *Handbook of Sensory Physiology*, vol. 2, W. D. Keidel and W. D. Neff (eds.). Berlin: Springer-Verlag, 461–480.

Green, K. P., and Norrix, L. W. 1997. Acoustic cues to place of articulation and the McGurk effect: The role of release bursts, aspiration, and formant transitions. *Journal of Speech, Language, and Hearing Research*, **40**, 646–665.

Greenberg, S., and Ainsworth, W. A. (eds.) 2006. *Listening to Speech: An Auditory Perspective*. Mahwah, NJ: Erlbaum. (Chapters on various topics were assembled to provide "a multi-tier framework" for understanding spoken language.)

Greenwood, D. D. 1961. Critical bandwidth and the frequency coordinates of the basilar membrane. *Journal of the Acoustical Society of America*, **33**, 1344–1356.

Greenwood, D. D. 1990. A cochlear frequency-position function for several species – 29 years later. *Journal of the Acoustical Society of America*, **87**, 2592–2605.

Greenwood, D. D. 1997. The mel scale's disqualifying bias and a consistency of pitch-difference equisections in 1956 with equal cochlear distances *and* equal frequency ratios. *Hearing Research*, **103**, 199–224.

Guttman, N., and Julesz, B. 1963. Lower limit of auditory periodicity analysis. *Journal of the Acoustical Society of America*, **35**, 610.

Hafter, E. R., and Carrier, S. C. 1972. Binaural interaction in low-frequency stimuli: The inability to trade time and intensity completely. *Journal of the Acoustical Society of America*, **51**, 1852–1862.

Hafter, E. R., Dye, R. H., Jr., and Gilkey, R. H. 1979. Lateralization of tonal signals which have neither onsets nor offsets. *Journal of the Acoustical Society of America*, **65**, 471–477.

Hafter, E. R., and Jeffress, L. A. 1968. Two-image lateralization of tones and clicks. *Journal of the Acoustical Society of America*, **44**, 563–569.

Hall, D. A., Haggard, M. P., Akeroyd, M. A., Palmer, A. R., Summerfield, Q. A., Elliott, M. R., Gurney, E. M., and Bowtell, R. W. 1999. "Sparse" temporal sampling in auditory fMRI. *Human Brain Mapping*, **7**, 213–223.

Hall, J. W., Haggard, M. P., and Fernandes, M. A. 1984. Detection in noise by spectro-temporal pattern analysis. *Journal of the Acoustical Society of America*, **76**, 50–56.

Hall, L. L., and Blumstein, S. E. 1978. The effect of syllabic stress and syllabic organization on the identification of speech sounds. *Perception & Psychophysics*, **24**, 137–144.

Halle, M., and Stevens, K. N. 1972. Speech recognition: A model and a program for research. In *The Structure of Language*, J. A. Fodor and J. J. Katz (eds.). Englewood Cliffs, NJ: Prentice Hall, 604–612.

Ham, L. B., and Parkinson, J. S. 1932. Loudness and intensity relations. *Journal of the Acoustical Society of America*, **3**, 511–534.

Harris, G. G. 1960. Binaural interactions of impulsive stimuli and pure tones. *Journal of the Acoustical Society of America*, **32**, 685–692.

Hartmann, W. M. 1983. Localization of sound in rooms. *Journal of the Acoustical Society of America*, **74**, 1380–1391.

Hartmann, W. M. 1998. *Signals, Sound, and Sensation*. New York: Springer-Verlag.

Hartmann, W. M., and Wittenberg, A. 1996. On the externalization of sound images. *Journal of the Acoustical Society of America*, **99**, 3678–3688.

Held, R. 1955. Shifts in binaural localization after prolonged exposures to atypical combinations of stimuli. *American Journal of Psychology*, **68**, 526–548.

Helmholtz, H. L. F. 1863. *Die Lehre von den Tonempfindunger als physiologische* Grundlage für die Theorie der Musik. Braunschweig: Fr. Viewig und Sohn.

Helmholtz, H. L. F. 1954. *On the Sensations of Tone as a Physiological Basis for the Theory of Music*. New York: Dover, 1954. (Reprint of 2nd English edition of 1885, A. J. Ellis, translator, based upon the 3rd German edition (1870) and rendered conformal with the 4th German edition (1877)).

Helson, H. 1964. *Adaptation Level Theory: An Experimental and Systematic Approach to Behavior*. New York: Harper & Row.

Henning, G. B. 1974. Detectability of interaural delay in high-frequency complex waveforms. *Journal of the Acoustical Society of America*, **55**, 84–90.

Hirano, M., Ohala, J., and Vennard, W. 1969. The function of laryngeal muscles in regulating fundamental frequency and intensity of phonation. *Journal of Speech and Hearing Research*, **12**, 616–628.

Hirsh, I. J. 1948a. The influence of interaural phase on interaural summation and inhibition. *Journal of the Acoustical Society of America*, **20**, 536–544.

Hirsh, I. J. 1948b. Binaural summation and interaural inhibition as a function of the level of the masking noise. *American Journal of Psychology*, **61**, 205–213.

Hirsh, I. J. 1959. Auditory perception of temporal order. *Journal of the Acoustical Society of America*, **31**, 759–767.

Hirsh, I. J., and Sherrick, C. E. 1961. Perceived order in different sense modalities. *Journal of Experimental Psychology*, **62**, 423–432.

Holcombe, A. O., Kanwisher, N., and Treisman, A. 2001. The midstream order deficit. *Perception & Psychophysics*, **63**, 322–329.

Holloway, C. M. 1970. Passing the strongly voiced components of noisy speech. *Nature*, **226**, 178–179.

Houtgast, T. 1972. Psychophysical evidence for lateral inhibition in hearing. *Journal of the Acoustical Society of America*, **51**, 1885–1894.

Houtgast, T. 1973. Psychophysical experiments on "tuning curves" and "two-tone inhibition." *Acustica*, **29**, 168–179.

Houtgast, T. 1974a. *Lateral Suppression in Hearing*. Unpublished Doctoral Dissertation, Free University, Amsterdam.

Houtgast, T. 1974b. Masking patterns and lateral inhibition. In *Facts and Models in Hearing*, E. Zwicker and E. Terhardt (eds.). Berlin: Springer-Verlag, 258–265.

Houtgast, T. 1974c. The slopes of masking patterns. In *Facts and Models in Hearing*, E. Zwicker and E. Terhardt (eds.). Berlin: Springer-Verlag, 269–272.

Houtgast, T. 1976. Subharmonic pitches of a pure tone at low S/N ratio. *Journal of the Acoustical Society of America*, **60**, 405–409.

Houtsma, A. J. M., and Goldstein, J. L. 1972. The central origin of the pitch of complex tones: Evidence from musical interval recognition. *Journal of the Acoustical Society of America*, **51**, 520–529.

Huey, E. B. 1968. *The Psychology and Pedagogy of Reading*. Cambridge, MA: MIT Press.

Huggins, A. W. F. 1964. Distortion of the temporal pattern of speech: Interruption and alternation. *Journal of the Acoustical Society of America*, **36**, 1055–1064.

Huizing, E. H., and Spoor, A. 1973. An unusual type of tinnitus. *Archives of Otolaryngology*, **98**, 134–136.

Hunt, H. V. 1978. *Origins in Acoustics: The Science of Sound from Antiquity to the Age of Newton*. New Haven, CT: Yale University Press.

Husain, F. T., Lozito, T. P., Ulloa, A., and Horwitz, B. 2005. Investigating the neural basis of the auditory continuity illusion. *Journal of Cognitive Neuroscience*, **17**, 1275–1292.

Jakobson, R., Fant, C. G. M., and Halle, M. 1963. *Preliminaries to Speech Analysis: The Distinctive Features and Their Correlates*. Cambridge, MA: MIT Press.

Javel, E. 1986. Basic response properties of auditory fibers. In *Neurobiology of Hearing: The Cochlea*, R. A. Altschuler, R. P. Bobbin, and D. W. Hoffman (eds.). New York: Raven Press, 213–245.

Johnstone, B. M., and Boyle, A. J. F. 1967. Basilar membrane vibration examined with the Mössbauer technique. *Science*, **158**, 389–390.

Johnstone, B. M., Taylor, K. J., and Boyle, A. J. 1970. Mechanics of the guinea pig cochlea. *Journal of the Acoustical Society of America*, **47**, 504–509.

Jones, M. R. 1978. Auditory patterns: Studies in the perception of structure. In *Handbook of Perception*, vol. 8, *Perceptual Coding*, E. C. Carterette and M. P. Friedman (eds.). New York: Academic Press, 255–288.

Jongkees, L. B. W., and van der Veer, R. A. 1957. Directional hearing capacity in hearing disorders. *Acta Oto-Laryngologica*, **48**, 465–474.

Joos, M. 1948. Acoustic phonetics. Supplement to *Language*, **24**, 1–136 (Language Monograph No. 23).

Jusczyk, P. W., Smith, L. B., and Murphy, C. 1981. The perceptual classification of speech. *Perception & Psychophysics*, **30**, 10–23.

Kaernbach, C. 1992. On the consistency of tapping to repeated noise. *Journal of the Acoustical Society of America*, **92**, 788–793.

Kaernbach, C. 1993. Temporal and spectral basis of the features perceived in repeated noise. *Journal of the Acoustical Society of America*, **94**, 91–97.

Kaernbach, C. 2004. The memory of noise. *Experimental Psychology*, **51**, 240–248.

Kashino, M., and Warren, R. M. 1996. Binaural release from temporal induction. *Perception & Psychophysics*, **58**, 899–905.

Kemp, D. T. 1978. Stimulated acoustic emissions from within the human auditory system. *Journal of the Acoustical Society of America*, **64**, 1386–1391.

Kiang, N. Y.-S. 1965. *Discharge Patterns of Single Fibers in the Cat's Auditory Nerve* (Research Monograph No. 35). Cambridge, MA: MIT Press.

Kim, D. O. 1980. Cochlear mechanics: Implications of electrophysiological and acoustical observations. *Hearing Research*, **2**, 297–317.

Kimura, D. 1967. Functional asymmetry of the brain in dichotic listening. *Cortex*, **3**, 163–178.

Kinney, J. A. S. 1961. Discrimination of auditory and visual patterns. *American Journal of Psychology*, **74**, 529–541.

Klatt, D. H. 1979. Speech perception: A model of acoustic-phonetic analysis and lexical access. *Journal of Phonetics*, **7**, 279–312.

Kluender, K. R., Diehl, R. L., and Killeen, P. R. 1987. Japanese quail can learn phonetic categories. *Science*, **237**, 1195–1197.

Klumpp, R. G., and Eady, H. R. 1956. Some measurements of interaural time-difference thresholds. *Journal of the Acoustical Society of America*, **28**, 859–860.

Kock, W. E. 1950. Binaural localization and masking. *Journal of the Acoustical Society of America*, **22**, 801–804.

Kohllöffel, L. U. E. 1972a. A study of basilar membrane vibrations. I. Fuzziness detection: A new method for the analysis of microvibrations with laser light. *Acustica*, **27**, 49–65.

Kohllöffel, L. U. E. 1972b. A study of basilar membrane vibrations. II. The vibratory amplitude and phase pattern along the basilar membrane (post mortem). *Acustica*, **27**, 66–81.

Kohllöffel, L. U. E. 1972c. A study of basilar membrane vibrations. III. The basilar membrane frequency response curve in the living guinea pig. *Acustica*, **27**, 82–89.

von Kries, J. 1962. Commentary. In *Helmholtz's Treatise on Physiological Optics*, vol. 3, J. P. C. Southall (ed.). New York: Dover, p. 239. (Translated from the 3rd German edition originally published in 1910.)

Kryter, K. D. 1960. Speech bandwidth compression through spectrum selection. *Journal of the Acoustical Society of America*, **32**, 547–556.

Kuhl, P., and Miller, J. D. 1974. Discrimination of speech sounds by the chinchilla: /t/ vs. /d/ in CV syllables. *Journal of the Acoustical Society of America*, **56**, S52 (Abstract).

Kuhl, P., and Miller, J. D. 1978. Speech perception by the chinchilla: Identification functions for synthetic VOT stimuli. *Journal of the Acoustical Society of America*, **63**, 905–917.

Kuhn, G. F. 1977. Model for the interaural time differences in the azimuthal plane. *Journal of the Acoustical Society of America*, **62**, 157–167.

Kunov, H., and Abel, S. 1981. Effects of rise/decay time on the lateralization of interaurally delayed 1-kHz tones. *Journal of the Acoustical Society of America*, **69**, 769–773.

Laird, D. A., Taylor, E., and Wille, H. H. 1932. The apparent reduction of loudness. *Journal of the Acoustical Society of America*, **3**, 393–401.

Lane, C. E. 1925. Binaural beats. *Physical Review*, **26**, 401–412.

Lane, H. L., Catania, A. C., and Stevens, S. S. 1961. Voice level: Autophonic scale, perceived loudness, and effects of sidetone. *Journal of the Acoustical Society of America*, **33**, 160–167.

Langmuir, I., Schaefer, V. J., Ferguson, C. V., and Hennelly, E. F. 1944. A study of binaural perception of the direction of a sound source. *OSRD Report No. 4079*, Publ. No. 31014. (Available from the United States Department of Commerce.)

Lashley, K. S. 1951. The problem of serial order in behavior. In *Cerebral Mechanisms in Behavior: The Hixon Symposium*, L. A. Jeffress (ed.). New York: Wiley, 112–136.

Lawrence, M. 1965. Middle ear muscle influence on binaural hearing. *Archives of Otolaryngology*, **82**, 478–482.

Lawrence, M., and Yantis, P. A. 1956. Onset and growth of aural harmonics in the overloaded ear. *Journal of the Acoustical Society of America*, **28**, 852–858.

Layton, B. 1975. Differential effects of two nonspeech sounds on phonemic restoration. *Bulletin of the Psychonomic Society*, **6**, 487–490.

Levelt, W. J. M. 1992. Accessing words in speech production: Stages, processes and representations. *Cognition*, **42**, 1–22.

Levelt, W. J. M., and Wheeldon, L. 1994. Do speakers have access to a mental syllabary? *Cognition*, **50**, 239–269.

Levy, E. T., and Butler, R. A. 1978. Stimulus factors which influence the perceived externalization of sound presented through headphones. *Journal of Auditory Research*, **18**, 41–50.

Lewis, B., and Coles, R. 1980. Sound localization in birds. *Trends in NeuroSciences*, **3**, 102–105.

Liberman, A. M., Cooper, F. S., Shankweiler, D. P., and Studdert-Kennedy, M. 1967. Perception of the speech code. *Psychological Review*, **74**, 431–461.

Liberman, A. M., Delattre, P., and Cooper, F. S. 1952. The role of selected stimulus-variables in the perception of the unvoiced stop consonants. *American Journal of Psychology*, **65**, 497–516.

Liberman, A. M., and Mattingly, I. G. 1985. The motor theory of speech perception revisited. *Cognition*, **21**, 1–36.

Liberman, I. Y., Shankweiler, D., Fischer, F. W., and Carter, B. 1974. Reading and the awareness of linguistic segments. *Journal of Experimental Child Psychology*, **18**, 201–212.

Licklider, J. C. R. 1951. A duplex theory of pitch perception. *Experientia*, **7**, 128–134.

Licklider, J. C. R. 1954. "Periodicity" pitch and "place" pitch. *Journal of the Acoustical Society of America*, **26**, 945 (Abstract).

Lieberman, P. 1963. Some effects of semantic and grammatical context on the production and perception of speech. *Language and Speech*, **6**, 172–187.

Lim, D. J. 1980. Cochlear anatomy related to cochlear micromechanics. A review. *Journal of the Acoustical Society of America*, **67**, 1686–1695.

Lindsay, P. H., and Norman, D. A. 1977. *Human Information Processing: An Introduction to Psychology*, 2nd edition. New York: Academic Press.

Litovsky, R. Y., Colburn, H. S., Yost, W. A., and Guzman, S. J. 1999. The precedence effect. *Journal of the Acoustical Society of America*, **106**, 1633–1654.

Locke, J. 1690. *Concerning Human Understanding*. London: Holt. Book 2, Chapter 14, Section 13 (Reprinted Oxford: Clarendon, 1894).

Luce, P. A., Goldinger, S. D., Auer, E. T. J., and Vitevitch, M. S. 2000. Phonetic priming, neighborhood activation, and PARSYN. *Perception & Psychophysics*, **62**, 615–662.

Luce, P. A., and Pisoni, D. B. 1998. Recognizing spoken words: The neighborhood activation model. *Ear and Hearing*, **19**, 1–36.

Luce, P. A., Pisoni, D. B., and Goldinger, S. D. 1990. Similarity neighborhoods of spoken words. In *Cognitive Models of Speech Processing: Psycholinguistic and Computational Perspectives*, G. T. M. Altmann (ed.). Cambridge, MA: MIT Press.

MacNeilage, P. F. 1970. Motor control of serial ordering in speech. *Psychological Review*, **77**, 182–196.

MacNeilage, P. F., and Ladefoged, P. 1976. The production of speech and language. In *Handbook of Perception*, vol. 7, E. C. Carterette and M. P. Friedman (eds.). New York: Academic Press, 75–120.

Mammano, F., and Ashmore, J. F. 1995. A laser interferometer for subnanometer measurements in the cochlea. *Journal of Neuroscience Methods*, **60**, 89–94.

Marks, L. E. 1978. *The Unity of the Senses: Interrelations Among the Modalities.* New York: Academic Press.

Massaro, D. W. 1987. *Speech Perception by Ear and Eye: A Paradigm for Psychological Inquiry.* Hillsdale, NJ: Erlbaum.

Massaro, D. W., and Cohen, M. M. 1995. Perceiving talking faces. *Current Directions in Psychological Science*, **4**, 104–109.

Matsumoto, M. 1897. Researches on acoustic space. *Studies from the Yale Psychological Laboratory*, **5**, 1–75.

Maxfield, J. P. 1930. Acoustic control of recording for talking motion pictures. *Journal of the Society of Motion Picture Engineers*, **14**, 85–95.

Maxfield, J. P. 1931. Some physical factors affecting the illusion in sound motion pictures. *Journal of the Acoustical Society of America*, **3**, 69–80.

McClelland, J. L. and Elman, J. L. 1986. The TRACE model of speech perception. *Cognitive Psychology*, **18**, 1–86.

McFadden, D., and Pasanen, E. G. 1975. Binaural beats at high frequencies. *Science*, **190**, 394–396.

McGurk, H., and MacDonald, J. 1976. Hearing lips and seeing voices. *Nature*, **264**, 746–748.

McKenna, T. M., Weinberger, N. M., and Diamond, D. M. 1989. Responses of single auditory cortical neurons to tone sequences. *Brain Research*, **481**, 142–153.

Meddis, R., and Hewitt, M. J. 1991a. Virtual pitch and phase sensitivity of a computer model of the auditory periphery. I. Pitch identification. *Journal of the Acoustical Society of America*, **89**, 2866–2882.

Meddis, R., and Hewitt, M. J. 1991b. Virtual pitch and phase sensitivity of a computer model of the auditory periphery. II. Phase sensitivity. *Journal of the Acoustical Society of America*, **89**, 2883–2894.

Meringer, R., and Mayer, C. 1895. *Versprechen und Verlesen: Eine psychologische-linguistische Studie.* Stuttgart: Göschensche Verlagsbuschhandlung.

Mershon, D. H., and King, L. E. 1975. Intensity and reverberation as factors in the auditory perception of egocentric distance. *Perception & Psychophysics*, **18**, 409–415.

Meyer, M. F. 1957. Aural harmonics are fictitious. *Journal of the Acoustical Society of America*, **29**, 749.

Micheyl, C., Carlyon, R. P., Shtyrov, Y., Hauk, O., Dodson, T., and Pullvermüller, F. 2003. The neurophysiological basis of the auditory continuity illusion: A mismatch negativity study. *Journal of Cognitive Neuroscience*, **15**, 747–758.

Miller, G. A. 1947. Sensitivity to changes in the intensity of white noise and its relation to masking and loudness. *Journal of the Acoustical Society of America*, **19**, 609–619.

Miller, G. A. 1962. Decision units in the perception of speech. *IRE Transactions on Information Theory*, **8**, 81–83.

Miller, G. A. 1991. *The Science of Words.* New York: Freeman.

Miller, G. A., and Licklider, J. C. R. 1950. The intelligibility of interrupted speech. *Journal of the Acoustical Society of America*, **22**, 167–173.

Miller, J. L., and Jusczyk, P. W. 1989. Seeking the neurobiological bases of speech perception. *Cognition,* **33**, 111–137.

Miller, R. L. 1947. Masking effects of periodically pulsed tones as a function of time and frequency. *Journal of the Acoustical Society of America,* **19**, 798–807.

Mills, A. W. 1958. On the minimum audible angle. *Journal of the Acoustical Society of America,* **30**, 237–246.

Mills, A. W. 1972. Auditory localization. In *Foundations of Modern Auditory Theory,* vol. 2, J. V. Tobias (ed.). New York: Academic Press, 303–348.

Mohrmann, K. 1939. Lautheitskonstanz im Entfernungswechsel. *Zeitschrift für Psychologie,* **145**, 145–199.

Møller, A. 2006. *Hearing: Anatomy, Physiology, and Disorders of the Auditory System,* 2nd edition. San Diego, CA: Academic Press.

Monroe, M. 1932. *Children who Cannot Read.* Chicago, IL: University of Chicago Press.

Moore, B. C. J. 1974. Relation between the critical bandwidth and the frequency-difference limen. *Journal of the Acoustical Society of America,* **55**, 359.

Moore, B. C. J. 2003. *An introduction to the Psychology of Hearing,* 5th edition. San Diego, CA: Academic Press.

Moore, M. W., and Bliss, J. C. 1975. The Optacon reading system. *Education of the Visually Handicapped,* **7**, 15–21.

Moore, T. J., and Mundie, J. R. 1971. Specification of the minimum number of glottal pulses necessary for reliable identification of selected speech sounds. *Aerospace Medical Research Laboratory Report,* TR-70-104.

Morais, J., Cary, L., Alegria, J., and Bertelson, P. 1979. Does awareness of speech as a sequence of phones arise spontaneously? *Cognition,* **7**, 323–331.

Morais, J., and Kolinsky, R. 1994. Perception and awareness in phonological processing: The case of the phoneme. *Cognition,* **50**, 287–297.

Müsch, H., and Buus, S. 2001a. Using statistical decision theory to predict speech intelligibility. I. Model structure. *Journal of the Acoustical Society of America,* **109**, 2896–2909.

Müsch, H., and Buus, S. 2001b. Using statistical decision theory to predict speech intelligibility. II. Measurement and prediction of consonant-discrimination performance. *Journal of the Acoustical Society of America,* **109**, 2910–2920.

Näätänen, R., and Winkler, I. 1999. The concept of auditory stimulus representation in cognitive neuroscience. *Psychological Bulletin,* **125**, 826–859.

Necker, L. A. 1832. Observations on some remarkable phenomena seen in Switzerland; and on an optical phenomenon which occurs on viewing of a crystal or geometrical solid. *Philosophical Magazine (Series 1),* **3**, 239–337.

Negus, V. E. 1949. *The Comparative Anatomy and Physiology of the Larynx.* New York: Grune & Stratton.

Neisser, U., and Hirst, W. 1974. Effect of practice on the identification of auditory sequences. *Perception & Psychophysics,* **15**, 391–398.

Newton, I. 1730. *Opticks, or a Treatise of the Reflections, Refractions, Inflections & Colours of Light,* 4th edition. London (Reprinted New York: Dover, 1952).

van Noorden, L. P. A. S. 1975. *Temporal Coherence in the Perception of Tone Sequences.* Unpublished Doctoral Dissertation, Eindhoven University of Technology.

van Noorden, L. P. A. S. 1977. Minimum differences of level and frequency for perceptual fission of tone sequences ABAB. *Journal of the Acoustical Society of America*, **61**, 1041–1045.

Nordmark, J. O. 1968. Mechanisms of frequency discrimination. *Journal of the Acoustical Society of America*, **44**, 1533–1540.

Norris, D. 1994. Shortlist: A connectionist model of continuous speech recognition. *Cognition*, **52**, 189–234.

Norris, D., McQueen, J. M., and Cutler, A. 2000. Merging information in speech recognition: Feedback is never necessary. *Behavioral and Brain Sciences*, **23**, 299–325.

Obusek, C. J., and Warren, R. M. 1973. Relation of the verbal transformation and the phonemic restoration effects. *Cognitive Psychology*, **5**, 97–107.

Oertel, D. 1999. The role of timing in the brain stem auditory nuclei of vertebrates. *Annual Review of Physiology*, **61**, 497–519.

Ohm, G. S. 1843. Ueber die Definition des Tones, nebst daran geknüpfter Theorie der Sirene und ähnlicher tonbildender Vorrichtungen. *Annalen der Physik und Chemie*, **59**, 513–565.

Ohm, G. S. 1844. Noch ein Paar Worte über die Definition des Tones. *Annalen der Physik und Chemie*, **62**, 1–18.

Öhman, S. E. G. 1966. Perception of segments of VCCV utterances. *Journal of the Acoustical Society of America*, **40**, 979–988.

Opheim, O., and Flottorp, G. 1955. The aural harmonics in normal and pathological hearing. *Acta Oto-Laryngologica*, **45**, 513–531.

Ortmann, O. 1926. On the melodic relativity of tones. *Psychological Monographs, **35** (1, No. 162).

Paivio, A. 1971. *Imagery and Verbal Processes.* New York: Holt, Rinehart & Winston.

Paivio, A., and Csapo, K. 1969. Concrete-image and verbal memory codes. *Journal of Experimental Psychology*, **80**, 279–285.

Patterson, J. H., and Green, D. M. 1970. Discrimination of transient signals having identical energy spectra. *Journal of the Acoustical Society of America*, **48**, 894–905.

Patterson, R. D. 1969. Noise masking of a change in residue pitch. *Journal of the Acoustical Society of America*, **45**, 1520–1524.

Patterson, R. D., and Wightman, F. L. 1976. Residue pitch as a function of component spacing. *Journal of the Acoustical Society of America*, **59**, 1450–1459.

Peake, W. T., and Ling, A., Jr. 1980. Basilar-membrane motion in the alligator lizard: Its relation to tonotopic organization and frequency selectivity. *Journal of the Acoustical Society of America*, **67**, 1736–1745.

Peterson, G. E. 1946. Influence of voice quality. *Volta Review*, **48**, 640–641.

Peterson, G. E., and Barney, H. L. 1952. Control methods used in a study of the vowels. *Journal of the Acoustical Society of America*, **24**, 115–184.

Petkov, C. I., O'Connor, K. N., and Sutter, M. I. 2003. Illusory sound perception in Macaque monkeys. *Journal of Neuroscience*, **23**, 9155–9161.

Philipchalk, R., and Rowe, F. J. 1971. Sequential and nonsequential memory for verbal and nonverbal auditory stimuli. *Journal of Experimental Psychology*, **91**, 341–343.

Pickles, J. O. 1988. *An Introduction to the Physiology of Hearing*, 2nd edition. San Diego, CA: Academic Press.

Pierce, A. H. 1901. *Studies in Auditory and Visual Space Perception*. New York: Longmans, Green.

Piston, W. 1947. *Counterpoint*. New York: Norton.

Plack, C. J., Oxenham, A. J., Fay, R., and Popper, A. N. (eds.) 2005. *Pitch: Neural Coding and Perception*. New York: Springer-Verlag.

Plateau, J. 1872. Sur la mesure des sensations physiques, et sur la loi qui lie l'intensité de ces sensations à l'intensité de la cause excitante. *Bulletins de l'Académie Royale des Sciences, des Lettres et des Beaux-Arts de Belgique*, **33**, 376–388 (Série 2).

Plenge, G. 1974. On the differences between localization and lateralization. *Journal of the Acoustical Society of America*, **56**, 944–951.

Plomp, R. 1964. The ear as a frequency analyzer. *Journal of the Acoustical Society of America*, **36**, 1628–1636.

Plomp, R. 1966. *Experiments on Tone Perception*. Unpublished Doctoral Dissertation, University of Utrecht.

Plomp, R. 1967a. Pitch of complex tones. *Journal of the Acoustical Society of America*, **41**, 1526–1533.

Plomp, R. 1967b. Beats of mistuned consonances. *Journal of the Acoustical Society of America*, **42**, 462–474.

Plomp, R. 1968. Pitch, timbre, and hearing theory. *International Audiology*, **7**, 322–344.

Plomp, R. 1976. *Aspects of Tone Sensation: A Psychophysical Study*. New York: Academic Press.

Plomp, R. 1981. Perception of sound signals at low signal-to-noise ratio. In *Auditory and Visual Pattern Recognition*, D. J. Getty and J. H. Howard (eds.). Hillsdale, NJ: Erlbaum, 27–35.

Plomp, R. 2002. *The Intelligent Ear*. Mahwah, NJ: Erlbaum (see Chapter 3 for a discussion on sequence perception).

Plomp, R., and Levelt, W. J. M. 1965. Tonal consonance and critical bandwidth. *Journal of the Acoustical Society of America*, **38**, 548–560.

Polanyi, M. 1958. *Personal Knowledge*. Chicago, IL: Chicago University Press.

Polanyi, M. 1968. Logic and psychology. *American Psychologist*, **23**, 27–43.

Pollack, I. 1952. On the measurement of the loudness of speech. *Journal of the Acoustical Society of America*, **24**, 323–324.

Potter, R. K., Kopp, G. A., and Kopp, H. G. 1947. *Visible Speech*. New York: Van Nostrand (Reprinted New York: Dover, 1966).

Poulton, E. C., and Freeman, P. R. 1966. Unwanted asymmetrical transfer effects with balanced experimental designs. *Psychological Bulletin*, **66**, 1–8.

Powers, G. L., and Wilcox, J. C. 1977. Intelligibility of temporally interrupted speech with and without intervening noise. *Journal of the Acoustical Society of America*, **61**, 195–199.

Pravdich-Neminsky, V. V. 1913. Ein Versuch der Registrierung der elektrischen Gehirnerscheinungen (in German). *Zentralblatt Physiology*, **27**, 951–960.

Preusser, D. 1972. The effect of structure and rate on the recognition and description of auditory temporal patterns. *Perception & Psychophysics*, **11**, 233–240.

Probst, R., Lonsbury-Martin, B. L., and Martin, G. K. 1991. A review of otoacoustic emissions. *Journal of the Acoustical Society of America*, **89**, 2027–2067.

Puel, J. L. 1995. Chemical synaptic transmission in the cochlea. *Progress in Neurobiology*, **47**, 449–476.

Pujol, R., Lenoir, M., Ladrech, S., Tribillac, F., and Rebillard, G. 1992. Correlation between the length of the outer hair cells and the frequency coding of the cochlea. In *Auditory Physiology and Perception*, Y. Cazals, K. Horner, and L. Demany (eds.). Oxford: Pergamon, 45–52.

Rasmussen, G. L. 1946. The olivary peduncle and other fiber projections of the superior olivary complex. *Journal of Comparative Neurology*, **84**, 141–219.

Rasmussen, G. L. 1953. Further observations of the efferent cochlear bundle. *Journal of Comparative Neurology*, **99**, 61–74.

Rayleigh, Lord 1907. On our perception of sound direction. *Philosophical Magazine*, **13**, 214–232.

Read, C. A., Zhang, Y., Nie, H., and Ding, B. 1986. The ability to manipulate speech sounds depends on knowing alphabetic writing. *Cognition*, **24**, 31–44.

Reisz, R. R. 1928. Differential sensitivity of the ear for pure tones. *Physical Review*, **31**, 867–875.

Relkin, E. M., and Ducet, J. R. 1997. Is loudness simply proportional to the auditory nerve spike count? *Journal of the Acoustical Society of America*, **101**, 2735–2740.

Remez, R. E. 1979. Adaptation of the category boundary between speech and nonspeech: A case against feature detectors. *Cognitive Psychology*, **11**, 38–57.

Remez, R. E., Rubin, P. E., Berns, S. M., Pardo, J. S., and Lang, J. M. 1994. On the perceptual organization of speech. *Psychological Review*, **101**, 129–156.

Repp, B. H. 1992. Perceptual restoration of a "missing" speech sound: Auditory induction or illusion. *Perception & Psychophysics*, **51**, 14–32.

Rhode, W. S. 1971. Observations of the vibration of the basilar membrane in squirrel monkeys using the Mössbauer technique. *Journal of the Acoustical Society of America*, **49**, 1218–1231.

Rhode, W. S. 1973. An investigation of post-mortem cochlear mechanics using the Mössbauer effect. In *Basic Mechanisms in Hearing*, A. R. M. Møller (ed.). New York: Academic Press, 49–67.

Rhode, W. S., and Robles, L. 1974. Evidence from Mössbauer experiments for non-linear vibration in the cochlea. *Journal of the Acoustical Society of America*, **55**, 588–596.

Richardson, L. F., and Ross, J. S. 1930. Loudness and telephone current. *Journal of General Psychology*, **3**, 288–306.

Riesen, A. H. (ed.) 1975. *The Developmental Neuropsychology of Sensory Deprivation*. New York: Academic Press.

Ritsma, R. J. 1962. Existence region of the tonal residue. I. *Journal of the Acoustical Society of America*, **34**, 1224–1229.

Ritsma, R. J. 1963. Existence region of the tonal residue. II. *Journal of the Acoustical Society of America*, **35**, 1241–1245.

Ritsma, R. J. 1970. Periodicity detection. In *Frequency Analysis and Periodicity Detection in Hearing*, R. Plomp and G. F. Smoorenburg (eds.). Leiden: Sijthoff, 250–266.

Roffler, S. K., and Butler, R. A. 1968. Factors that influence the localization of sound in the vertical plane. *Journal of the Acoustical Society of America*, **43**, 1255–1259.

Rose, J. E., Brugge, J. F., Anderson, D. J., and Hind, J. E. 1967. Phase-locked response to low-frequency tones in single auditory nerve fibers of the squirrel monkey. *Journal of Neurophysiology*, **30**, 769–793.

Rose, J. E., Hind, J. E., Anderson, D. J., and Brugge, J. F. 1971. Some effects of stimulus intensity on response of auditory nerve fibers in the squirrel monkey. *Journal of Neurophysiology*, **34**, 685–699.

Rosen, S. M. 1979. Range and frequency effects in consonant categorization. *Journal of Phonetics*, **7**, 393–402.

Rosen, S. M., Fourcin, A. J., and Moore, B. C. J. 1981. Voice pitch as an aid to lipreading. *Nature*, **291**, 150–152.

Roth, G. L., Kochhar, R. K., and Hind, J. E. 1980. Interaural time differences: Implications regarding the neurophysiology of sound localization. *Journal of the Acoustical Society of America*, **68**, 1643–1651.

Rowe, E. J., and Cake, L. J. 1977. Retention of order information for sounds and words. *Canadian Journal of Psychology*, **31**, 14–23.

Rowley, R. R., and Studebaker, G. A. 1969. Monaural loudness-intensity relationships for a 1,000-Hz tone. *Journal of the Acoustical Society of America*, **45**, 1186–1192.

Royer, F. L., and Garner, W. R. 1970. Perceptual organization of nine-element auditory temporal patterns. *Perception & Psychophysics*, **7**, 115–120.

Rozin, P., Poritsky, S., and Sotsky, R. 1971. American children with reading problems can easily learn to read English represented by Chinese characters. *Science*, **171**, 1264–1267.

Sachs, C. 1953. *Rhythm and Tempo*. New York: Norton.

Sams, M., Hari, R., Rif, J., and Knuutila, J. 1993. The human auditory trace persists about 10s: Neuromagnetic evidence. *Journal of Cognitive Neurosciences*, **5**, 363–370.

Samuel, A. G. 1987. Lexical uniqueness effects on phonemic restoration. *Journal of Memory and Language*, **26**, 36–56.

Sandel, T. T., Teas, D. C., Feddersen, W. E., and Jeffress, L. A. 1955. Localization of sound from single and paired sources. *Journal of the Acoustical Society of America*, **27**, 842–852.

Sasaki, T. 1980. Sound restoration and temporal localization of noise in speech and music sounds. *Tohoku Psychologica Folia*, **39**, 79–88.

Savin, H. B. 1972. What the child knows about speech when he starts to learn to read. In *Language by Ear and by Eye*, J. F. Kavanagh and I. G. Mattingly (eds.). Cambridge, MA: MIT Press, 319–329.

Savin, H. B., and Bever, T. G. 1970. The nonperceptual reality of the phoneme. *Journal of Verbal Learning and Verbal Behavior*, **9**, 295–302.

Sawusch, J. R., and Nusbaum, H. C. 1979. Contextual effects in vowel perception. l: Anchor-induced contrast effects. *Perception & Psychophysics*, **25**, 292–302.

Scharf, B. 1970. Critical bands. In *Foundations of Modern Auditory Theory*, vol. I, J. V. Tobias (ed.). New York: Academic Press, 157–202.

Schouten, J. F. 1938. The perception of subjective tones. *K Akademie van Wetenschappen, Amsterdam. Afdeeling Natuurkunde (Proceedings)*, **41**, 1086–1093.

Schouten, J. F. 1939. Synthetic sound. *Philips Technical Review*, **4**, 153–180.

Schouten, J. F. 1940a. The residue, a new component in subjective sound analysis. *K. Akademie van Wetenschappen, Amsterdam. Afdeeling Natuurkunde (Proceedings)*, **43**, 356–365.

Schouten, J. F. 1940b. The perception of pitch. *Philips Technical Review*, **5**, 286–294.

Schouten, J. F. 1940c. The residue and the mechanism of hearing. *K. Akademie van Wetenschappen, Amsterdam. Afdeeling Natuurkunde (Proceedings)*, **43**, 991–999.

Schouten, J. F. 1970. The residue revisited. In *Frequency Analysis and Periodicity Detection in Hearing*, R. Plomp and G. F. Smoorenburg (eds.). Leiden: Sijthoff, 41–58.

Schouten, J. F., Ritsma, R. J., and Cardozo, B. L. 1962. Pitch of the residue. *Journal of the Acoustical Society of America*, **34**, 1418–1424.

Schreiner, C., Gottlob, D., and Mellert, V. 1977. Influences of the pulsation threshold method on psychoacoustical tuning curves. *Acustica*, **37**, 29–36.

Schröger, E. 1996. Interaural time and level differences: Integrated or separated processing? *Hearing Research*, **96**, 191–198.

Schultz, D. P. 1965. *Sensory Restriction: Effects on Behavior*. New York: Academic Press.

Searle, C. L., Jacobson, J. Z., and Rayment, S. G. 1979. Stop consonant discrimination based on human audition. *Journal of the Acoustical Society of America*, **65**, 799–809.

Seebeck, A. 1841. Beobachtungen über einige Bedingungen der Enstehung von. Tönen. *Annalen der Physik und Chemie*, **53**, 417–437.

Seebeck, A. 1843. Ueber die Sirene. *Annalen der Physik und Chemie*, **60**, 449–481.

Seebeck, A. 1844. Ueber die Definition des Tones. *Annalen der Physik und Chemie*, **63**, 353–368.

Sellick, P. M., Patuzzi, R., and Johnstone, B. M. 1982. Measurement of basilar membrane motion in the guinea pig using the Mössbauer technique. *Journal of the Acoustical Society of America*, **72**, 131–141.

Semal, C., and Demany, L. 1990. The upper limit of "musical" pitch. *Music Perception*, **8**, 165–176.

Severance, E., and Washburn, M. F. 1907. Minor studies from the psychological laboratory of Vassar College. IV. The loss of associative power in words after long fixation. *American Journal of Psychology*, **18**, 182–186.

Shankweiler, D., and Liberman, I. Y. 1972. Misreading: A search for causes. In *Language by Ear and by Eye*, J. F. Kavanaugh and I. G. Mattingly (eds.). Cambridge, MA: MIT Press, 293–317.

Shattuck, S. R. 1975. *Speech Errors and Sentence Production*. Unpublished Doctoral Dissertation, Massachusetts Institute of Technology.

Shaxby, J. H., and Gage, F. H. 1932. Studies in the localisation of sound. *Medical Research Council Special Report*, Series No. 166, 1–32.

Sherman, G. L. 1971. *The Phonemic Restoration Effect: An Insight into the Mechanisms of Speech Perception.* Unpublished Master's Thesis, University of Wisconsin-Milwaukee.

Shigenaga, S. 1965. The constancy of loudness and of acoustic distance. *Bulletin of the Faculty of Literature, Kyushu University*, **9**, 289–333.

Shore, S. E., Godfrey, D. A., Helfert, R. H., Altschuler, R. A., and Bledsoe, S. C., Jr. 1992. Connections between the cochlea nuclei in guinea pig. *Hearing Research*, **62**, 16–26.

Shriberg, E. E. 1992. Perceptual restoration of filtered vowels with added noise. *Language and Speech*, **35**, 127–136.

Shutt, C. E. 1898. Experiments in judging the distance of sound. *Kansas University Quarterly*, **7A**, 1–8.

Siegel, R. J. 1965. A replication of the mel scale of pitch. *American Journal of Psychology*, **78**, 615–620.

Silverman, S. R., and Hirsh, I. J. 1955. Problems related to the use of speech in clinical audiometry. *Annals of Otology, Rhinology, and Laryngology*, **64**, 1234–1245.

Simmons, F. B. 1964. Perceptual theories of middle ear function. *Annals of Otology, Rhinology, and Laryngology*, **73**, 724–740.

Simon, H. J., and Studdert-Kennedy, M. 1978. Selective anchoring and adaptation of phonetic and nonphonetic continua. *Journal of the Acoustical Society of America*, **64**, 1338–1357.

Sinnott, J. M., Beecher, M. D., Moody, D. B., and Stebbins, W. C. 1976. Speech sound discrimination by monkeys and humans. *Journal of the Acoustical Society of America*, **60**, 687–695.

Small, A. M., Jr., and Campbell, R. A. 1961. Masking of pulsed tones by bands of noise. *Journal of the Acoustical Society of America*, **33**, 1570–1576.

Smith, R. L. 1988. Encoding of sound intensity by auditory neurons. In *Auditory Function: Neurological Bases of Hearing*, G. M. Edelman, W. E. Gall, and W. M. Cowan (eds.). New York: Wiley, 243–274.

Sorkin, R. D. 1987. Temporal factors in the discrimination of tonal sequences. *Journal of the Acoustical Society of America*, **82**, 1218–1226.

Sperling, G., and Reeves, G. 1980. Measuring the reaction time of a shift of visual attention. In *Attention and Performance VIII*, R. S. Nickerson (ed.). Hillsdale, NJ: Erlbaum, 347–360.

Spiegel, M. F. 1981. Thresholds for tones in maskers of various bandwidths as a function of signal frequency. *Journal of the Acoustical Society of America*, **69**, 791–795.

Springer, S. P., and Deutsch, G. 1993. *Left Brain, Right Brain*, 4th edition. New York: Freeman.

Starch, D., and Crawford, A. L. 1909. The perception of the distance of sound. *Psychological Review*, **16**, 427–430.

Starr, A., and Don, M. 1988. Brain potentials evoked by acoustic stimuli. In *Human Event-Related Potentials*, vol. 3, T. W. Picton (ed.). Amsterdam: Elsevier, 97–157.

Steeneken, H. J. M., and Houtgast, T. 1980. A physical method for measuring speech - transmission quality. *Journal of the Acoustical Society of America*, **67**, 318–326.

Steeneken, H. J. M., and Houtgast, T. 2002. Phoneme-group specific octave-band weights in predicting speech intelligibility. *Speech Communication*, **38**, 399–411.

Stein, B. E., and Meredith, M. A. 1993. *The Merging of the Senses*. Cambridge, MA: MIT Press.

Steinberg, J. C., and Snow, W. B. 1934. Physical factors. *Bell System Technical Journal*, **13**, 245–258.

Stevens, K. N. 1960. Toward a model of speech recognition. *Journal of the Acoustical Society of America*, **32**, 47–55.

Stevens, K. N. 1971. The role of rapid spectrum changes in the production and perception of speech. In *Form and Substance: Festschrift for Eli Fischer-Jørgensen*, L. L. Hammerlich and R. Jakobson (eds.). Copenhagen: Akademisk Forlag, 95–101.

Stevens, K. N., and Blumstein, S. E. 1981. The search for invariant acoustic correlates of phonetic features. In *Perspectives on the Study of Speech*, P. D. Eimas and J. L. Miller (eds.). Hillsdale, NJ: Erlbaum, 1–38.

Stevens, K. N., and Halle, M. 1967. Remarks on analysis by synthesis and distinctive features. In *Models for the Perception of Speech and Visual Form*, W. Wathen-Dunn (ed.). Cambridge, MA: MIT Press, 88–102.

Stevens, S. S. 1936. A scale for the measurement of a psychological magnitude: Loudness. *Psychological Review*, **43**, 405–416.

Stevens, S. S. 1955. The measurement of loudness. *Journal of the Acoustical Society of America*, **27**, 815–829.

Stevens, S. S. 1961. The psychophysics of sensory function. In *Sensory Communication*, W. A. Rosenblith (ed.). New York: Wiley, 1–33.

Stevens, S. S. 1972. Perceived level of noise by Mark VII and decibels (E). *Journal of the Acoustical Society of America*, **51**, 575–601.

Stevens, S. S. 1975. *Psychophysics: Introduction to its Perceptual, Neural and Social Prospects*. G. Stevens (ed.). New York: Wiley.

Stevens, S. S., and Davis, H. 1938. *Hearing, its Psychology and Physiology*. New York: Wiley.

Stevens, S. S., and Guirao, M. 1962. Loudness, reciprocality and partition scales. *Journal of the Acoustical Society of America*, **34**, 1466–1471.

Stevens, S. S., and Newman, E. B. 1936. The localization of actual sources of sound. *American Journal of Psychology*, **48**, 297–306.

Stevens, S. S., Volkmann, J., and Newman, E. B. 1937. A scale for the measurement of the psychological magnitude pitch. *Journal of the Acoustical Society of America*, **8**, 185–190.

Stuart, A., Kalinowski, J., Rastatter, M. P., and Lynch, K. 2002. Effect of delayed auditory feedback on normal speakers at two speech rates. *Journal of the Acoustical Society of America*, **111**, 2237–2241.

Stuhlman, O., Jr. 1943. *An Introduction to Biophysics*. New York: Wiley.

Sugita, Y. 1997. Neuronal correlates of auditory induction in the cat cortex. *Cognitive Neuroscience and Neuropsychology, NeuroReport*, **8**, 1155–1159.

Supa, M., Cotzin, M., and Dallenbach, K. M. 1944. "Facial vision": The perception of obstacles by the blind. *American Journal of Psychology*, **57**, 133–183.

Swisher, L., and Hirsh, I. J. 1972. Brain damage and the ordering of two temporally successive stimuli. *Neuropsychologia*, **10**, 137–152.

Tallal, P., and Piercy, M. 1973. Defects of non-verbal auditory perception in children with developmental aphasia. *Nature*, **241**, 468–469.

Talley, C. H. 1937. A comparison of conversational and audience speech. *Archives of Speech*, **2**, 28–40.

Teranishi, R. 1977. Critical rate for identification and information capacity in hearing system. *Journal of the Acoustical Society of Japan*, **33**, 136–143.

Terhardt, E. 1974. Pitch, consonance, and harmony. *Journal of the Acoustical Society of America*, **55**, 1061–1069.

Thomas, I. B., Cetti, R. P., and Chase, P. W. 1971. Effect of silent intervals on the perception of temporal order for vowels. *Journal of the Acoustical Society of America*, **49**, 85 (Abstract).

Thomas, I. B., Hill, P. B., Carroll, F. S., and Garcia, B. 1970. Temporal order in the perception of vowels. *Journal of the Acoustical Society of America*, **48**, 1010–1013.

Thompson, R. K. R. 1976. *Performance of the Bottlenose Dolphin (Tursiops truncatus) on Delayed Auditory Sequences and Delayed Auditory Successive Discriminations.* Unpublished Doctoral Dissertation, University of Hawaii.

Thompson, S. P. 1882. On the function of two ears in the perception of space. *The London, Edinburgh, and Dublin Philosophical Magazine and Journal of Science (Series 5)*, **13**, 406–416.

Thurlow, W. R. 1957. An auditory figure-ground effect. *American Journal of Psychology*, **70**, 653–654.

Thurlow, W. R. 1963. Perception of low auditory pitch: A multicue, mediation theory. *Psychological Review*, **70**, 461–470.

Thurlow, W. R., and Elfner, L. F. 1959. Continuity effects with alternately sounding tones. *Journal of the Acoustical Society of America*, **31**, 1337–1339.

Thurlow, W. R., and Erchul, W. P. 1978. Understanding continuity effects with complex stimuli. *Journal of the American Auditory Society*, **4**, 113–116.

Thurlow, W. R., and Jack, C. E. 1973. Certain determinants of the "ventriloquism" effect. *Perceptual and Motor Skills*, **36**, 1171–1184.

Thurlow, W. R., and Marten, A. E. 1962. Perception of steady and intermittent sound with alternating noise-burst stimuli. *Journal of the Acoustical Society of America*, **34**, 1853–1858.

Thurlow, W. R., and Rosenthal, T. M. 1976. Further study of the existence regions for the "ventriloquism" effect. *Journal of the American Audiological Society*, **1**, 280–286.

Titchener, E. B. 1915. *A Beginner's Psychology.* New York: Macmillan.

Tobias, J. V., and Schubert, E. D. 1959. Effective onset duration of auditory stimuli. *Journal of the Acoustical Society of America*, **31**, 1595–1605.

Tonndorf, J. 1960. Shearing motion in scala media of cochlear models. *Journal of the Acoustical Society of America*, **32**, 238–244.

Tonndorf, J. 1970. Cochlear mechanics and hydro-dynamics. In *Foundations of Modern Auditory Theory*, vol. I, J. V. Tobias (ed.). New York: Academic Press, 203–254.

Tonndorf, J., and Khanna, S. M. 1972. Tympanic-membrane vibrations in human cadaver ears studied by time-averaged holography. *Journal of the Acoustical Society of America*, **52**, 1221–1233.

Vernon, J. 1963. *Inside the Black Room*. New York: Potter.

Verschuure, J. 1978. *Auditory Excitation Patterns: The Significance of the Pulsation Threshold Method for the Measurement of Auditory Nonlinearity*. Unpublished Doctoral Dissertation, Erasmus University, Rotterdam.

Verschuure, J., Rodenburg, M., and Maas, A. J. J. 1974. Frequency selectivity and temporal effects of the pulsation threshold method. In *Proceedings of the 8th International Congress on Acoustics (London)*, **1**, 131.

Vicario, G. 1960. L'effetto tunnel acustico. *Rivista di Psicologia*, **54**, 41–52.

Voldrich, L. 1978. Mechanical properties of basilar membrane. *Acta Oto-Laryngologica*, **86**, 331–335.

Ward, W. D. 1954. Subjective musical pitch. *Journal of the Acoustical Society of America*, **26**, 369–380.

Warfield, D., Ruben, R. J., and Glackin, R. 1966. Word discrimination in cats. *Journal of Auditory Research*, **6**, 97–119.

Warren, R. M. 1958. A basis for judgments of sensory intensity. *American Journal of Psychology*, **71**, 675–687.

Warren, R. M. 1961a. Illusory changes of distinct speech upon repetition – the verbal transformation effect. *British Journal of Psychology*, **52**, 249–258.

Warren, R. M. 1961b. Illusory changes in repeated words: Differences between young adults and the aged. *American Journal of Psychology*, **74**, 506–516.

Warren, R. M. 1962. Are 'autophonic' judgments based on loudness? *American Journal of Psychology*, **75**, 452–456.

Warren, R. M. 1968a. Vocal compensation for change in distance. In *Proceedings of the 6th International Congress of Acoustics (Tokyo)*, A, 61–64.

Warren, R. M. 1968b. Relation of verbal transformations to other perceptual phenomena. *Conference Publication No. 42, Institution of Electrical Engineers (London)*, Supplement No. 1, 1–8.

Warren, R. M. 1968c. Verbal transformation effect and auditory perceptual mechanisms. *Psychological Bulletin*, **70**, 261–270.

Warren, R. M. 1969. Visual intensity judgments: An empirical rule and a theory. *Psychological Review*, **76**, 16–30.

Warren, R. M. 1970a. Elimination of biases in loudness judgments for tones. *Journal of the Acoustical Society of America*, **48**, 1397–1403.

Warren, R. M. 1970b. Perceptual restoration of missing speech sounds. *Science*, **167**, 392–393.

Warren, R. M. 1971. Identification times for phonemic components of graded complexity and for spelling of speech. *Perception & Psychophysics*, **9**, 345–349.

Warren, R. M. 1972. Perception of temporal order: Special rules for initial and terminal sounds of sequences. *Journal of the Acoustical Society of America*, **52**, 167 (Abstract).

Warren, R. M. 1973a. Quantification of loudness. *American Journal of Psychology*, **86**, 807–825.

Warren, R. M. 1973b. Anomalous loudness function of speech. *Journal of the Acoustical Society of America*, **54**, 390–396.

Warren, R. M. 1974a. Auditory temporal discrimination by trained listeners. *Cognitive Psychology*, **6**, 237–256.

Warren, R. M. 1974b. Auditory pattern discrimination by untrained listeners. *Perception & Psychophysics*, **15**, 495–500.

Warren, R. M. 1976. Auditory perception and speech evolution. In *Origins and Evolution of Language and Speech*, S. R. Harnad, H. D. Steklis, and J. Lancaster (eds.). New York: New York Academy of Sciences, 708–717.

Warren, R. M. 1977a. Subjective loudness and its physical correlate. *Acustica*, **37**, 334–346.

Warren, R. M. 1977b. Les illusions verbales. *La Recherche*, **8**, 538–543.

Warren, R. M. 1981a. Measurement of sensory intensity. *Behavioral and Brain Sciences*, **4**, 175–189 (target article); 213–223 (response to open peer commentaries).

Warren, R. M. 1981b. Perceptual transformations in vision and hearing. *International Journal of Man-Machine Studies*, **14**, 123–132.

Warren, R. M. 1984. Perceptual restoration of obliterated sounds. *Psychological Review*, **96**, 371–385.

Warren, R. M. 1985. Criterion shift rule and perceptual homeostasis. *Psychological Review*, **92**, 574–584.

Warren, R. M. 1988. Perceptual basis for the evolution of speech. In *The Genesis of Language: A Different Judgement of Evidence*, M. E. Landsberg (ed.). Berlin: Mouton de Gruyter, 101–110.

Warren, R. M., and Ackroff, J. M. 1976a. Two types of auditory sequence perception. *Perception & Psychophysics*, **20**, 387–394.

Warren, R. M., and Ackroff, J. M. 1976b. Dichotic verbal transformations and evidence of separate processors for identical stimuli. *Nature*, **259**, 475–477.

Warren, R. M., and Bashford, J. A., Jr. 1976. Auditory contralateral induction: An early stage in binaural processing. *Perception & Psychophysics*, **20**, 380–386.

Warren, R. M., and Bashford, J. A., Jr. 1981. Perception of acoustic iterance: Pitch and infrapitch. *Perception & Psychophysics*, **29**, 395–402.

Warren, R. M., and Bashford, J. A., Jr. 1988. Broadband repetition pitch: Spectral dominance or pitch averaging? *Journal of the Acoustical Society of America*, **84**, 2058–2062.

Warren, R. M., and Bashford, J. A., Jr. 1993. When acoustic sequences are not perceptual sequences: The global perception of auditory patterns. *Perception & Psychophysics*, **54**, 121–126.

Warren, R. M., and Bashford, J. A., Jr. 1999. Intelligibility of 1/3-octave speech: Greater contribution of frequencies outside than inside the nominal passband. *Journal of the Acoustical Society of America*, **106**, L47–L52.

Warren, R. M., Bashford, J. A., Jr., Cooley, J. M., and Brubaker, B. S. 2001. Detection of acoustic repetition for very long stochastic patterns. *Perception & Psychophysics*, **63**, 175–182.

Warren, R. M., Bashford, J. A., Jr., and Gardner, D. A. 1990. Tweaking the lexicon: Organization of vowel sequences into words. *Perception & Psychophysics*, **47**, 423–432.

Warren, R. M., Bashford, J. A., Jr., and Healy, E. W. 1992. The subtractive nature of auditory continuity: Reciprocal changes in alternating sounds. *Journal of the Acoustical Society of America*, **91**, 2334 (Abstract).

Warren, R. M., Bashford, J. A., Jr., Healy, E. W., and Brubaker, B. S. 1994. Auditory induction: Reciprocal changes in alternating sounds. *Perception & Psychophysics*, **55**, 313–322.

Warren, R. M., Bashford, J. A., Jr., and Lenz, P. W. 2004. Intelligibility of bandpass filtered speech: Steepness of slopes required to eliminate transition band contributions. *Journal of the Acoustical Society of America*, **115**, 1292–1295.

Warren, R. M., Bashford, J. A., Jr., and Lenz, P. W. 2005. Intelligibility of 1-octave rectangular bands spanning the speech spectrum when heard separately and paired. *Journal of the Acoustical Society of America*, **118**, 3261–3266.

Warren, R. M., Bashford, J. A., Jr., and Wrightson, J. M. 1979. Infrapitch echo. *Journal of the Acoustical Society of America*, **65**, S38 (Abstract).

Warren, R. M., Bashford, J. A., Jr., and Wrightson, J. M. 1980. Infrapitch echo. *Journal of the Acoustical Society of America*, **68**, 1301–1305.

Warren, R. M., Bashford, J. A., Jr., and Wrightson, J. M. 1981. Detection of long interaural delays for broadband noise. *Journal of the Acoustical Society of America*, **69**, 1510–1514.

Warren, R. M., and Byrnes, D. L. 1975. Temporal discrimination of recycled tonal sequences: Pattern matching and naming of order by untrained listeners. *Perception & Psychophysics*, **18**, 273–280.

Warren, R. M., and Gardner, D. A. 1995. Aphasics can distinguish permuted orders of phonemes – but only if presented rapidly. *Journal of Speech and Hearing Research*, **38**, 473–476.

Warren, R. M., Gardner, D. A., Brubaker, B. S., and Bashford, J. A., Jr. 1991. Melodic and nonmelodic sequence of tones: Effects of duration on perception. *Music Perception*, **8**, 277–290.

Warren, R. M., and Gregory, R. L. 1958. An auditory analogue of the visual reversible figure. *American Journal of Psychology*, **71**, 612–613.

Warren, R. M., Hainsworth, K. R., Brubaker, B. S., Bashford, J. A., Jr., and Healy, E. W. 1997. Spectral restoration of speech: Intelligibility is increased by inserting noise in spectral gaps. *Perception & Psychophysics*, **59**, 275–283.

Warren, R. M., Healy, E. W., and Chalikia, M. H. 1996. The vowel-sequence illusion: Intrasubject stability and intersubject agreement of syllabic forms. *Journal of the Acoustical Society of America*, **100**, 2452–2461.

Warren, R. M., and Obusek, C. J. 1971. Speech perception and phonemic restorations. *Perception & Psychophysics*, **9**, 358–362.

Warren, R. M., and Obusek, C. J. 1972. Identification of temporal order within auditory sequences. *Perception & Psychophysics*, **12**, 86–90.

Warren, R. M., Obusek, C. J., and Ackroff, J. M. 1972. Auditory induction: Perceptual synthesis of absent sounds. *Science*, **176**, 1149–1151.

Warren, R. M., Obusek, C. J., Farmer, R. M., and Warren, R. P. 1969. Auditory sequence: Confusion of patterns other than speech or music. *Science*, **164**, 586–587.

Warren, R. M., Riener, K. R., Bashford, J. A., Jr., and Brubaker, B. S. 1995. Spectral redundancy: Intelligibility of sentences heard through narrow spectral slits. *Perception & Psychophysics*, **57**, 175–182.

Warren, R. M., Sersen, E., and Pores, E. 1958. A basis for loudness-judgments. *American Journal of Psychology*, **71**, 700–709.

Warren, R. M., and Sherman, G. L. 1974. Phonemic restorations based on subsequent context. *Perception & Psychophysics*, **16**, 150–156.

Warren, R. M., and Warren, R. P. 1958. Basis for judgments of relative brightness. *Journal of the Optical Society of America*, **48**, 445–450.

Warren, R. M., and Warren, R. P. 1963. A critique of S. S. Stevens' "New psychophysics." *Perceptual and Motor Skills*, **16**, 797–810.

Warren, R. M., and Warren, R. P. 1966. A comparison of speech perception in childhood, maturity, and old age by means of the verbal transformation effect. *Journal of Verbal Learning and Verbal Behavior*, **5**, 142–146.

Warren, R. M., and Warren, R. P. 1968. *Helmholtz on Perception: Its Physiology and Development*. New York: Wiley.

Warren, R. M., and Warren, R. P. 1970. Auditory illusions and confusions. *Scientific American*, **223**, 30–36 (December).

Warren, R. M., and Wrightson, J. M. 1981. Stimuli producing conflicting temporal and spectral cues to frequency. *Journal of the Acoustical Society of America*, **70**, 1020–1024.

Watson, C. S. 1987. Uncertainty, informational masking, and the capacity of immediate memory. In *Auditory Processing of Complex Sounds*, W. A. Yost and C. S. Watson (eds.). Hillsdale, NJ: Erlbaum, 267–277.

Watson, C. S., Kelly, W. J., and Wroton, H. W. 1976. Factors in the discrimination of tonal patterns. II. Selective attention and learning under various levels of stimulus uncertainty. *Journal of the Acoustical Society of America*, **60**, 1176–1186.

Watson, C. S., Wroton, H. W., Kelly, W. J., and Benbassat, C. A. 1975. Factors in the discrimination of tonal patterns. I. Component frequency, temporal position, and silent intervals. *Journal of the Acoustical Society of America*, **57**, 1175–1185.

Wegel, R. L., and Lane, C. E. 1924. The auditory masking of one pure tone by another and its probable relation to the dynamics of the inner ear. *Physical Review*, **23**, 266–285.

Weinberger, N. M., and McKenna, T. M. 1988. Sensitivity of single neurons in auditory cortex to contour: Toward a theory of neurophysiology of music perception. *Music Perception*, **5**, 355–390.

Welford, A. T. 1958. *Ageing and Human Skill*. London: Oxford University Press.

Wever, E. G. 1949. *Theory of Hearing*. New York: Wiley.

Wever, E. G., and Bray, C. 1930. Action currents in the auditory nerve in response to acoustical stimulation. In *Proceedings of the National Academy of Sciences* (USA), **16**, 344–350.

Wheeldon, L. R., and Levelt, W. J. M. 1995. Monitoring the time course of phonological encoding. *Journal of Memory and Language*, **34**, 311–334.

Whitfield, I. C. 1970. Central nervous system processing in relation to spatio-temporal discrimination of auditory patterns. In *Frequency Analysis and Periodicity Detection in Hearing*, R. Plomp and G. F. Smoorenburg (eds.). Leiden: Sijthoff, 136–152.

Whitworth, R. H., and Jeffress, L. A. 1961. Time vs. intensity in the localization of tones. *Journal of the Acoustical Society of America*, **33**, 925–929.

Wickelgren, W. A. 1969. Context-sensitive coding, associative memory, and serial order in (speech) behavior. *Psychological Review*, **76**, 1–15.

Wiener, F. 1947. On the diffraction of a progressive wave by the human head. *Journal of the Acoustical Society of America*, **19**, 143–146.

Wightman, F. L. 1973. The pattern transformation model of pitch. *Journal of the Acoustical Society of America*, **54**, 407–416.

Wightman, F. L., and Kistler, D. J. 1989a. Headphone simulation of free-field listening. I: Stimulus synthesis. *Journal of the Acoustical Society of America*, **85**, 858–867.

Wightman, F. L., and Kistler, D. J. 1989b. Headphone simulation of free-field listening. II: Psychophysical validation. *Journal of the Acoustical Society of America*, **85**, 868–878.

Wilcox, G. W., Neisser, U., and Roberts, J. 1972. Recognition of auditory temporal order. *Paper presented at the Eastern Psychological Association, Boston, MA (Spring)*.

Wiley, R. L. 1968. *Speech Communication using the Strongly Voiced Components Only*. Unpublished Doctoral Dissertation, Imperial College, University of London.

Willey, C. F., Inglis, E., and Pearce, C. H. 1937. Reversal of auditory localization. *Journal of Experimental Psychology*, **20**, 114–130.

Wilson, J. P., and Johnstone, J. R. 1975. Basilar membrane and middle-ear vibration in guinea pig measured by capacitive probe. *Journal of the Acoustical Society of America*, **57**, 705–723.

Winckel, F. 1967. *Music, Sound and Sensation: A Modern Exposition*. New York: Dover.

Winkler, I., Korzyukov, O., Gumenyuk, V., Cowan, N., Linkenkaer-Hansenk, K., Illmoniemi, R. J., Alho, K., and Näätänen, R. 2002. Temporary and longer term retention of acoustic information. *Psychophysiology*, **39**, 530–534.

Winslow, R. L., and Sachs, M. B. 1988. Single-tone intensity discrimination based on auditory-nerve rate responses in backgrounds of quiet, noise, and with stimulation of the crossed olivocochlear bundle. *Hearing Research*, **35**, 165–190.

Wohlgemuth, A. 1911. On the after-effect of seen movement. *British Journal of Psychology, Monograph Supplement*. Cambridge: Cambridge University Press.

Woodworth, R. S. 1938. *Experimental Psychology*. New York: Holt.

Worchel, P., and Dallenbach, K. M. 1947. "Facial vision": Perception of obstacles by the deaf-blind. *American Journal of Psychology*, **60**, 502–553.

Worden, F. G. 1971. Hearing and the neural detection of acoustic patterns. *Behavioral Science*, **16**, 20–30.

Wright, D., Hebrank, J. H., and Wilson, B. 1974. Pinna reflections as cues for localization. *Journal of the Acoustical Society of America*, **56**, 957–962.

Wrightson, J. M., and Warren, R. M. 1981. Incomplete auditory induction of tones alternated with noise: Effects occurring below the pulsation threshold. *Journal of the Acoustical Society of America*, **69**, 5105–5106 (Abstract).

Yates, A. J. 1963. Delayed auditory feedback. *Psychological Bulletin*, **60**, 213–232.

Yost, W. A., and Hill, R. 1978. Strength of pitches associated with ripple noise. *Journal of the Acoustical Society of America*, **64**, 485–492.

Yost, W. A., and Hill, R. 1979. Models of the pitch and pitch strength of ripple noise. *Journal of the Acoustical Society of America*, **66**, 400–410.

Yost, W. A., Hill, R., and Perez-Falcon, T. 1978. Pitch and pitch discrimination of broadband signals with rippled power spectra. *Journal of the Acoustical Society of America*, **63**, 1166–1173.

Young, P. T. 1928. Auditory localization with acoustical transposition of the ears. *Journal of Experimental Psychology*, **11**, 399–429.

Yund, E. W., and Efron, R. 1974. Dichoptic and dichotic micropattern discrimination. *Perception & Psychophysics*, **15**, 383–390.

Zemlin, W. R. 1998. *Speech and Hearing Science: Anatomy and Physiology*, 4th edition. Needham Heights, MA: Allyn & Bacon.

Zimmerman, G., Brown, C., Kelso, J. A. S., Hurtig, R., and Forest, K. 1988. The association between articulatory events in a delayed auditory feedback paradigm. *Journal of Phonetics*, **16**, 437–451.

Zurek, P. M. 1981. Spontaneous narrowband acoustic signals emitted by human ears. *Journal of the Acoustical Society of America*, **69**, 514–523.

Zwicker, E. 1970. Masking and psychological excitation as consequences of the ear's frequency analysis. In *Frequency Analysis and Periodicity Detection in Hearing*, R. Plomp and G. F. Smoorenburg (eds.). Leiden: Sijthoff, 376–396.

Zwislocki, J. J. 1980. Five decades of research on cochlear mechanics. *Journal of the Acoustical Society of America*, **67**, 1679–1685.

Zwislocki, J. J., and Kletsky, E. J. 1979. Tectorial membrane: A possible effect on frequency analysis in the cochlea. *Science*, **204**, 639–641.

Index